# Religion and the COVID-19 Pandemic in Southern Africa

This book investigates the role of religion in the context of the COVID-19 pandemic in Southern Africa.

Building on a diverse range of methodologies and disciplinary approaches, the book reflects on how religion, politics and health have interfaced in Southern African contexts, when faced with the sudden public health emergency caused by the pandemic. Religious actors have played a key role on the frontline throughout the pandemic, sometimes posing roadblocks to public health messaging, but more often deploying their resources to help provide effective and timely responses. Drawing on case studies from African indigenous knowledge systems, Islam, Rastafari and various forms of Christianity, this book provides important reflections on the role of religion in crisis response.

This book will be of interest to researchers across the fields of African Studies, Health, Politics and Religious Studies.

**Fortune Sibanda** (DPhil) is a Professor of Religious Studies in the Department of Philosophy and Religious Studies, Great Zimbabwe University, Masvingo.

**Tenson Muyambo** (DPhil) lectures in the Department of Teacher Development at Great Zimbabwe University in Masvingo, Zimbabwe.

**Ezra Chitando** (DPhil) serves as a Professor in History and Phenomenology of Religion at the University of Zimbabwe, and Theology Consultant on HIV and AIDS in Africa for the World Council of Churches.

*Routledge Studies on Religion in Africa and the Diaspora*

1 **Community and Trinity in Africa**
*Ibrahim S. Bitrus*

2 **Contextualizing Eschatology in African Cultural and Religious Beliefs**
*Ibigbolade S. Aderibigbe*

3 **Politics and Religion in Zimbabwe**
The Deification of Robert G. Mugabe
*Edited by Ezra Chitando*

4 **Personality Cult and Politics in Mugabe's Zimbabwe**
*Edited by Ezra Chitando*

5 **Race, Class and Christianity in South Africa**
Middle-Class Moralities
*Ibrahim Abraham*

6 **Religion and the COVID-19 Pandemic in Southern Africa**
*Edited by Fortune Sibanda, Tenson Muyambo and Ezra Chitando*

# Religion and the COVID-19 Pandemic in Southern Africa

Edited by
Fortune Sibanda, Tenson Muyambo and
Ezra Chitando

Routledge
Taylor & Francis Group
LONDON AND NEW YORK

First published 2022
by Routledge
4 Park Square, Milton Park, Abingdon, Oxon OX14 4RN

and by Routledge
605 Third Avenue, New York, NY 10158

*Routledge is an imprint of the Taylor & Francis Group, an informa business*

*British Library Cataloguing-in-Publication Data*
A catalogue record for this book is available from the British Library

*Library of Congress Cataloging-in-Publication Data*
Names: Sibanda, Fortune, editor, author. | Muyambo, Tenson, editor, author. | Chitando, Ezra, editor, author.
Title: Religion and the COVID-19 pandemic in southern Africa / edited by Fortune Sibanda, Tenson Muyambo and Ezra Chitando.
Description: New York : Routledge, 2022. | Includes bibliographical references and index.
Identifiers: LCCN 2021042620 (print) | LCCN 2021042621 (ebook) | ISBN 9781032147833 (hardback) | ISBN 9781032147857 (paperback) | ISBN 9781003241096 (ebook)
Subjects: LCSH: COVID-19 (Disease)—Africa, Southern—Religious aspects. | Crisis management—Africa, Southern—Religious aspects. | Public health administration—Africa, Southern.
Classification: LCC RA644.C67 R456 2022 (print) | LCC RA644.C67 (ebook) | DDC 362.1962/41400968—dc23
LC record available at https://lccn.loc.gov/2021042620
LC ebook record available at https://lccn.loc.gov/2021042621

ISBN: 978-1-032-14783-3 (hbk)
ISBN: 978-1-032-14785-7 (pbk)
ISBN: 978-1-003-24109-6 (ebk)

DOI: 10.4324/9781003241096

Typeset in Times New Roman
by codeMantra

# Contents

*Short Biography of Corresponding Editor*                                   vii

1  **Introduction: religion and public health in the shadow of
   COVID-19 pandemic in Southern Africa**                                     1
   FORTUNE SIBANDA, TENSON MUYAMBO AND EZRA CHITANDO

2  **Exploring the ethics of *Ubuntu* in the era of COVID-19**               25
   BEATRICE OKYERE-MANU AND STEPHEN NKANSAH MORGAN

3  **Social distancing in the context of COVID-19 in Zimbabwe:
   perspectives from Ndau religious indigenous knowledge systems**          37
   TENSON MUYAMBO

4  **Coping with the coronavirus (COVID-19): resources from
   Ndau indigenous religion**                                               52
   MACLOUD SIPEYIYE

5  **Living with COVID-19 in Zimbabwe: a religious and scientific
   healing response**                                                       72
   BERNARD PINDUKAI HUMBE

6  **Religion, law and COVID-19 in South Africa**                           89
   HELENA VAN COLLER AND IDOWU A. AKINLOYE

7  **Tele-evangelism, tele-health and cyberbullying in the wake of
   the outbreak of COVID-19 in Zimbabwe**                                  103
   LUCIA PONDE-MUTSVEDU AND SOPHIA CHIRONGOMA

8  **The role of religion in response to COVID-19 pandemic
   challenges in Tanzania**                                                115
   PASKAS WAGANA

9 COVID-19 containment measures and 'prophecies' in Kenya 126
JULIUS GATHOGO

10 Christian religious understandings and responses to
COVID-19 in Eswatini 141
SONENE NYAWO

11 Standing together in faith through the time of COVID-19: the
responses of Church umbrella bodies in Zambia 155
NELLY MWALE AND JOSEPH CHITA

12 Churches and COVID-19 in Botswana 172
TSHENOLO J. MADIGELE AND JAMES N. AMANZE

13 The coronavirus pandemic and persons with disabilities:
towards a liberating reading of the Bible for Churches in
Southern Africa 186
MAKOMBORERO ALLEN BOWA

14 The influence of health perceptions on Zimbabwe Muslim
responses to COVID-19 restrictions over Ramadan,
pilgrimages and funeral rites in 2020 202
EDMORE DUBE

15 Repositioning the agency of Rastafari in the context of
COVID-19 crisis in Zimbabwe and Malawi 213
FORTUNE SIBANDA

16 'When a pandemic wears the face of a woman': intersections of
religion and gender during the COVID-19 pandemic in Zimbabwe 232
MOLLY MANYONGANISE

17 Religion and COVID-19 in Southern Africa: implications for
the discourse on religion and development 244
EZRA CHITANDO

*Index* 257

# Short Biography of Corresponding Editor

**Fortune Sibanda (DPhil)** is a Professor of Religious Studies in the Department of Philosophy and Religious Studies, Great Zimbabwe University, Masvingo. His research interests include new religious movements, indigenous knowledge systems, human rights issues, religion and the environment, law and religion, religion and health. Professor Sibanda is a member of a number of academic associations including the American Academy of Religion (AAR) and African Consortium for Law and Religion Studies (ACLARS).

## Short Biographies of Co-Editors

**Ezra Chitando (DPhil)** serves as a Professor in History and Phenomenology of Religion at the University of Zimbabwe and Theology Consultant on HIV and AIDS in Africa for the World Council of Churches. His broad research and publication interests include religion and method and theory, health, gender, security, politics, development, climate change, sexuality and others.

**Tenson Muyambo (PhD)** lectures in the Department of Teacher Development at Great Zimbabwe University in Masvingo, Zimbabwe. He is a Doctor of Philosophy (Gender and Religion) graduate and aluminus of University of KwaZulu Natal, South Africa. His research and publication interests include indigenous knowledge systems, religion, African identity, education, COVID-19, gender and African Spirituality.

## Short Biographies of Authors to the Edited Volume

**Idowu A. Akinloye (PhD)** currently lectures in the Faculty of Law, Ajayi Crowther University, Nigeria. He is a self-supporting priest in the Anglican Church both in Nigeria and South Africa and also a barrister and solicitor of the Supreme Court of Nigeria. He has a PhD in Law from Rhodes University, focusing on law and religion.

**Makomborero Allen Bowa** is a Lecturer in the Department of Philosophy, Religion and Ethics at the University of Zimbabwe, where he teaches Old Testament studies. He is a registered DPhil candidate with the University of Zimbabwe and his research interrogates the nexus between disability and poverty in contemporary Zimbabwe from a Biblical perspective. His approach to the Old Testament is not confessional but scientific in that he treats Old Testament themes as models for Africa, to either emulate or reject in addressing its religious, socio-economic and political challenges. As such, he is profoundly interested in the appropriation of biblical themes in the analysis of issues relating to poverty, disability, gender, social death, violence, politics, human rights and many other contemporary challenges bedevilling African societies.

**Sophia Chirongoma (PhD)** is a Senior Lecturer in the Religious Studies Department at Midlands State University, Zimbabwe. She is also an Academic Associate/Research Fellow at the Research Institute for Theology and Religion (RITR) in the College of Human Sciences, University of South Africa (UNISA).

**Joseph Chita** is a Lecturer in the Department of Religious Studies at the University of Zambia. His research interests are in religion and society, and some of his publications cut across disciplines. He is a member of the African Association for the Study of Religions (AASR), and Association for the Study of Religion in Southern Africa (ASRSA).

**Edmore Dube (PhD**, University of Zimbabwe) is a Senior Lecturer in the Department of Philosophy and Religious Studies, Great Zimbabwe University. His research interests are in the areas of religion, health and justice resonating with the common good.

**Julius Gathogo (PhD)** is a Senior Lecturer in Kenyatta University and is a Distinguished Professor at ANCCI University. He is also a Research Fellow at UNISA, Pretoria, South Africa. He is one of Africa's prolific writers in ecclesiastical history, theology and missiology in African context.

**Bernard Pindukai Humbe** is a PhD holder in Religion Studies from the University of Free State, South Africa. He is a Lecturer in the Department of Philosophy and Religious Studies at Great Zimbabwe University, Masvingo. His areas of research interest include African indigenous religious knowledge systems, contemporary meaning of African traditional religion, symbolism of animals in African indigenous religion, onomastics, traditional law and social development, religion and entrepreneurship, religion and social transformation, and religion and power.

**Tshenolo Jennifer Madigele (BA, MA and PhD)** is a Theology Lecturer at the University of Botswana. Her research interests include human sexuality, with a particular focus on the LGBTI communities, gerontology and Botho Pastoral Care and Counseling.

**Molly Manyonganise** holds a PhD in Biblical and Religious Studies from the University of Pretoria. She is a Senior Lecturer in the Department of Religious Studies and Philosophy at the Zimbabwe Open University. She is a Research Associate in the Department of Religion Studies, Faculty of Theology and Religion of the University of Pretoria. She is currently a Georg Forster Postdoctoral Research Fellow run under the Alexander von Humboldt Foundation. Her research interests include religion and politics, gender and religion, religion and sexuality, African indigenous religion(s) and African Christianity.

**Stephen Nkansah Morgan (PhD)** is currently a Lecturer with the Department of Philosophy and Classics of the University of Ghana where he teaches a wide range of philosophical courses at both graduate and undergraduate level. Stephen holds a PhD in Ethics Studies from the University of KwaZulu-Natal in South Africa.

**Nelly Mwale (PhD)** is a Lecturer in the Department of Religious Studies at the University of Zambia. Her research interests include religion and education, religion in the public sphere, church history and African indigenous religions.

**Amanze James Nathaniel (PhD)** is a Professor of Systematic Theology in the Department of Theology and Religious Studies, University of Botswana. He has published academic books, book chapters and articles in refereed journals and books.

**Sonene Nyawo (PhD)** is a Senior Lecturer and Head of Department in the Department of Theology and Religious Studies, Faculty of Humanities, University of Eswatini. She holds a Doctorate of Philosophy (Gender and Religion) from the University of KwaZulu-Natal.

**Beatrice Okyere-Manu (PhD)** is a Senior Lecturer in the School of Religion, Philosophy and Classics at the University of KwaZulu-Natal. She is the Programme Director for Applied Ethics. Her research interest is in development ethics.

**Lucia Ponde-Mutsvedu** holds a Bachelors' degree in Counselling from Zimbabwe Open University and a Master's degree in Child Rights from Africa University. She also holds a certificate in Strategic Management in HIV/AIDS from the University of Zimbabwe. She is currently teaching at a private school in Harare.

**Macloud Sipeyiye (PhD)** is an Academic Associate/Research Fellow with the Research Institute for Theology and Religion (RITR) in the College of Human Sciences, University of South Africa (UNISA). He is also a Senior Lecturer in the Department of Religious Studies and Ethics at the Midlands State University (MSU), Zimbabwe. His research interests revolve around the interface of spirituality and development issues that include health and human flourishing, ecological conservation, politics and conflict management and transformation.

**Helena van Coller (PhD)** is an Associate Professor and Deputy Dean in the Faculty of Law at Rhodes University, South Africa. She obtained her LLD on the topic of Administrative Law and Religious Organisations in 2012. Her main field of research is administrative law and aspects of law and religion.

**Paskas Wagana (PhD)** is a Lecturer in the Department of Sociology at St. Augustine University of Tanzania. He holds a PhD in Gerontology from the University of Vechta in Germany. He also holds MA in Social Work and BA in Economics, both from the University of Madras in India.

# 1 Introduction

## Religion and public health in the shadow of COVID-19 pandemic in Southern Africa

*Fortune Sibanda, Tenson Muyambo and Ezra Chitando*

### Introduction

Sweeping across the globe and causing death, untold suffering and unprecedented disruption, the COVID-19 pandemic announced its presence in a staggering manner in 2020 and 2021. Within a short period of time, the pandemic became the world's most pressing emergency, exposing the limitations of bio-medicine and highlighting the vulnerability of human beings in different parts of the world. This included those in the Global North who had generally tended to associate pandemics with the Global South. Confirming the earlier observation by the historian of religions, Mircea Eliade (1959) that human beings are essentially *homo religiosus* (human existence is inherently religious), religion featured prominently in making sense of the pandemic, across different cultures and contexts. Even the global appeal of the South African massive hit song, "Jerusalema" (Master KG featuring Nomcebo with its accompanying dance challenge) that went viral in 2020 confirmed humanity's search for healing in the middle of death and anxiety. It was in this context that religion in Africa sought to interface with COVID-19 and to be a positive force in society. Different religions played different roles in diverse African settings, intersecting with politics and shaping how people experienced and responded to COVID-19. As we elaborate below, this volume seeks to paint vivid images of such interactions, as well as to analyse them in depth.

Although several epidemics have been recorded in human history since time immemorial (Barry 2004), there has been limited work on the interface of religion and public health in the African context. As this volume was being finalised, the world was grappling with a health emergency caused by COVID-19 and it seemed timely to provide a scholarly introspection into the responses and impact of this pandemic in society. First identified in December 2019 in Wuhan, China, COVID-19 was declared a public health concern by the World Health Organization on 11 March 2020. This was because this viral disease had reached alarming levels in terms of its spread and severity given that many people were infected whilst others died. Although some

DOI: 10.4324/9781003241096-1

work on religion and the COVID-19 pandemic has begun to appear (among others, Dein et al. 2020; Kowalczyk et al. 2020; Parish 2020; Sonntag et al. 2020; Wildman et al. 2020), with additional publications on this theme to be expected in future, there is limited material emerging from the Southern African context. Given the speed and impact of the pandemic, we are anticipating an avalanche of literature on religion and COVID-19, perhaps similar to, if not exceeding, the interest in religion and other pandemics such as Ebola and HIV and AIDS.

This particular volume seeks to trace the diverse effects and responses to the pandemic across the broad spectrum of society including the religious, socio-cultural and public health fraternities. A lot of questions remain unanswered since the pandemic has affected people differently and has been responded to in a heterogeneous manner in the Global South, particularly in Southern Africa. Some of the key questions include: How have faith communities in Southern Africa acted as both a help and a hindrance (Mtata 2013) in response to COVID-19? What is the interface between religion and public health in the face of the pandemic in Southern Africa? As others are rethinking the entire Humanities curriculum in the wake of COVID-19 (Du Preez et al. 2020; Mendy and Madiope 2020; Ramrathan et al. 2020), how can the curriculum of Religious Studies and Theology in Southern Africa be transformed to equip graduates to be better able to handle pandemics in future?

In order to better understand possible responses to the pandemic, it is imperative to conceptualise how religion is understood in this volume. The use of the term "religion" follows an age-old debate on its elusiveness, culture specificity, flexibility, non-normativity and non-universality (Smith 1964, 1987; Cox 1996; Chitando 1997). In other words, the term is fluid and at times associated with misleading connotations because it is binding and confessional. For that reason, Smith (1964) suggests that we should jettison the term "religion" and replace it with two concepts, namely "personal faith" and "cumulative traditions". In the same quandary with Smith (1964), Ninian Smart (1969) asserts that it is not prudent to expend our efforts in trying to define religion, but rather proposes its dimensions, to which he identifies six or seven in all. In fact, Smart (1969) cited by Sharma (2011:44) prefers the term "worldviews" over "religion", which is more inclusive and beneficial. For Smart (1969) the separation of religion and the secular is unnecessary because essentially what we deal with is the religious and the symbolic aspect of human life – rituals, ultimate beliefs, myths and so on. Given these conceptions, contributors in this volume utilise a broad understanding of religion where the term "worldview" gives a new and more relevant view on religion. Smart quoted in Sharma (2011:49) had this to say:

> I would argue that there are gains in stretching scope of religious studies and so in effect the definition of religion. It is of course awkward in ordinary conversation. So I use the term 'worldview' and the phrase

'worldview analysis' for what we do. It is not the best of words, but the English and other languages are very poor in vocabulary for discussing beliefs, ideologies as the like. Often the vocabulary of a people simply reflects its own religious history and that is typically not good for describing other systems.

Given the above insights, we learn that religion is a complex and variegated phenomenon which requires a "worldview analysis". This does justice to the various religious traditions under discussion in this volume.

Writing as far back as the late 1960s, the Kenyan-born African Christian theologian, John S. Mbiti asserted that "Africans are notoriously religious" (1969:1). This has become a basis of understanding the spirituality and religiosity of Africans testified in the global shift of the centre of gravity of Christianity from the Northern to the Southern hemisphere (Kalu 2003:215; Sibanda 2018:8). In the context of COVID-19, the spirituality of Africans has been undoubtedly a prominent feature among the religious and non-religious personalities of various stripes, including politicians and public health practitioners. For instance, John Magufuli, the late President of Tanzania, claimed that the virus was a "devil's tool" and went on to encourage people to continue visiting their places of worship at a time when other countries were stepping up measures to curb gatherings. Magufuli proclaimed that: "These Holy places are where God is. [...]Coronavirus cannot survive in the body of Christ, it will burn" (Taylor 2020). Here, Magufuli was self-presenting as a faithful devotee of the Christian faith. His decision to reject the lockdown route that gained momentum in most countries in the world, including Africa, set him apart from other African leaders. Magufuli, with an unorthodox approach to the office of president, was projecting the image of a pious and independent African leader who was implementing a uniquely African solution to respond to a global challenge. During the second wave of the pandemic in early 2021, Magufuli persisted with his ultra-conservative stance, saying:

> We will also continue to take health precautions including the use of steam inhalation. You inhale while you pray to God, you pray while farming maize, potatoes, so that you can eat well and corona fails to enter your body. They will scare you a lot, my fellow Tanzanians, but you should stand firm.
>
> (Reuters 2021)

Contributors to this volume have approached their chapters with flexible definitions of politics, but leaning more towards appreciating politics as the exercise of power (Heywood 1997; Modebadze 2010), with an impact on development (Oloruntoba and Falola 2018) in Southern Africa. They seek to examine how actors in the fields that have traditionally been demarcated as religious (dealing with spiritual issues, indigenous knowledge systems, beliefs and practices that fall within their worldview in space and time), political (dealing with decision-making and relating to the distribution of resources) and public health (dealing with the allopathic and alternative medical services for human flourishing) have interacted in the wake of a global pandemic in Africa. Whereas one of the most prominent sociologists of African Pentecostalism, Asonzeh Ukah, makes the bold claim that, "COVID-19 could as much lay bare where the real power and resources of Africa and Africans lie: in religion or the political economy of the postcolonial state" (2020:459), we contend that an "either/or" approach is inadequate and misses the complexity of the interface between religion, public health and politics in Southern Africa. Contributors, therefore, seek to provide more nuanced analyses of how COVID-19 offers fresh insights into the religion, public health and politics conundrum in Southern African settings. Anthropologist Francis Nyamnjoh and historian Joel Carpenter have articulated an informative interpretation of the role of religion in society and we cite their observation below:

> The fact that religion does not occur in a social, political and cultural vacuum should necessarily alert the attention of scholars – who provide for and are sensitive to the suggested approach – to the categorical imperative of the role of power, money, poverty and the cultures they engender and perpetuate in what form religion and religiosity assume in the lives of individuals and in the institutions and everyday relations of a given society.
>
> (Nyamnjoh and Carpenter 2018:290)

In this way, the volume makes several assumptions that point to the role of religion in its variegated form as it interacts with public health and politics. The assumptions include:

a   that religion as an independent institution plays a vital role in health matters of the population, whether positively or negatively;
b   that religion facilitates in a positive way how states respond to the pandemic;
c   and that religion and politics are interrelated and, in some ways, interconnected to Africa's development.

The foregoing assumptions are anchored on theoretical and methodological considerations that undergird this volume. Theoretically, the volume encompasses a wide range of theories on which contributors ground their chapters. By and large, the volume mirrors an Afrocentric thinking and experience where Southern Africa is the focus. In other words, contributors in this volume present the COVID-19 experiences of different communities, nations and states. Given the complex nature and severity of the pandemic, analogies/metaphors of collective consciousness become handy.

It is in this context that we adopt "the theory of the hut on fire" (Kurian 2001; Dube 2009:83) metaphor to explain the diverse and varied responses to the COVID-19 pandemic. This "hut on fire" theory was originally used by Kurian (2001) and further adopted by Dube (2009) to explain the different types of responses to the HIV and AIDS pandemic and we find it helpful in the context of COVID-19. As the nations feel the impact of COVID-19, they become the "burning hut" that members of the village provide varied responses to, which responses include (a) some villagers jumping into action to douse the fire and save the hut; (b) some villagers standing still, putting their hands on their heads and crying helplessly; (c) some villagers ignore the burning hut and remain indifferent taking it as none of their business, while (d) other villagers blame it on the victims whose hut is on fire saying that "those who play with fire get their fingers burnt".

All these responses are indicative of the diverse standpoints of responses to COVID-19, positively or negatively. Contributors in this volume present many forms of responses to the "burning hut" due to COVID-19 along the lines of gender, religious, class and national identities. Using "the theory of a hut on fire", the different chapters recognise that individuals, communities and the nations in Southern Africa under the shadow of COVID-19 can better understand the problem at hand and its possible solutions. Methodologically, contributors in this volume utilise various methods for data gathering and analysis from different paradigms. Due to COVID-19 crisis, the studies in this volume were carried out in the midst of the pandemic thereby leading contributors to adopt data collecting techniques amenable to COVID-19 containment measures.

Geographically, the book covers countries in Southern Africa whose boundaries largely follow those of the Southern African Development Community (SADC). Initially, we sought to do an Africa-wide volume with all linguistic regions represented. Unfortunately, due to the COVID-19-induced disruptions, we could not get contributors from the Lusophone and Francophone countries in SADC. However, chapters in this volume do not cover all the countries in the SADC region. The inclusion of a chapter from Tanzania is informed by Tanzania's status as a member of the SADC. However, we included a chapter from Tanzania's neighbour, Kenya, although Kenya is outside the SADC.

## Background: religion, COVID-19 and politics

As COVID-19 took its toll in Western countries before coming to the African continent, one politician from Zimbabwe claimed that the virus was God's way of punishing the Global North for imposing economic sanctions on Zimbabwe. God and COVID-19 were being roped into the sanctions discourse or "political football" (Chingono 2010). This shows the influence of religion in the public sphere. Some claimed that ancient prophecies of African Traditional Religions and relatively new ones within African

Pentecostalism were being confirmed through this pandemic. Therefore, whereas many religious leaders, governments and communities were taking decisive measures guided by public health officials to slow the spread of the virus such as halting congregational services and offering private and public spiritual guidance, others, however, were generating and circulating messianic and apocalyptic messages, which downplayed the value of official public health guidance, and offering religious panaceas that were running contrary to good public health practice (Dein 2021). On this basis, the volume presents chapters that show the ambivalent influence of religion (see Appleby 2000) across various sections of society in the era of COVID-19 in Southern Africa.

As part of the politics of public health, the histories of national and international responses to epidemic events tell us a lot about the interplay of power, religion, science and geopolitics. In the era of COVID-19, religion joined with science amid the virus crisis as people would "pray and wash" (VOA News 2020). Therefore, instead of magnifying the warfare theory of faith's relationship to science, evoking the theory of religion and science as dialogue partners became urgent to test in the face of COVID-19 in Southern Africa. It can be asked: How far did religion complement public health in curbing the spread of COVID-19? Furthermore, instead of solely relying on biomedical strategies to deal with the crisis by combining epidemiological, clinical, and behavioural aspects, attention should also be duly accorded to the use of indigenous knowledge systems to understand, prevent, manage and reduce the impact of symptomatic elements of the disease. What has been the role of (non-) herbal remedies (Dandara et al. 2020) and African religion in this maze?

As human interaction had largely been turned into a virtual affair because of the COVID-19 crisis, new intervention strategies became critical. For instance, the lockdown made tele-health a useful mitigating measure to reduce the risk between patients and medical health personnel in the shadow of COVD-19 in Southern Africa. Even religious institutions began to seriously consider the viability of intensifying the use of online religion and religion online (Asamoah-Gyadu 2015) in times of COVID-19 and beyond. What were the politics of accessing online platforms and how did these shape religious identities in Southern Africa? Did this advantage those forms of religious expression that were already techno savvy, such as Pentecostalism, while disadvantaging those that were not as adept at embracing information and communication technologies such as mainline and African Initiated Churches (AICs)?

The government and public health call of social distancing was meant to reduce the spread of this pandemic. Some critics and contributors in this volume have questioned how amenable people were to the rules of lockdown and social distancing in the African context. To what extent is *unhu/ ubuntu* ethics (Sambala et al. 2019) relevant when dealing with the infected in times of COVID-19 in Southern Africa? This reminds us of the attitude of accompaniment and solidarity, which were helpful to those infected by HIV and AIDS (Chitando 2007), notwithstanding that COVID-19 stressed the social distancing rule. For some, social distancing, using hand sanitisers and staying at home were privileges accessible only to the affluent, whilst the poor majority did not have spacious living space, money to buy sanitisers and yet others were homeless. Did religious leaders, who are expected to have a prophetic voice, challenge some of the policies and vicious enforcement of the lockdown regulations by the police in the different Southern African countries? Did religious leaders denounce the corruption that characterised some of the disbursements of COVID-19 funds in various contexts? Such questions lead us to reflect on these dynamics below (as well as in some of the chapters in this volume).

## Politicians, religious leaders and COVID-19 in Southern Africa

With the COVID-19 pandemic gathering momentum, many African political leaders began to cajole the religious constituency to play an important role in responding to COVID-19. In many countries, including South Africa and Zimbabwe, Days of National Prayer were held, where political leaders ceded space to religious leaders to lead nations in prayers of supplication, as well as to mobilise their constituencies and beyond to respond to the pandemic. As chapters in this volume illustrate, this was achieved with varying degrees of success. For the purposes of this introduction, we seek to draw attention to a few major themes.

First, we approach the religion-politics-public health interface in the face of COVID-19 with a very specific model of interaction. We conceptualise this in terms of the relations between these spheres as being: (i) cordial, (ii) tense and (iii) mixed, with moments of cordiality being interspaced with those where there was tension. In the case of cordial relations among the spheres, actors from the religious, political and public health sectors share programmes, collaborate on joint actions, promote development and have front-door entry policies. In those instances where relationships are tense, there is constant criticism among the spheres. Relations are generally toxic and there is hardly any collaboration. In the third form of engagement, relations move between being cordial and being tense across different, but within short periods of time (see, among others, Ellis and Ter Haar 1998; Fox 2008, 2018 for other reviews of religion and politics). We have sought to interpret the religion-politics-public health interface in times of COVID-19 in Southern Africa within this scheme.

Second, it became clear in most cases that there was generally good rapport between the more prominent religious leaders and politicians who were running the different governments in Southern Africa. Thus, the dominant type of religion-politics-public health interaction that we identified was that of cordial relations, as in our model above. Most African political leaders have often sought not to antagonise religious leaders. Recognising the strategic importance of religious leaders, and the faith-based organisations that are often related to faith communities, political leaders have deemed it helpful to have religious leaders on their side. Further, they acknowledge the religious social capital (Maselko et al. 2011) that the religious leaders bring to the table. Adopting an interfaith approach, they mobilised the religious leaders, gave them prominent positions at the meetings to respond to COVID-19, acknowledged their role in social transformation and sought to make them feel relevant and appreciated.

While we do not wish to suggest that politicians running governments adopted an instrumentalist approach in their interface with religious leaders in the face of COVID-19 in Southern Africa, it is fair to say that they sought to make religious leaders feel relevant. On their part, most religious leaders, particularly from the mainline churches and Muslim traditions, undertook to uphold and promote the COVID-19 protocols that were being popularised and enforced by African governments and public health officials. In these transactions between politicians and religious leaders, the ideal of securing the common good was prioritised. Thus, both the politicians and religious leaders presented themselves as selfless individuals keen to promote human security (Tarusarira and Chitando 2020) in the wake of a devastating pandemic.

Third, we observe that in some Southern African countries tension emerged between political and religious leaders over three main issues that we will need to summarise due to space considerations. In the first instance, there were some religious leaders, particularly from independent and charismatic movements (mainly Christian) that are not affiliated to any ecumenical group (Protestant or Pentecostal) that insisted on going ahead with large gatherings for religious purposes. Some Muslim groups also fall into this category (see, for example, Kindzeka 2020). Due to various religious and political reasons, they felt the need to resist the lockdown restrictions. In the second instance, some ecumenical bodies such as the South African Council of Churches (SACC) launched an anti-corruption campaign against the looting of COVID-19 funds. The SACC used strong language, describing the looting of COVID-19 funds as genocide (WCC 2020). Finally, there was also tension over some religious leaders' active resistance to vaccines in Southern Africa. For instance, the Rastafarian religious communities in Southern Africa were/are sceptical about the use of "Babylon" manufactured COVID-19 vaccines, as illustrated by Fortune Sibanda in this volume.

Overall, however, our central observation and submission regarding the religion-politics-public health interface in Southern Africa's engagement with COVID-19, and which has relevance in analysing future pandemics is this: pre-existing patterns and models of interaction determined the interface. This learning is critical in terms of preparing for future pandemics in Southern Africa (and probably elsewhere). Although pandemics have the capacity to generate new forms of interacting and disrupting previous types of engagement, the most dominant trend or pattern will in large measure be shaped by previous and ongoing ways of interfacing between politicians and religious leaders in public health matters.

## Public health, religion, and politics in the context of COVID-19 in Southern Africa

The previous section has highlighted the patterns of interaction between politicians and religious leaders in the face of COVID-19 in many Southern African countries. The main request by politicians was for religious leaders to act responsibly and adhere to the public health messages that were being disseminated by the authorities. This leads us to a discussion on religion, public health and politics in the era of COVID-19 in Southern Africa.

There is limited literature on religion and public health in general, and in Southern Africa particularly. However, following the devastating impact of HIV and AIDS, there have been efforts to understand the interface (see, for example, Azetsop 2016). The picture that is emerging suggests that religious leaders are very well placed to influence their constituents in matters relating to health. For example, the insistence on exclusive claims to faith healing by some neo-Pentecostal prophets has had a negative impact on the uptake of antiretroviral therapy in the context of HIV and AIDS. The inverse is true: where religious leaders have overcome stigma and have actively promoted antiretroviral therapy, adherence has been impressive. Therefore, religious leaders are strategic in communicating and supporting public health messages in Southern Africa.

In the context of COVID-19, most mainstream Christian, Muslim and traditional leaders were forthcoming in promoting public health messages that emphasised foregoing coming together for worship, sanitising and observing social distance. In this regard, they sought to complement public health officials and politicians in preaching messages of prevention. Religious leaders were simultaneously increasing or enhancing their social standing by saying the right things in the face of a devastating pandemic. This was not the result of some feigned "political correctness" (Fairclough 2003), but out of their commitment towards making a difference. Major religious activities such as the massive Easter gatherings for Christians and the Eid al-Fitr at the end of the month of Ramadan for Muslims were inconspicuous in 2020/2021.

By promoting public health messages to prevent and mitigate the impact of COVID-19, religious leaders in Southern Africa were subscribing to the ideology of religion-state partnership, or the cordiality model that we articulated above. In the face of a highly threatening pandemic, competition and tension with the state would result in missed opportunities when time would have been of utmost essence. However, the politics of gender still came out to the fore as illustrated by Molly Manyonganise's chapter in this volume. In different settings and mirroring pre-existing gender norms, the faces of religion and politics responding to COVID-19 in Africa were mostly those of middle-aged to older men. Images of God as the father tend to justify male dominance in religion and society (Modise and Wood 2016), resulting in male dominance. As the Ugandan feminist and legal scholar, Sylvia Tamale (2020) has cogently argued that colonial and missionary regimes have coalesced to give rise to male dominance in various spheres of life in Africa.

There was a general sacralisation of the COVID-19 public health messages. Although such an approach would be deemed problematic or even as compromising the clarity of public health messages in other parts of the world, this was not the case in Southern Africa. Thus, the COVID-19 messages of frequent hand washing, sanitising and keeping social distance were "baptised" and embraced as God's very own strategy of protecting humanity. Here, the assumption that there must be or there is an inherent conflict or tension between religion and science was defused, as Bernard Pindukai Humbe illustrates in his chapter. Presenting the public messages in religious garb made it easier for the various communities of faith to embrace and implement them. Thus, for example, staying at home and not going to a religious gathering became a sign of obedience to a divine command, and not only accepting public health messages.

In keeping with the dynamics of upholding COVID-19 protocols, many religious activities moved online. This move benefitted mostly African Pentecostal churches, who have always been media savvy from the beginning (see, for example, Hackett 1998; Togarasei 2012) and are influencing other forms of religious expression such as groups steeped in African Traditional Religions (De Witte 2018). This transition to tele-evangelism and tele-health is extensively dealt with in Lucia Ponde Mutsvedu and Sophia Chirongoma's chapter in this volume.

Although the picture of collaboration between religious and political actors in communicating COVID-19 prevention measures in Southern Africa is largely an accurate one, we concede that there were also some religious leaders who refused to heed public health messages, let alone to popularise them. For example, some "ultra conservatives" within the African Initiated Churches (AICs) refused to put on masks and continued to have their open air meetings in different countries in Southern Africa. For instance, the Johane Marange Apostolic Church in Zimbabwe has been castigated for flouting COVID-19 gathering restrictions by holding their Annual Pascal Festival for 21 days in July 2021 (NewsDay 2021). This was consistent with the underlying AIC ideology that biomedical approaches are part of the Western, colonising agenda. In reality, therefore, the resistance to public health messages by some AICs must be located within the discourse of decoloniality (Ndlovu-Gatsheni 2020). In this regard, AICs prefigure the concern with African epistemologies and jettisoning Western/colonial approaches to health and healing. AICs would stridently oppose the tendency to associate indigenous practices with facilitating the spread of pandemics (Jaja et al. 2020).

It must be admitted, though, that the lockdown left many religious practitioners battling for survival in economic terms. Once the weekly offerings were no longer coming due to the strict lockdowns imposed by many governments across the continents, many religious leaders felt the impact. It became clear that most faith communities are not well prepared to face emergencies. In an effort to mitigate the impact, some religious leaders sought to play politics to try and arm-twist their governments into including them on the "privileged list" of those who were providing "essential services" during the COVID-19 pandemic. This confirmed the transactional nature of the interface between politicians and religious leaders. Although this demand/request was not met in most instances, the fact that religious leaders felt confident that they could lobby governments to grant them special favours suggests that they sense that they can always get concessions from the politicians.

## Revelations, contestations and explaining COVID-19

Related to the foregoing discussion is the theme of the politics of making sense of COVID-19. How were citizens in Southern Africa to explain COVID-19? What were the frames that politicians (and especially religious leaders) going to deploy to account for the pandemic? Although the first wave of the pandemic had left Africa relatively unscathed, the devastation of the second and the more vicious third waves, particularly in Southern Africa, saw the retrieval and use of images of apocalypticism (as we elaborate below). Consequently, the public space was awash with multiple interpretations of the origin of the pandemic, its signification and routes of resolution. For example, what, if any, would be the place of (a) vaccine/s? It would require a longer narrative to do justice to these themes than can be undertaken in this introduction. However, we shall raise a few salient points.

With COVID-19 paralysing in person religious gatherings and feeling that their authority was diminishing, some African Pentecostal leaders sought to reclaim authority by making pronouncements on the pandemic. If they could not retain prominence through healing claims, they would seek to do so by providing narratives that re-placed them at the centre. Thus, prominent African Pentecostal leaders such as Chris Oyakhilome, founder-owner of Christ Embassy Church and LoveWorld Television Network (Ukah 2020:454, note 89) and Emmanuel Makandiwa in Zimbabwe sought to explain the origins of the pandemic and to reassure their followers of divine protection. The late T. B. Joshua, well known for his claim to make accurate prophecies, had suggested that the epidemic would be over very quickly and had to change course when it persisted in 2020 (Orjinmo 2020).

Conspiracy theories, either generated from, or getting lubricated within, African Pentecostalism (but enjoying currency well beyond), gained momentum once the issue of rolling out vaccines became prominent from early 2021. However, efforts to account for the global pandemic, or what was said to be God's unique plans to protect Africa from the pandemic, how to prevent COVID-19 and other issues constituted key issues in the public discourse on COVID-19. Ukah provides a helpful outline when he writes:

> Some of the information, sermons, messages, and interpretations circulating from church leaders indicate different perceptions, perspectives, and practices regarding how churches and their leaders are coping with and adapting to the new and unusual circumstances of COVID-19. Interpreted as a plague, the COVID-19 pandemic is seen as understandable and controllable as divine retribution that prescribes a course of action as a remedy: return to God, prayers, acknowledgement of God in human affairs, and so forth. Some claim that the pandemic is not caused by a virus but is a byproduct of 5G telecommunications technology.
>
> (Ukah 2020:453–454)

The discourse persisted in relation to whether Africans/members of specific faith communities could trust vaccines that had been developed in the Global North to respond to COVID-19. This was a highly contentious issue, with some Pentecostal leaders fomenting resistance to the vaccines. There were insinuations that some devilish plan was underway to exterminate Africans, or that the vaccines were designed to alter the DNA of those who would be injected, thereby tampering with God's plan and form regarding humans. The influence of Pentecostalism on strategically placed individuals became clear when the South African Chief Justice, MogoengMogoeng linked COVID-19 vaccines to a satanic agenda (Reuters Staff 2020). To be sure, this segment of Africans was not alone in questioning the efficacy of COVID-19 vaccines. The problem of vaccine scepticism also came to the fore in Zambia where Dr. Nevers Mumba, a Pentecostal politician, emphasised the need to provide a strenuous verification and validation of vaccines before using them on Zambians lest people would die like fools. For him, vaccines would be declared unsafe until they were scientifically proven by local medical experts, not foreigners. In the United States, some Evangelical Christians, many of whom were supporters of former president Donald Trump, also challenged COVID-19 vaccines (DW, n.d.). Some African governments fell prey to self-interests that bordered on the lack of responsible leadership.

Processing the meaning of pandemics is a task that no generation has been able to complete. Religious leaders and their followers went through different stages in trying to decipher what COVID-19 meant. African Traditional Religions, Christianity, Islam, Rastafari and other religions all offered different explanations of the pandemic. Indeed, there were internal variations within these diverse faith groups, as well as overlaps in how they sought to make COVID-19 intelligible and to enable individuals and communities to cope amidst its devastating impact. This goes some way in confirming the notion that religion is a meaning-making framework to cope with stress (Park 2005). Faced with a highly disruptive pandemic, followers of different religions fell back on their faith traditions to extract meaning. In the case of Christians, the Bible was available for consultation.

## The politics of reading the Bible in the context of COVID-19

The other form of politics that emerged from the religious engagement with COVID-19 relates to biblical interpretation. Across history and different settings, there has never been one, binding and universally agreed upon interpretation of the Bible. For example, there have been attempts to bring together African and European readers of the Bible in the quest for a shared meaning (de Wit and West 2009). It is clear, however, that there were multiple interpretations of the Bible in the wake of COVID-19. Further, it would appear that as there was HIV biblical hermeneutics (see, for example, Dube 2008; Muneja 2012), we can talk of COVID-19 biblical hermeneutics unravelling.

While a separate study is required to do justice to the theme of the politics of biblical interpretation in the context of COVID-19, it is possible to identify some key dimensions. For example, the dominant hermeneutical strand in readings of the Bible during COVID-19 in Africa was on security. As media images of overflowing hospitals and mortuaries in the Global North were being displayed, many Africans sought refuge in the Bible. This was accentuated during the second and third waves of the pandemic in early and mid-2021 when the death rate went up significantly in Southern Africa. The politics of reading in this regard were around "reading for security and individual/communal salvation." The popular passages tended to be from the Old Testament (Hebrew Bible). Many social media posts sought to reassure individuals, families, communities, nations and the continent that the promises of God to protect and guide God's people were still relevant. For example, the passage in Numbers 31: 49, "and said to Moses 'Your servants counted the warriors who are under our command, and not one of us is missing'" was popular due to its suggestion that all those who were in quarantine would come out alive and be counted, without any one of them missing.

When the death rate increased during the second and third waves, there were calls for prayer and fasting from within different sectors. Thus, Ezra 8: 21–23, which refers to fasting, was popular with some religious leaders. Other readers of the Bible understood the COVID-19 as representing the end of time. Reflecting on the theme from a different context, Dein (2020) has explored the politics of interpreting COVID-19 as the apocalypse. In this scheme, the pandemic represents the end of time, where God is now acting decisively to bring history to a close. Indeed, the authors of this chapter encountered numerous social media posts by Christians from different confessional backgrounds that suggested that the pandemic was a sure sign that time was coming to an end through God's intervention. Evoking the earlier association of the HIV epidemic as punishment from God, yet others read the COVID-19 pandemic as a sign that God was punishing a generation that had turned away from the Creator (Pieterse and Landman 2021). But, to be fair, some Pentecostal leaders, such as Pastor Mensa Ottabil from Ghana, refused to endorse the popular reading of COVID-19 as punishment from evil or a form of demonic attack.[1]

In heavily polarised societies, some citizens embraced COVID-19 deaths among the political leaders. They regarded this as divine judgement on those who denied citizens their rights. They too appealed to the Bible. For example, they cited the following text, "When the righteous prosper, the city rejoices; when the wicked perish, there are shouts of joy" (Proverbs 11:10). All these developments highlight both the interface between the Bible and politics in Africa (Gunda and Kügler 2012), as well as the politics of interpreting the Bible in the context of COVID-19.

## The status of African indigenous knowledge systems in the context of COVID-19

As the Western medical system struggled to address COVID-19 and its pretensions were exposed, it was almost inevitable that discourses on indigenous knowledge systems (IKS) gained ground in Africa. For long trivialised, minimised and de-valorised by Western ways of knowing (Mawere 2014), IKS resurfaced with vigour in the face of COVID-19. Again, this theme requires more space than is available in this chapter. We highlight some of the key issues.

First, some countries such as Madagascar, Cameroon, Tanzania and others announced that traditional medicines would play a significant role in their COVID-19 responses. In particular, Madagascar's president, Andriy Rojoelin, a promoted herbal tea which he said was effective against COVID-19. This generated considerable debate, with the World Health Organization (WHO) questioning the efficacy of the herbal tea. On their part, African ideologues challenged the WHO of sustaining a colonial agenda by refusing to accept solutions from Africa. The politics of "the centre versus the periphery" were being played out yet again, with some African intellectuals contending that the WHO needed to be decolonised. However, it must be conceded that there was need for the efficacy of African alternative therapies to be proven, even by alternative scientific paradigms, since lives were at stake.

Second, the increasing death rates from the second and third waves of COVID-19, particularly in Southern Africa, generated the increased use of traditional practices and medicines. For example, steaming and inhalation gained popularity, alongside traditional herbs. What is clear is that most Africans realised that they could not wait for the Global North to think about them in cruel race for vaccines where rich and developed nations would buy vaccines in excess at the expense of developing nations, dubbed "vaccine apartheid". Vaccine nationalism would be the order of the day, where citizens of the Global North would receive priority, while Africans and others in the Global South would literally have only God on their side.

Third, the resurgence of IKS in the wake of COVID-19 in Africa confirms that the dominance of the foreign ideologies might only be superficial. Whereas the Christian and Muslim influences are real and Western paradigms dominate at the official level across most parts of the continent, it is worth noting the resilience of IKS. Going forward, IKS will continue to shape the responses of many Africans to pandemics. Investing in greater understanding of the role of IKS among Africans from diverse backgrounds remains highly strategic.

## Chapters in this volume

Africa, Southern Africa in particular, is a rich terrain for the exploration of the complex relationships and new ways of understanding the interplay of religious beliefs, practices, state and society in the context of public health. On this basis, writing from a perspective of the indigenous knowledge systems (IKS), chapters constituting the first part of this volume point out the extent to which individuals and communities utilised this heritage-based philosophy in responding to COVID-19. In Chapter 2, Beatrice Okyere-Manu and Stephen N. Morgan explore the implications the ethics of *Ubuntu* have on public health in the era of COVID-19 in Southern Africa. *Ubuntu* is a widespread concept used in diverse African contexts. The authors situated their contribution in context by stating that "*Ubuntu,* the ethical theory that lies at the very heart of traditional African values, can be explored to meet the challenges brought about as a result of the outbreak of COVID-19." Given that the COVID-19 pandemic has presented a new order to the African way of life, the duo critically explores ways in which the African ethics of *Ubuntu* can remain relevant in this new way of life confronting Southern African communities. They emphatically ask in wonder: how can the fundamental moral principles of *Ubuntu* be appropriated in the African community today? Thus, their chapter reflects on such principles of *Ubuntu* as good human relationship, the show of solidarity, high regard for family, respect for authorities and elders, and a sense of religion to demonstrate how the ethics of *Ubuntu* can inform the best ways to live and relate to one another amid the COVID-19 pandemic.

Similarly, in Chapter 3, Tenson Muyambo, arguing from a Ndau indigenous knowledge system, examines the social distancing strategy as an indigenous knowledge systems of the Ndau people helpful in the contexts of pandemics and epidemics in Zimbabwe. His research sought to establish the respondents' experiences and views on social distancing as a prevention and control measure against the spread of COVID-19 from past experiences of epidemics. Using the Sankofa approach, the chapter argues that pandemics like COVID-19 do not only demand unique and unusual strategies that may go against a people's indigenous knowledge, but use that available indigenous knowledge as building blocks to minimise the spread and severity of such pandemics. Muyambo established that while the Ndau people appreciated social distancing not necessarily as a new measure to prevent the spread of COVID-19, it equally compromised and went against the dictates of *ubuntu*, which was then difficult to practice within the framework of African spirituality. The chapter recommends that a community-based task force led by traditional leadership and medical health officials is essential to educate the communities, in accessible languages and media, on the need to utilise both indigenous and Western epistemics concomitantly in the face of pandemics as deadly as COVID-19.

Still on the Ndau people, Macloud Sipeyiye in Chapter 4, explores the promises and challenges of the Ndau indigenous religion in the context of the pandemic with a view to finding how resources embedded within it can transform death-dealing behaviours in current and future times. Employing Carkoglu's (2008) spiritual capital theory, he examines how religious ideas and activities inspire adherents to transform their lives and that of others beyond their immediate comfort zone. Therefore, the chapter is an empirical qualitative phenomenological study that seeks to access the meaning embedded in the religious activities of the Ndau in the context of religion, public health and COVID-19. Bernard P. Humbe's call in Chapter 5 is to integrate religion and science as a response to COVID-19 pandemic in Zimbabwe. For him, the COVID-19 pandemic has reignited a long-standing debate on the relationship between religion and science. His chapter can also be located in the scheme where African indigenous knowledge systems and religions are taken into account because they provide the spectacles that the majority of citizens use to frame their understanding of disasters or development initiatives.

In Chapter 6, Helena Van Coller and Idowu A. Akinloye's provide a critical examination of the state regulatory response in containing the spread of COVID-19 in light of the constitutionally guaranteed human rights, including the rights to freedom of movement, freedom of association, freedom of religion and the right to human dignity in South Africa. By using a doctrinal research approach through analysis of literature, statutes and case examples, the chapter evaluates the state regulations enacted to curb the spread of the COVID-19 in South Africa vis-à-vis the constitutional provisions protecting freedom of religion in the country in order to determine the constitutional justification of the regulations. They argue that parts of the regulations that provide for the total or partial ban of religious gatherings in the wake of the outbreak of the COVID-19 are permissible limitations of religious freedom. The chapter resonates with the view that law and religion can invoke restorative and therapeutic roles following a proper diagnosis of the problem at hand (Green 2014:214).

From the role of the law and religion in society, the volume moves on to Chapter 7, by Lucia Ponde-Mutsvedu and Sophia Chirongoma. This chapter draws insights from Bronfenbrenner's ecological model and the African ethic of *Ubuntu/Unhu* as lenses for reflecting on how COVID-19 has impacted on social relationships, particularly family interactions in African communities. The authors tackled the cutting edge issue of the media and its considerable power with special reference to the Karanga-Shona people in Zimbabwe. They argue that people have tried to bridge the gap created by social distancing measures through the increased use of Information and Communication Technology (ICT), particularly social media, tele-evangelism and tele-health services, which has also inadvertently unleashed the problem of cyberbullying. This resonates with Green's (2014) observation that the new media has power to shape perceptions that become new social sources of value and normativity through mediated religion, health and social hostilities on social media. The chapter concludes by foregrounding the need for African communities to continue preserving and practising the principles of *Ubuntu/Unhu* whilst embracing realistic and practical adjustments so as to protect and preserve lives in the wake of the COVID-19 epidemic.

Paskas Wagana's Chapter 8 examines the role of religion in response to the COVID-19 pandemic challenges in Tanzania. Tanzania provides a unique case study of religion, politics and health because (at the time of writing) it was the only African country in the region to defy the advice to institute quarantine and national lockdown to curb the spread of COVID-19. Instead, under the leadership of the late President John Magufuli, Tanzania incorporated religion as a major tool in its own national guidelines to counteract both the spread of the disease and to mitigate the social and psychological effects brought by the traumatic COVID-19. The chapter employed the theory of governmentality whilst grappling with the question: how effective is religion in combating the spread of epidemics? Wagana concludes that Tanzania has been exemplary in evaluating its strengths, social structures and localizing standard measures of COVID-19 according to local conditions and resources available, including religion.

The next chapter by Julius Gathogo (Chapter 9) on "COVID-19 Containment Measures and 'Prophecies' in Kenya" explores the nature, impact, and progression of COVID-19 in Kenya during its first two months (March–April 2020). It provides the government of Kenya's initial response and that of religious leaders to the pandemic. Gathogo argues that while the State strove hard to play its role in addressing the pandemic, the resultant "prophecies" from some religious leaders were problematic. He also surveys the chronological events from 13 March to 25 April so as to understand the initial trends, the setbacks, and the progression of the pandemic.

In Chapter 10, Sonene Nyawo explores the Christian religious understandings and responses to COVID-19 in the Kingdom of Eswatini. The chapter shows how religious communities, influenced by a traditional cosmological orientation, understand and interpret this phenomenon. Beyond interpreting COVID-19 as a biological warfare, as some conspiracy theories would claim, the chapter argues that some contended that it is a spiritual warfare between two kingdoms, which calls for a spiritual intervention to restore the disturbed equilibrium in the spiritual and natural milieu of human life. In addition, other people regarded COVID-19 to be God's punishment for sin and as a fulfilment of biblical prophecies about the end times. However, the chapter demonstrates that such understandings and responses can bind the nation together and contribute to successful coping with the pandemic, but may also lead to low perception of risk and create a fatalistic attitude in the face of the virus.

Nelly Mwale and Joseph Chita's Chapter 11 engages with how the Church mother bodies in Zambia, namely, Council of Churches in Zambia, Evangelical Fellowship of Zambia, Zambia Conference of Catholic Bishops and Independent Churches of Zambia responded to COVID-19. Drawing on Content Analysis of interviews, press statements and communications in the media from the Church Mother bodies, the chapter shows that the responses were characterised by both submission and defiance. Church Mother bodies reinterpreted their Christian dogma on worship to prevent and manage COVID-19. Additionally, they provided spiritual and public health education, material support and advocated for accountability and support towards society's vulnerable groups. Contrary to using religion as a barrier in the context of the pandemic, Mwale and Chita argue that the Mother bodies used religion as a resource to mobilise its members for the good of human life.

From the responses of the mother bodies in Zambia, the volume includes Tshenolo J. Madigele and James N. Amanze's Chapter 12 on the Churches and COVID-19 in Botswana. By using reports from Church Organizations under the Botswana Network of Christian Communities (BONECO), interviews with pastors and leaders of churches and literature available on the Internet, the chapter provided an overview of how the religious fraternity in Botswana has responded to COVID-19. The authors identified the strengths and challenges of the responses of churches under BONECO and outlining lessons learnt from the interface of epidemics, religion and politics. The chapter refers to *diaconia* as a vital responsibility of the church whilst the government is blameworthy for not giving the Church an ample opportunity to mobilise their members to take part in relieving those who were financially affected by COVID-19. The authors conclude that dealing with marginalization and social inequality may consequently bring sustainable long-term development under the guise of Christian ministry and work in complementing the government.

Makomborero Allen Bowa's Chapter 13 explores the challenges faced by persons with disabilities in Zambia, Zimbabwe and South Africa. He points out that in general, navigating many community and institutional barriers is a challenge for persons with disabilities in normal times. These include physical and environment barriers that are inaccessible, communication barriers, and attitudinal barriers, which negatively impact on them. In the context of a pandemic, these barriers become even more complex and heightened. Essentially, it is clear that this pandemic is negatively impacting on the health and economic well-being of persons with disabilities in the Southern African context. For him, there is need for a more comprehensive and inclusive response from the Church in partnership with other stakeholders if the retrogressive impact of this pandemic is to be minimised, especially in the context of disability. He further asserts that the Church in Zambia, Zimbabwe and South Africa should take appropriate action to guard against the further marginalisation and stigmatisation of persons with disabilities during and especially after this pandemic through a liberative reading of the Bible. This chapter therefore assesses the potential risks for persons with disabilities during the pandemic and articulates the measures that the Church in collaboration with other stakeholders can put in place to mitigate processes that may further marginalise persons with disabilities from the mainstream structures of society and expose them to poverty.

Edmore Dube's Chapter 14 argues that Muslim public health perceptions had immense influence on the way Zimbabwe Muslims coped with COVID-19 restrictions. Such perceptions are centred on the Quran and the Sunnah of the Prophet; with the central maxim legalizing lockdowns coming from the *hadith* stating: "When you hear about a break of plague in any area, do not enter there and when it has broken in a land where you are, then do not run away from it [and spread elsewhere]." This and other sacred texts helped Muslims comprehend restrictions barring them from prayer houses during the invaluable Ramadan. They were equally enabled to accept science and anthropological research works barring them from their religious shrines, where they touched and kissed parts of the shrines. They understood the decrees of the religious laws proscribing them from being in areas where their presence could exacerbate epidemics. It was easy to take the results from Shia shrines, because history had a number of plagues in the holy shrines. Funeral rites appeared to be the only challenges for Zimbabwe Muslims, as elsewhere. The spontaneity and outpouring grief could not be contained leading to disregard for social distancing. The need to prove the social media wrong, as well as religious completion worsened the chances for breaking the law, even in the face of strong religious morality. Since funeral rites have the tenacity to resist regulation, which endangers the whole community, state security agents should work closely with religious leadership and the health sector during funerals.

In a heavily polarised society along creedal, gender, political, racial and class divides, it becomes urgent to shun hegemonic tendencies that stigmatise, demonise and criminalise, without justice. On this basis, Fortune Sibanda's Chapter 15 examines the responses of selected Rastafari communities in Africa. The chapter argues that Rastafari, an often stigmatised, demonised and criminalised minority religious movement located on the margins, navigated around hegemonic attitudes, *politricks* and conspiracy theories of *Babylon* system in order to reposition their agency in the context of COVID-19 crisis in Africa. The chapter examines the Rastafari communities' responses to COVID-19 crisis in Africa. The chapter argues that Rastafari, an often stigmatised, demonised and criminalised minority religious movement located on the margins, has navigated around hegemonic attitudes, politricks and conspiracy theories of Babylon system in order to reposition their agency in the context of COVID-19 crisis in Africa. By using Afrocentricity perspective as theoretical framework, the chapter further demonstrates that Rastafari cultural identities such as music, Ital foodways, wholistic natural herbalism and environmentalism as well as spiritual and physically balanced lives engender creative and unique parameters that promote public health and human flourishing. The chapter concludes that Rastafari Afro-epistemological strategies in response to COVID-19 defy Western epistemological hegemonic tendencies and biomedical approaches. In the final analysis, Rastafari foregrounds the embracement of human diversity and the practice of One love, One aim, One people and One human race to drive positive complementary actions in the face of pandemics in Africa and beyond.

In Chapter 16, Molly Manyonganise explores how religion has to a large extent influenced the various experiences of women during COVID-19 in Zimbabwe. The chapter utilizes African Womanist theory as a way of starting constructive conversations on how men and women can negotiate their way through the pandemic as a collective. Data for the chapter were collected through social media, namely, Twitter, Facebook and WhatsApp.

In the last and concluding Chapter 17, Ezra Chitando synthesises the responses by religions to COVID-19 in Southern Africa in the context of the discourse on religion and development. He argues that whereas the dominant narrative in scholarly analyses of religion and development has been to insist on whether religion is a positive or negative social force, the chapters in this volume call for an acknowledgement of the fact that the picture is far more complex than this. The chapter provides a brief exploration of the growth of the religion and development sub-field within the academic study of religion in order to place the discussion into its proper historical and theoretical perspectives. It then states its central argument, namely, that the relationship between religion and development is more complicated than saying whether religion is a positive or negative factor in the quest for development. The chapter is a review of the chapters in this volume and illustrates how religion has been both a positive and negative factor in responding to COVID-19 in Southern Africa. It then draws some conclusions for the discourse on religion and development.

## Conclusion

This volume represents an important repository of the responses of various religious actors to COVID-19 in Southern Africa. It describes how different religions in the region sought to prevent the spread of the pandemic, collaborate with politicians and public health officials and to mitigate its impact. In some instances, the responses by religious actors were helpful, such as when they complemented public health messages to prevent the spread of the pandemic. However, in other instances their interventions were counterproductive. This includes when they adopted militant attitudes towards the call to stop in person meetings, or proclaiming messages that discouraged the uptake of vaccines. Overall, this volume invites scholars and readers from diverse disciplines to appreciate the complex interface between religion and COVID-19 in Southern Africa.

## Note

1 The Christian Response to COVID-19, Time with Pastor Mensa Otabil, Streamed live on 24 March 2020. YouTube, viewed on 26 January 2021.

## References

Appleby, R. Scott. (2000). *Ambivalence of the Sacred: Religion, Violence, and Reconciliation*. Lanham, MD: Rowman and Littlefield.

Asamoah-Gyadu, J.K. (2015). We are on the Internet: Contemporary Pentecostalism in Africa and the new culture of online religion. R.J. Hackett and B.F. Soares (eds.). New *Media and Religious Transformations in Africa*. Bloomington: Indiana University Press, 157–170.

Azetsop, J. (2016). *HIV and AIDS in Africa: Christian Reflection, Public Health, Social Transformation*. Maryknoll, NY: Orbis Books.

Barry, J.M. (2004). *The Great Influenza: The Epic Story of the Deadliest Plague in History*. New York: Penguin Viking.

Çarkoğlu, A. (2008). Social vs. spiritual capital in explaining philanthropic giving in a Muslim setting: The case of Turkey. A. Day. (ed.). *Religion and the Individual: Belief, Practice, Identity. Theology and Religion in Interdisciplinary Perspective*. London: Ashgate, pp. 111–126.

Chingono, H. (2010). Zimbabwe sanctions: An analysis of the "Lingo" guiding the perceptions of the sanctioners and sanctionees. *African Journal of Political Science and International Relations* 4(2): 66–74.

Chitando, E. (1997). A curse of western heritage? Imagining religion in an African context. *Journal for the Study of Religion* 10(2): 75–98.

Chitando, E. (2007). *Living with Hope: African Churches and HIV/AIDS*. Geneva: World Council of Churches.

Cox, J.L. (1996). *Expressing the Sacred: An Introduction to the Phenomenology of Religion*. Harare: University of Zimbabwe Publications.

Dandara, C., Dzobo, K., & Chirikure, S. (2020). COVID-19 Pandemic and Africa: From the situation in Zimbabwe to a case for precision herbal medicine. *OMICS A Journal of Integrative Biology* 24: 1–4.

De Wit, H. & West, G.O. (2009). *African and European Readers of the Bible in Dialogue: In Quest of a Shared Meaning*. Pietermaritzburg: Cluster.

De Witte, M. (2018). Pentecostal forms across religious divides: Media, publicity, and the limits of an anthropology of global Pentecostalism. *Religions* 9(217). doi:10.3390/rel9070217

Dein, S. (2021). Covid19 and the apocalypse: Religious and secular perspectives. *Journal of Religion and Health.* doi:10.1007/s10943-020-01100-w

Dein, S. et al. (2020). COVID-19, mental health and religion: An agenda for future research. *Mental Health, Religion & Culture* 23(1): 1–9.

Du Preez, P., Ramrathan, L. & Simmonds, S. (2020). Editorial: On curriculum philosophy, thinking, and theorising in South African higher education transformation. *Alternation Special Edition* 31: 1–5.

Dube, M.W. (2008). *The HIV/AIDS Bible: Selected Essays.* Scranton, PA: University of Scranton Press.

Dube, M.W. (2009). On being firefighters: Insights on curriculum transformation in HIV and AIDS contexts. *Studia Historiae Ecclessiasticae* 35: 83–98.

DW. (n.d.). Americas: American evangelicals and the resistance to COVID vaccines. https://www.dw.com/en/american-evangelicals-and-the-resistance-to-covid-vaccines/a-55957915. Accessed 26 January 2021.

Eliade, M. (1959). *The Sacred and the Profane: The Nature of Religion.* New York: Harper and Row.

Ellis, S. & Ter Haar, G. (1998). Religion and politics in sub-Saharan Africa. *The Journal of Modern African Studies* 36(2): 175–201.

Fairclough, N. (2003). 'Political correctness': The politics of culture and language. *Discourse & Society* 14(1): 17–28.

Fox, J. (2008). *A World Survey of Religion and the State.* Cambridge: Cambridge University Press.

Fox, J. (2018). *An Introduction to Religion and Politics: Theory and Practice.* Second edition. London: Routledge.

Green, M.C. (2014). From social hostility to social media: Religious pluralism, human rights and democratic reform in Africa. *African Human Rights Law Journal* 14: 93–125.

Gunda, M.R. & Kügler, J. (eds.) (2012). *The Bible and Politics in Africa.* Bamberg: University of Bamberg Press.

Hackett, R.I.J. (1998). Charismatic/Pentecostal appropriation of media technologies in Nigeria and Ghana. *Journal of Religion in Africa* 28(3): 258–277.

Heywood, A. (1997). *Politics.* London: Macmillan.

Jaja, I.F., Anyanwu, M.U. & Jaja, C-J.I. (2020). Social distancing: How religion, culture and burial ceremony undermine the effort to curb COVID-19 in South Africa. *Emerging Microbes & Infections* 9(1): 1077–1079. doi:10.1080/22221751.2020.1769501

Kalu, O.U. (2003). Globecalisation and religion. The Pentecostal model in contemporary Africa. J.L. Cox and G. Ter Haar (eds.). *Uniquely African? African Christian Identity from Cultural and Historical Perspectives.* Trenton: Africa World Press, 215–240.

Kindzeka, M.E. (2020). Cameroonian Muslims defy coronavirus prayer restrictions. 28 March. https://www.voanews.com/science-health/coronavirus-outbreak/cameroonian-muslims-defy-coronavirus-prayer-restrictions. Accessed 25 January 2021.

Kowalczyk, O. et al. (2020). Religion and faith perception in a pandemic of COVID19. *Journal of Religion and Health* 59: 2671–2677.

Kurian, M. (2001). *Report of the Church Leaders' Consultation on the Approach to HIV/AIDS Crisis.* Nairobi: AACC.

Maselko, J. et al. (2011). Religious social capital: Its measurement and utility in the study of the social determinants of health. *Social Science and Medicine* 73(5): 759–767.

Mawere, M. (2014). *Culture, Indigenous Knowledge and Development in Africa: Reviving Interconnections and Sustainable Development*. Bamenda, Cameroon: RPICG.

Mbiti, J.S. (1969). *African Religions and Philosophy*. London: Macmillan.

Mendy, J. & Madiope, M. (2020). Curriculum transformation: A case in South Africa. *Perspectives in Education* 38(2). doi:10.18820/2519593X/pie.v38.i2.01

Modebadze, V. (2010). The term politics reconsidered in the light of recent theoretical developments. *IBSU Scientific Journal (IBSUSJ)* (International Black Sea University, Tbilisi) 4(1): 39–44.

Modise, L. & A. Wood. (2016). The relevance of the metaphor of god as father in a democratic, non-sexist and religious society. *Stellenbosch Theological Journal* 2(1): 285–304.

Mtata, Kenneth. (ed.). (2013). *Religion: Help or Hindrance to Development?* Leipzig: EVA.

Muneja, M. (2012). *HIV/AIDS and the Bible in Tanzania: A Contextual Re-reading of 2 Samuel 13: 1–14:33*. Bamberg: University of Bamberg Press.

Ndlovu-Gatsheni, S.J. (2019). Discourses of decolonisation/decoloniality. *Papers of Languages and Literature* 55(3): 201–226.

NewsDay (2021). Are Johane Marange followers above the law? https://www.newsday.co.zw/2021/07/are-johane-marange-followers-above-the-law/. Accessed: 10 November 2021.

Nyamnjoh, F. & Carpenter, J. (2018). Religious innovation and competition in contemporary African Christianity. *Journal of Contemporary African Studies* 36(3): 289–302.

Odozi, A. (2020). Coronavirus cannot survive in the body of Jesus—Tanzania's president (video). 25 March. https://www.informationng.com/2020/03/coronavirus-cannot-survive-in-the-body-of-jesus-tanzanias-president-video.html.

Oloruntoba, S.O. & Falola, T. (eds.) (2018). *The Palgrave Handbook of African Politics, Governance and Development*. New York: Palgrave Macmillan.

Oloyede, I.O. (2014). Theologising the mundane, politicising the divine: The cross-currents of law, religion and politics in Nigeria. *African Human Rights Law Journal* 14: 178–202.

Orjinmo, N. (2020). Coronavirus: Nigeria's mega churches adjust to empty auditoriums. *BBC News*, Lagos. 08 April. https://www.bbc.com/news/world-africa-52189785. Accessed 26 January 2020.

Parish, H. (2020). The absence of presence and the presence of absence: Social distancing, sacraments, and the virtual religious community during the COVID-19 pandemic. *Religions* 11(276). doi:10.3390/rel11060276

Park, C.L. (2005). Religion as a meaning-making framework in coping with life stress. *Journal of Social Issues* 61(4): 707–729.

Pieterse, T. & Landman, C. (2021). Religious views on the origin and meaning of COVID-19. *HTS Teologiese Studies/Theological Studies* 77(3): a6283. https://doi.org/10/.4102/hts.v77i3.6283, accessed 08 July 2021.

Ramrathan, L., Ndimande-Hlongwa, N. Mkhize, N. & Smit, J.A. (2020). *Re-Thinking the Humanities Curriculum in the Time of COVID-19*, Vol. 1. Durban: CSSALL Publishers (Pty) Ltd.

Reuters. (2021). Decrying vaccines, Tanzania leader says, 'God will protect from COVID-19.' 27 January. https://www.yahoo.com/news/decrying-vaccines-tanzania-leader-says-152726339.html. Accessed 29 January 2021.

Reuters Staff. (2020). South Africa's chief justice unrepentant linking vaccines to Satanism. 11 December. https://www.rueters.com/article/health-coronovirus-saafrica-vaccine-idUSL8N21R2VW. Accessed 23 February 2021.

Sambala, E., Cooper, S., & Manderson, L. (2019). Ubuntu as a framework for ethical decision making in Africa: Responding to epidemics. *Ethics and Behaviour* 30(1): 1–13.

Sharma, A. (2011). *Problematising Religious Freedom*. London: Springer Dordrecht Heidelberg.

Sibanda, F. (2018). Background and history of Pentecostalism in Zimbabwe. In T.P. Mapuranga (ed.). *Powered by Faith: Pentecostal Businesswomen in Harare*. Eugene, OR: Wipf & Stock Publishers, 8–28.

Smart, N. (1969). *The Religious Experience of Mankind*. Englewood Cliffs, NJ: Prentice Hall.

Smith, B.K. (1987). Exorcising the transcendent: Strategies for defining Hinduism and religion. *History of Religion* 27(1): 32–55.

Smith, W.C. (1964). *The Meaning and End of Religion*. London: SPCK.

Sonntag, E., Frost, M. & Ohlmann, P. (2020). Religious leaders' perspectives on corona – Preliminary findings. *Policy Brief*, https://jliflc.com/resources/religious-leaders-perspectives-on-corona-preliminary-findings/. Accessed 20 February 2021.

Tamale, S. (2020). *Decolonization and Afro-Feminism*. Ottawa: Daraja Press.

Tarusarira, J. & Chitando, E. (eds.) (2020). *Themes in Religion and Human Security in Africa*. London: Routledge.

Taylor, B. (2020) Tanzania's Gamble: Anatomy of a totally novel coronavirus response. https://africanarguments.org/2020/05/tanzania-gamble-anatomy-totally-novel-coronavirus-response/. Accessed 20 February 2021.

Togarasei, L. (2012). Mediating the gospel: Pentecostal Christianity and media technology in Botswana and Zimbabwe. *Journal of Contemporary Religion* 27(2): 257–274.

Ukah, A. (2020). Prosperity, prophecy and the COVID-19 pandemic: The healing economy of African Pentecostalism. *Pneuma* 42(3 & 4): 430–459.

VOA News. (2020). Pray and wash: Religion joins with science amid virus crisis. 12 March. https://www.voanews.com/science-health/coronavirus-outbreak/pray-and-wash-religion-joins-science-amid-virus-crisis. Accessed 24 February 2021.

WCC. (2020). South African church leaders say COVID-19 corruption kills, as they campaign against it. 23 September. https://www.oikoumene.org/news/south-african-church-leaders-say-covid-19-corruption-kills-as-they-campaign-against-it. Accessed 20 January 2021.

Wildman, W. et al. (2020). Religion and COVID-19 pandemic. *Religion Brain and Behaviour* 10(2): 115–117.

# 2 Exploring the ethics of *Ubuntu* in the era of COVID-19

*Beatrice Okyere-Manu and*
*Stephen Nkansah Morgan*

## Introduction

Since the outbreak of the coronavirus disease 2019 (COVID-19), which is known to have started in the Wuhan City, Hubei province of China in December 2019, the disease has had a global spread and led to many deaths. As on 23 May 2020, the total number of infections globally was at 5,331,427 with associated 340,560 deaths (COVID-19 Coronavirus Pandemic, 2020). Egypt was the first African country to confirm a case of the coronavirus in Africa on 14th February 2020 involving a Chinese national. Since that first infection, the disease has emerged and spread throughout the continent, and the number of infections keeps rising daily to date. The total number of infections in Africa as on 23 May 2020 was 106,299 with 3,205 deaths. South Africa, at this time, has the highest number of infections at 20,125, with 397 deaths, followed by Egypt at 15,786 with 707 deaths (COVID-19 Coronavirus Pandemic, 2020).

Although, as the numbers indicate, Africa has a very low number of infections and deaths globally, the devastating effect and impact of the disease are no less felt on the African continent. Just as it is for the rest of the world, the COVID-19 pandemic has brought with it so much socio-economic hardship on the African people. It is estimated that the African continent is going to feel the economic impact the most due to its already existing poor and below-average socio-economic conditions even before the advent of the pandemic. Billionaire Bill Gates, for example, warned that the coronavirus pandemic could have more 'dramatic effect' in Africa than in China due to Africa's weak health system, which he believed may become overwhelmed (Wasserman & Monynihan, 2020). The World Health Organization also cautioned that the coronavirus has the potential to 'smolder' in Africa for many years and bring with it a high death toll across the continent (Burke & Akinwotu, 2020).

The ensuing governments' nationwide or partial lockdowns in affected African states and governments' regulations of social distancing, self-isolation, ban on large gatherings, closure of schools and churches, ban on funerals, and other social gatherings as measures to combat the spread of

DOI: 10.4324/9781003241096-2

the virus have affected the daily lives of the African people. Considering all these restrictions, there exist the tendency for panic and the disregard for positive cultural values that have held the people together. It is purposely because of this that the authors believe that the ethics of *Ubuntu* can present the African people some valuable moral values that bring to bear their germaneness in the COVID-19 period. This would ensure that the African does not abandon these values that, which in no small extent, mark out their Africanness.

The significance of cultural values to a society cannot be overemphasized. Sub-Saharan Africa is known for its rich values. These identifiable prevailing norms and values are widespread across the continent, although they may be expressed quite differently from one place to another. Traditional Africa is known for its conservativeness and slowness to change. Custodians of African cultures do their very best to often pass on their beliefs and values from one generation to another in a bid to ensure the continuity and preservation of their inherited traditions, which, often, is traced to generations before them in their respective histories. Nevertheless, cultural practices, beliefs, and values, as we know them, are often born out of necessities and as attempts to grapple with social, political, economic, and environmental exigencies of the group at a particular point in time. So that as these exigencies change, one would naturally expect that the group adjust, adapt or invent new approaches and values to tackle them.

Values are, more so, regarded as the moral and social ideals of a group of people that guide their everyday behavior, including what they hold as true, good, evil, taboo, beautiful, and just. Benson Igboin considers values as "the standard which members of the community adhere to in their personal and communal interaction towards the achievement of the goals" (Igboin, 2013, p. 98). He also regards them to be that which determine members who deserve praise or admonishment for their actions. Value can, in a way, denote that which is desirable (Igboin, 2013). For Gabriel Idang (2015), values can be perceived as a set of beliefs held about what is right and wrong and what is taken to be essential in life. He regards them as a point of view or convictions that people live with or live by and can even die for. These characterizations of values show how important values are to a people and perhaps the extent at which they are willing to go to defend or keep them. Idang points out further that since values are central to every culture and culture is what gives a people an identity, it stands to mean that these values they hold are mainly those which distinguish them from others.

Ruth Bulus Iganus and Andrew Haruna note that

> through modern changes in this globalized world, the African traditional setting or ways of managing crisis cannot remain intact, but they are by no means extinct. In times of crisis, they often come to surface or people revert to them in secret.
>
> (2017, p. 1)

Thus, it suffices to ask whether the African ethics of *Ubuntu* is robust enough to adapt and remain relevant during this COVID-19 pandemic. If it is, what moral principles therein are useful to assist Africans, and by extension, the rest of the world to navigate through this pandemic successfully? Idang (2015) believes that cultures always try to preserve values that are essential for the survival of their people. James Lassiter (2000) similarly asserts that many African scholars have many times pointed out that the use of these widely shared values, themes, and adaptive responses are vital in the attainment of feasible and sustainable African national and community development so much that some consider this effort as an important one for the crucial survival of Africa and its cultures.

The African ethics of *Ubuntu* has not only existed and guided the moral behavior of traditional African people but has shown itself to be relevant to modern African societies and adaptive to current socio-political challenges of the African people and beyond. As a result, the chapter aims to test the resilience of the ethics of *Ubuntu* in the face of the COVID-19 pandemic. By so doing, it critically explores ways in which the African ethics of *Ubuntu* remains relevant in the lives of African people who are confronted with a way of life quite different from what they are used to. Ultimately, the question being asked is how the principles of *Ubuntu* can influence an ethical outlook that can help the African people cope, manage, and survive the COVID-19 pandemic. The work is entirely non-empirical and relies entirely on already published works in its assessments, analyses, and recommendations.

## The African ethics of *Ubuntu*

The concept of *Ubuntu* is dominant in sub-Sahara communitarian Africa. This concept is also referred to as *Boto, Ukama, Umundu, Bumuntu*, amongst different people in Southern Africa. This singular word is embedded with such rich philosophical and metaphysical principles that have been argued to be the cultural, ethical, social, and political driving force of the African people. It does indeed embody the very identity of the African people and informs what they do, how they live, and their relationship with each other and others. It reflects their communitarian attitude, and their communitarian attitude reflects it. Barbara Nussbaum defines it as "the underlying social philosophy of African culture" (Nussbaum, 2009, p. 100), while Mogobe Ramose (2002) describes it as the root and basis of African philosophy, the wellspring flowing with African ontology and epistemology. Due to its richness in value, *Ubuntu* has been used in socio-political policies and theorization as well as in prescribing moral values to confront modern African challenges, and in defining the African sense of a good life. Again, due to its richness, a direct English translation of the word *Ubuntu* does not come readily. The closest English word commonly associated with it is *humanness* (Metz, 2007; Ramose, 2009) and perhaps rightly so if one should take the various related moral principles often extracted and extrapolated from it into account.

It is the moral connotations or underpinnings of *Ubuntu* that define what could be termed as *the ethics of Ubuntu*, albeit it is not any radically different from its socio-political connotations. The ethics of *Ubuntu* reflects on the human relationship with others, which is a relationship that highlights the interconnectedness of all humans, and that this interconnectedness is needed for individuals' self-realization. In other words, a person is not *complete* without others; an important reason why Africans tend to lay more emphasis on community solidarity rather than individual personal pursuits. As a result of this unavoidable inter-human relationship, one is to pursue a moral life that enforces or lead to common accord and social harmony with others. Thus, Mluleki Munyaka and Mokgethi Motlhabi refer to *Ubuntu* as "a way of life that seeks to promote and manifest itself and is best realized or made evident in harmonious relations within society" (Munyaka & Motlhabi, 2009, p. 65). To make this common accord and social harmony possible requires each person to consider the wellbeing of others in the pursuant of their wellbeing. Subsequently, to consider the wellbeing of others is also accomplished through the show of care and brotherliness/sisterliness for others and making the needs of others one's concern. In other words, a person's wellbeing is only laudable if it is linked with the overall wellbeing of the brother/sister community. In recent times, many scholars such as Mangena (2009), have critiqued term ubuntu, nevertheless, the fact still stands that its values are obtainable in the era of COVID-19.

Thus, the remainder of the chapter reflects on some of these ethical principles of *Ubuntu* such as the show of solidarity and good human relationship, strong regard for family and family values, and elevated respect for authorities and elders to demonstrate how the ethics of *Ubuntu* can inform the best ways to live and relate with each other amidst the COVID-19 pandemic.

### Solidarity and good human relationship

The humanistic feature of African ethics is well known and documented. Kwame Gyekye defines it as "the doctrine that sees human needs, interests, and dignity as fundamental" (1995, p. 43). Egbunu Fidelis Eleojo (2014) understands it as an attitude which does not only elevate the overall good of the human person but also the good of the African person as the purpose of all actions. It involves a constant concern for his or her wellbeing as the central object of policy. There is a famous saying among the Akans of Ghana that *onipa na ehia*, which means that it is the human being that matters. The implication of this is evident; it is to say that actions, behaviors, habits, attitudes, and characters that lead to the betterment of human life and wellbeing is paramount, required, preferred, and always encouraged rather than the amassing of wealth and properties or actions that bring about human misery and pain. This should foster a sense of good human-to-human relationship among people, a relationship where there is a demonstration of care for others and not only for oneself. Macaulay Kanu (2010) asserts that maintaining this type of relationship between individuals shows recognition of their worth as human beings without having recognition only for what they own or what one can receive from the other in return. It is essentially a fundamental recognition of the dignity of every person regardless of their position or status in life. This ought to be considered the starting point of all other values. Kanu writes further that in these traditional African societies:

> Help for one another is not based on immediate or an exact equivalent remuneration. Everyone is mindful that each person has something to contribute to his welfare, no matter the degree. The arrangement of human relation is that of being one's brother's keeper or caring for each other's welfare. Every man is obliged to assist those who need help. The needy and the helpless are taking care of and assisted.
>
> (Kanu, 2010, p. 153)

The value of a good human relationship remains very relevant during this pandemic. Surely, as nations and regions go under either partial or full lockdown, not everyone in the society has the financial means to get involved in the panic buying that was reported all over the continent. The poor and the destitute in our societies cannot stock food and groceries, and there are many of whom the order to stay at home will be of no effect because the streets are their homes. The way we can employ this virtue to help the vulnerable among us during this pandemic is to offer them a helping hand in any way that we can, either by offering them food and other essential groceries, hand sanitizers, and teaching them to observe social distancing. We will not be exhibiting the value of good human relationship if a few of us lock ourselves in the room with all we need while the poor are left on the streets in hunger and at the mercies of the disease.

For instance, the Human Right Watch reported on May 20 2020 that the South African government was ignoring the plight of refugees and asylum seekers who were confined in their homes and unable to work to provide for themselves due to the pandemic. It urged the government to take crucial steps to provide needed support for refugees and asylum seekers with little access to food and other basic necessities during the nationwide lockdown (Human Rights Watch, 2020). Evidently, any act that excludes a particular group of people does not foster good inter-human relationship. Ubuntu promotes integration rather than exclusion.

Related to the above value of a good human relationship is the value of community and solidarity. African societies are communitarian, a feature that leads to a shared social way of life. As such, members of the community join efforts in the attainment of the community's good and the good of the individual members, although the latter is often submerged within the former. The community's good or interest is mostly referred to as the common good, that is, the good that is mutually beneficial to all. This communitarian attitude and social way of life are highly primarily motivated by the value of solidarity and community. These values of solidarity and community suggest that one must always seek the good of the larger society rather than for one's self-interests. The good of the society is that action which promotes the overall wellbeing of the community. Out of the value of communalism comes other virtues such as looking out for others, caring for others, being benevolent and altruistic, being social, interdependence, co-operation, reciprocity, and being sympathetic.

A portrayal of solidarity is the vehicle towards the display of community. At the core of a communal society is a strong expression of solidarity. Solidarity is an authentic show of concern and empathy with others and an actual manifestation of these concerns with deeds that do not have conditions attached to them except for the desire to see others do well and the desire to ensure community's progress. An important aspect of community and the show of solidarity is recognizing that one's success is not truly a success if others do not succeed as well. Solidarity is a strong ideal expressed within the principles of *Ubuntu* and underscores the primacy of the human person and a strong need for everyone to join their individual forces to help alleviate or ameliorate the needs and suffering of others.

Gyekye (1995) posits that in the pursuit of human wellbeing, there is a need to adequately consider the distribution of the material and social benefits of the society, the adequacy and fairness of its legal system, and social justice, equality, equitable distribution of goods, and human rights. That said, the sense of community and solidarity is best expressed during this pandemic when we work together as a community to end the spread of the coronavirus. Resultantly, there is a need to pay heed to the directives of health experts and practice social distancing, self-isolation, and staying home when we can. It is indeed one of the rare occasions where we show solidarity and community by avoiding social gatherings. This is very important in the African context because sociability as well as physical and tactile social interactions are the hallmarks of traditional African societies and tend to manifest in almost every aspect of their socio-cultural lives. This means that there is a need to find new ways of showing solidarity, a sense of community, or community participation aside mass social gatherings to observe rites of passage (naming ceremonies, puberty rites, marriage rites, and funerals), festivals, among others.

The first step in doing this is by playing our part to end the spread of the virus, although the conditions may be unusual, unfamiliar, and uncomfortable to us. It is, therefore, not consistent with the values of solidarity and community, the actions of those who defile directives to stay at home or to put themselves in self-quarantine or those who agitate against government's lockdown directives. Such acts are best described as self-centered and individualistic. These individuals do not show *Ubuntu* nor have the common good of the society at heart.

Secondly, the pandemic has deepened and continues to deepen the yawning gap between the rich and poor in African societies. Already existing inequalities have been made worse with many people losing their jobs. This means more people are going to end up with nothing to eat as the lockdown extends. Plan International, as of May 2020, tells us that more than 5.8 million people in Zimbabwe and 2 million in Mozambique have been affected by food insecurity as a result of climate change, and political and economic instability. The situation in the two countries has been made dire in the wake of the COVID-19 pandemic (Plan International, 2020). Given these unfortunate situations, the pandemic presents a great opportunity for *ubuntu* to go to work, a test of the African's capability to solidarize with the vulnerable in society.

So far, some have been up to the task. A couple of individuals and some cooperation and institutions have made donations of food and clothes to the poor, and Personal Protective Equipment (PPEs) for the frontline health workers and health facilities. In South Africa, for example, the government set up a fund it calls 'The Solidarity Fund' on 23 March 2020 to provide an avenue for both public and private sectors, individuals and groups to donate in support of government initiatives. The fund has received large endorsement and support from both local and international quarters. Direct Relied, a nonprofit humanitarian organization, for example donated 1 million dollars to the Fund for the purchase of PPEs. Direct Relief President and CEO Thomas Tighe, who also serves as Managing Director of Direct Relief South Africa said that, "South Africa's Solidarity Fund is exactly the type of unifying, pragmatic approach that makes sense in the face of a pandemic that threatens everyone" (Sherer, 2020).

Similarly, private firms like SPAR South Africa and SPAR Zimbabwe partnered with NGOs such as Operation Hunger, Miracle Missions, and We2ndChance, and made separate donations of assorted food items to less fortunate families in their respective countries. Workers of SPAR and individual volunteers helped with the packaging of the food items in beautiful show of solidarity. According to Brett Botten, Managing Director of the SPAR South Rand Distribution Centre: "The donation aims to inspire people to be and do more. It is during times like these that we need to work together and support each other" (SPAR South Africa, 2020). Similar donations are reported throughout the continent as a practical show of solidarity among the people.

## Strong regards for family and family values

The expression of community and solidarity as well as virtues such as interdependency and concern for other people's wellbeing start at the family level. The notion of family in the traditional African context includes all members of the extended family. The family is a composition of people who share common blood or ancestry. There are, of course, many positive benefits that the individual enjoy by belonging to a family or a clan. The family, for example, gives to the individual identity, support in times of need, and a sense of belonging. Gyekye (1996) notes that one of the well-regarded values in traditional African societies is the social security or economic insurance that the extended family system offers. The security, he notes, covers family members who are old, poor, deprived and those struggling to make it in life despite their efforts. Wealthier and more successful members hold it as a duty to take care of the vulnerable members among them: first, for the fact that they are their blood and kin and, second, because they are the ones going to be there for them when they are also in need. The extended family system, therefore, provides a safety net where all of its members can run to when all odds fail or are against them. It is a place where members come to at any time to seek comfort and safety and recuperation from the challenges of their world. Consequently, the ethics of *Ubuntu*, which is altruistic and others-serving ethics, underscore the need for one to care for their family needs. Greediness and self-centeredness are actions that are frowned upon and eschewed.

While commenting on Southern African experience, Vhumani Magezi (2018) draws our attention to what he calls 'strongly enunciated rules about kin, responsibility and co-residence' that are passed down from the older generations to the younger generations. The extended family bond, Magezi maintains, is so strong that even when a member moves to work and settle elsewhere, they are expected to keep faith with the instructions, norms and values that have been handed down to them from the elders. He indicates that it is less likely for an individual to abandon who they are because they have moved to the city, for to abandon the values and norms passed on from the older generation is to deny oneself as an extension of the rural community (Magezi, 2018). Just line most Southern Africa countries, Iganus and Haruna (2017) indicate that among the Babur-Bura of Nigeria, to be considered in high esteem, one must partake in the beliefs and be involved in the cultural practices such as ceremonies, rituals, festivals of joy or suffering. As a result of these, they note that one cannot afford to exist without the family.

How then do we apply the principles in the value that Africans have for the family in the context of the COVID-19 pandemic? Here, family members need to identify the vulnerable and needy members among themselves and extend a helping hand. While the tendency for self-preservation, that is, to look within and to cater for only oneself and one's immediate family members, is high due to the loss of many jobs and reduction in income, it is here one needs to demonstrate a high moral fortitude and exhibit the spirit of *Ubuntu* the most by rising to the occasion. There is a need to extend a helping hand to every member of the extended family who may be faced with a job loss due to job cuts and retentions and those who may fall victim to the virus and become sick and bedridden.

Iganus and Haruna (2017) indicate that in preserving the extended family structure, some vital coping strategies used were the fellowship of sharing joy and suffering, faith and hopes. Consequently, it is crucial to bring to bear the act of sharing with others during the pandemic by caring for the sick and providing for the needy and giving family members hope when they are in despair. More so, the family must be there for members who may lose their lives to the pandemic and make sure that children who lose their parents or guardians to the virus are brought within their care. It is part of the African culture to show up and show solidarity when it is most needed in time of crises, and the coronavirus pandemic should not be an exception. The extended family system provides a bigger network of people who are more closely connected and can rely upon each other in these times.

## Elevated respect for authorities and elders

In traditional African societies, age is very significant and not considered a mere number. The number of years one has attained is often the measurement of the level of one's experience and wisdom. Older people, are, as a result, often conferred with for advice on life choices and life challenges. They are also consulted to resolve conflicts and personal feuds and on major decisions to be taken by the family or by the community. Elders are highly respected, and it is believed that disrespecting an elder, stranger or not, is asking for curses upon one's self. On the contrary, anyone who assists an elderly receives blessings of goodwill, good health, and long life. According to Kanu (2010), the significance of the African value of respect for elders is reflected in an Igbo saying that translates in English as: 'He who listens to an elder is like one who consults an oracle'. He explains that by this, the Igbo people liken the words of the elders to that of the oracles who are held to offer indubitable and sound truths. This implies that since the elders are regarded as the leaders and authorities in the community and the repository of wisdom, adhering to their words and instructions will not lead one astray. This is because the elders, just like the oracles, are considered to always look out for the good of their members and the community at large.

As the experts tell us, COVID-19 puts people of old age and poor health at a more significant risk than those of the younger and healthier population. True to this, the statistics on deaths caused by the virus show that more people in these two categories make the higher numbers. That said, there is a need to offer specialized care and a show of support for these groups of people. For the sake of their health and lives, those who are sick need to take self-isolation and self-quarantine seriously. As Kanu points out, if the respect given to the elders has practical effect in the maintenance of custom and tradition, then we can also somewhat say, although with some reservation, that our national authorities and leaders (governments) by their directives and lockdown protocols seek the social good and welfare of all citizens. Thus, it is worth sacrificing a few of our luxury and freedoms to pay heed to their directives. It is within the ethics of *Ubuntu* to think beyond self-interest and consider the greater good of the community in all of one's actions.

Furthermore, although the elders of societies are highly regarded for their wisdom and experiences, they are also known to be physically weaker due to their age. It, therefore, call on the community to protect them since they are most at risk of dying from the virus. The ethics of *Ubuntu* require that those who are stronger and better off protect and provide for the weak and vulnerable in society. The idea of old people's home, which is prevalent in the West, is foreign in traditional Africa because old people are not considered in traditional African societies as a burden. It is more of a blessing to have an old person in one's home because they enforce good moral behavior among the young and the passing on of traditional values to the younger generations. At the same time, caring for older family members is a moral duty of the younger generation. This virtue of care embedded in the ethics of *Ubuntu* must be emphasized and brought to bear in this period of coronavirus.

## Conclusion

Although changes in culture often occur slowly and sometimes even unintentionally, there are certain instances in history where certain events, episodes or happenings accelerate cultural change. The 2020 COVID-19 pandemic will pass as one of such occasions. Again, although it is evident that not every cultural value remains useful during this time, there are, within the same culture, some values that can be adopted in different ways to meet the new challenge. Thus, Gyekye (1995) was on point to have noted that the social, non-individualistic character of traditional African ethics, the traditional African conceptions of the value of man and the relationship between people in a society, and the sense of community and solidarity, and mutual responsibility are very needful in modern-day culture. They are, he noted, able to offer an adequate foundation for any social and ethical way of life today. The coronavirus pandemic provides a unique opportunity for Africans to revitalize these positive traditional values and demonstrate to the world the relevance, applicability, robustness, adaptiveness of African traditional cultural values.

Thus, the preoccupation of this chapter has been to highlight that the African ethics of *Ubuntu* contains in it such values or virtues that remain relevant and adaptive in times of the Coronavirus pandemic. These virtues include the show of solidarity and good human relationship, the strong regard for family and family values, and the elevated respect for authorities and elders. From these we postulate an ethic of care, brotherhood/sisterhood, social cohesion, and above all the pursuant of the community good or welfare. The chapter strongly holds that if the various virtues found within the ethics of *Ubuntu* are fully embraced, the African community can stand steadfastly in the fight against the COVID-19 pandemic.

## References

Burke, Jason and Akinwotu, Emmanuel. 2020. *Coronavirus could 'smoulder' in Africa for several years, WHO warns.* Retrieved May 23, 2020 from https://www.theguardian.com/world/2020/may/08/coronavirus-could-smoulder-in-africa-for-several-years-who-warns

COVID-19 Coronavirus Pandemic. 2020. Retrieved May 5, 2020 from https://www. worldometers.info/coronavirus/?utm_campaign=homeAdUOA?Si

Eleojo, Fidelis Egbunu. 2014. Africans and African humanism: What prospects? *American International Journal of Contemporary Research*, 4(1), 297–308.

Gyekye, Kwame. 1995. *An essay on African philosophical thought: The Akan conceptual scheme* (Revised ed.). Philadelphia: Temple University Press.

Gyekye, Kwame. 1996. *African cultural values: An Introduction.* Accra: Sankofa Publishing Company.

Human Rights Watch. 2020. *South Africa: End bias in Covid-19 food aid.* Retrieved June 16, 2020 from https://www.hrw.org/news/2020/05/20/south-africa-end-bias-covid-19-food-aid

Idang, Gabriel. E. 2015. African culture and values. *Phronimon*, 16(2), 97–111.

Iganus, Ruth Bulus and Haruna, Andrews. 2017. The strength of African culture in managing family crisis in a globalized world. *Anthropology*, 5(4), 1–5.

Igboin, Benson. O. 2013. Colonialism and African cultural values. *African Journal of History and Culture*, 3(6), 96–103.

Kanu, Macaulay A. 2010. The indispensability of the basic social values in African tradition: A philosophical appraisal. *OGIRISI: A New Journal of African Studies*, 7, 149–161.

Lassiter, James. E. 2000. African culture and personality: Bad social science, effective social activism, or a call to reinvent ethnology? *African Studies Quarterly*, 3(3), 1–21.

Magezi, Vhumani. 2018. Changing family patterns from rural to urban and living in the in-between: A public practical theological responsive ministerial approach in Africa. *HTS Teologiese Studies/Theological Studies.* Retrieved from http://www. scielo.org.za/pdf/hts/v74n1/42.pdf.

Mangena, Fainos. 2009. The search for an African feminist ethic: A Zimbabwean perspective. *Journal of International Women's Studies* 11(2), 18–30.

Metz, Thaddeus. 2007. Towards an African moral theory. *The Journal of Political Philosophy*, 15(3), 321–334.

Munyaka, Mluleki and Motlhabi, Motlhabi. 2009. Ubuntu and its socio-moral significance. In Felix Munyaradzi Murove (Eds.), *African ethics: An anthology of comparative and applied ethics.* Scottsville: University of KwaZulu-Natal Press, 63–84.

Nussbaum, Barbara. 2009. Reflections of a South African on our common humanity. In Felix. Munyaradzi Murove (Eds.), *African ethics: An anthology of comparative and applied ethics.* Scottsville: University of KwaZulu-Natal Press, 100–109.

Plan International. 2020. *Millions trapped between hunger and covid-19 in Zimbabwe and Mozambique.* Retrieved June 16, 2020 from https://plan-international.org/news/2020-05-13-zimbabwe-and-mozambique-catastrophe-hunger-and-covid

Ramose, Mogobe. B. 2002. The philosophy of *ubuntu* and *ubuntu* as a philosophy. In P. H. Coetzee and A. P. J. Roux (Eds.), *The African philosophy reader* (2nd ed.). New York: Routledge, 230–238.

Ramose, Mogobe. B. 2009. Ecology through *Ubuntu.* In Felix Munyaradzi Murove (Eds.), *African ethics: An anthology of comparative and applied ethics.* Scottsville: University of KwaZulu-Natal Press, 308–314.

Sherer, Paul. M. 2020. *Overcoming Covid-19 in South Africa: Direct relief donates $1 million, serves as U.S. fiscal agent for solidarity fund.* Retrieved June 16, 2020 from https://www.directrelief.org/2020/08/overcoming-covid-19-in-south-africa/

SPAR South Africa. 2020. *SPAR South Africa and operation hunger donate 3,000 food parcels to families in need.* Retrieved June 16, 2021 from https://spar-international.com/news/spar-south-africa-and-operation-hunger-donate-3000-food-parcels-to-families-in-need/

Wasserman, Helena and Moynihan, Qayyah. 2020. *Bill Gates warned the coronavirus could hit Africa worse than China.* Retrieved February 25, 2020, from https://www.businessinsider.com/bill-gates-warns-coronavirus-could-hit-africa-with-dire-consequences-2020-2?IR=T

# 3 Social distancing in the context of COVID-19 in Zimbabwe

## Perspectives from Ndau religious indigenous knowledge systems

*Tenson Muyambo*

### Introduction and background

The coronavirus that causes the COVID-19 pandemic has affected all spheres of human life. Jaja *et al.* (2020:1077) admit that "The 2019 novel coronavirus (2019-nCoV) has altered the way we live, interact and socialize". The pandemic was first discovered in the town of Wuhan in China in December 2019 and declared a public health concern by the World Health Organization (WHO) on 11 March 2020. At the time of writing this chapter, it had spread to the whole world, with Italy, Spain, United States, United Kingdom and China being the most affected statistically. In Africa, South Africa has the highest number of people affected followed by Algeria and Egypt. Zimbabwe had recorded 18 cases and three deaths as of 14 April 2020 as reported by the Ministry of Health and Child Care (MoHCC) (MoHCC 2020a).

In response to the fast spread of the coronavirus and the concomitant death trail in neighbouring South Africa, Zimbabwe promulgated the Statutory Instrument 83 of 2020: Public Health (COVID-19 Prevention, Containment and Treatment), which effectively closed all public and private institutions and instituted nationwide travel restrictions except for essential service providers (MoHCC 2020b). While at home, communities were encouraged to quarantine, stay indoors, constantly wash hands with soap on clean running water, avoid touching the face, use face masks, face shields and practice social distancing whenever outside the home (MoHCC 2020c, 2020d). The Statutory Instrument 83 of 2020 provided that those diagnosed and suspected of having COVID-19 should be quarantined at home and in health institutions to contain the virus. In quarantine centres, COVID-19 patients received a combination of drugs, often used to treat influenza and severe respiratory illnesses (WHO 2020). In extreme cases, seriously ill patients ended up in Intensive Care Unit, with ventilators to assist in their breathing (MoHCC 2020d). All these measures were/are meant to be the safety nets against the pandemic.

In this chapter, I focus on social distancing as one of the many containment measures introduced by the Zimbabwean government. I conceptualise social distancing, analyse its efficacy and establish whether it is a new

DOI: 10.4324/9781003241096-3

strategy or not among rural communities of south-eastern Zimbabwe. To do this, I identify the problem statement, give the theoretical lens that undergirds the chapter, briefly discuss social distancing or physical distancing, present the study's findings and sum up the chapter by way of a conclusion and recommendations.

## Statement of the problem

Admittedly, COVID-19 took the world by surprise and was declared a world health pandemic. Its declaration must be understood in the context that previously there were pandemics of either a similar nature or of more profound magnitude; yet the level of shock and pandemonium shown by governments was one of hopelessness, to say the least. While WHO came up with laudable recommendations such as social distancing as prevention and control measures, governments implemented it in an *ad hoc* manner without recourse to how humanity dealt with pandemics of similar nature that befell them in the past and how local communities in their unique circumstances responded to such pandemics. WHO guidelines were and are still being implemented under the "one size-fits-all approach" without taking recognition that contexts ravaged by COVID-19 are varied and different. Such an omission, coupled with lack of community-based COVID-19 education and deep-seated principles of *ubuntu* may account for the lack of complete compliance to social distancing in Zimbabwe.

## Theoretical framework

The chapter is underpinned by the Sankofa perspective. The Sankofa perspective is derived from an Akan story in Ghana of a mythical bird that moves forward while its head is turned backward toward the golden egg on its back (Slater 2019). The golden egg is symbolic of the treasure of historical wisdom. Loosely translated, the Sankofa simply means "Go back and get it/ Go back and take it" (Slater 2019:2). In other words, the perspective refers to the idea that it is not a taboo to go back and take that which is at risk of being left out yet is essential for survival. It is an approach similar to Cabral's *Return to the source* (1973) when confronted by new challenges.

The use of this Sankofa lens in this chapter is a clarion call for Africans, Zimbabweans in particular, to rediscover and reclaim historical wisdom to address contemporary problems and challenges. With the advent of COVID-19, the Sankofa perspective is urging Africans to retrace their footsteps into the past in order to understand the present holistically and chart the way forward. Put differently, the Sankofa perspective is of the view that while Africans (though it can be applied anywhere in the world for there is no human race without its historical wisdom) embrace WHO recommendations to curb the spread of COVID-19, such as social distancing, they need to equally look back into the past and rediscover how the past generations dealt with pandemics of a similar nature. According to Slater (2019), the Sankofa is interpreted and re-interpreted in several different ways. For the Akan people, Sankofa symbolises Africa's search for knowledge based on critical reasoning, as well as intelligent and patient investigation of the past. This thinking inspired the considerations of this chapter whose thesis is that as humanity searches for measures to curb the spread of COVID-19, it needs to go back to the past and take lessons learnt from past pandemics and epidemics and utilise them to complement and reinforce WHO recommendations for effective prevention and control of the highly infectious COVID-19. Social distancing, as one of such measures, must not be divorced from the religious indigenous knowledge systems of the communities it is meant to serve and save.

## Social distancing: a bird's eye view

Since it is agreed that the coronavirus pandemic does not move but is moved from one locality to another by human beings, social distancing, which "is a method to minimize crowd interactions and prevent the spread of disease within groups of people" (Aslam 2020), is viewed as reducing the rate at which infection takes place. This is a common practice which has been carried out over generations. During the 1918 influenza pandemic, 50–100 million deaths were reported worldwide. Although social distancing was not implemented back in 1918, majority of the population took reactive social distancing measures that made it possible to escape the disease outbreak (Aslam 2020). This behavioural practice followed by several millions led to the pandemic limiting the damage after World War 1 in several European countries. With this in mind, many governments, at the advice and direction of WHO, put in place social distancing or rather physical distance into place. This ranges from one metre to two metres. This recommended distance is believed to curb the transmission of the coronavirus from one person, who could be infected, to another.

Social distancing practices allow individuals to maintain distances from each other for a period of time to ensure the spread of the disease is minimized (Aslam 2020). This would reduce the basic reproduction number (R0) of the virus which would minimize the disease spread (Aslam 2020). A study carried out by Prem *et al.* (2020) identified that if social distancing practices were carried out properly, an estimate of 92% of cases would be lowered by the end of 2020. An individual affected with COVID-19 has the ability to spread it to 2–3 people which will go on until they are distanced from each other. There are two common practices followed using social distancing; one of them is social distancing and maintaining a distance of nearly one metre when in public and the other being staying indoors at home. This practice has been successful in the past and in the present as well where Wuhan was able to flatten the disease spread by following these practices.

Reluga (2010:1) argues that social distancing is a zero-cost method that is entirely dependent on behavioural patterns of individuals where most of them do not abide by the rules put out in the country. If social distancing methods are ignored the effect could last on for the upcoming generations as the COVID-19 virus will be able to develop different strains where till to date eight different strains of the virus has been discovered by scientists (https://www.news- medical.net/news/20200331/Eight- strains-of-coronavirus-afflicting-the- world.aspx).

Given the above benefits that accrue due to social distancing, why do most people (globally) resist the practice of social distancing? This question is fundamental when we look at Southern African countries where the people are not only 'notoriously religious' but whose economies, which are largely informal, are shrunk, where people eke a living through vending and other associated businesses. It is also essential to argue that social distancing has come camouflaged by WHO as a new strategy yet Africans in general and Zimbabweans in particular had used and still use social distance when confronted by eventualities beyond their comprehension.

## Methodology

The study adopted a qualitative approach with descriptive study, desk research (Travis 2016), and document analysis (Bowen 2009). Primary data were gathered using face-to-face interviews with ten traditional leaders (five males and five females), five academics (three females and two males), and ten ward councillors of two constituencies in Chipinge district. These purposively selected face-to-face interviewees were opinion leaders in their communities and gathering their views was essential for this study. Since this study was conducted during the lockdown imposed on Zimbabwe as a preventive and control measure, COVID-19 control measures were observed during all the face-to-face interviews. The researcher and the interviewees wore face masks (most of whom were improvisations of home-made masks) and observed social/physical distancing of a least one metre. With a few exceptions where the researcher's hand sanitiser was used for sanitising the hands, hand washing was done using ashes and clean running water before and after the interviews to mitigate any possible infections from the COVID-19. The interviewees' consent was obtained by having them either sign a consent form (for those who could write) or verbally consent (for those who could not write) to ensure that they willingly engaged in the study without coercion. To protect the privacy of the study participants, pseudo identification was utilised to treat all personal information of study participants in anonymity. The study also relied on observations of people's behaviour as they interacted with each other with the intent to take note of the people's uptake (or lack of it) of social distancing as a prevention and control measure against COVID-19.

The gathered data (both primary and secondary) were thoroughly analysed thematically based on the research questions for the study. After the transcription of the interviews, they were verified and validated through member checking with ten selected study participants.

# Results

Having conducted the study, data were analysed and culminated in the following thematic areas:

## Social distancing as "old wine in new wine skins"

To check whether social distancing as a containment measure against the spread of the COVID-19 pandemic was really a new measure among the indigenous Ndau people of south-eastern Zimbabwe, the following findings were revealed by the participants. Twenty (80%) of the participants indicated that social distancing was not new to them. The elderly and traditional leaders were quite conversant with the need to keep a distance from someone who has a contagious disease. They cited the following as some of the ailments that they had to contend with in the past.

## *Maperembudzi* (leprosy)

Just like the biblical perception of leprosy (Leviticus 13) most Shona people in general, the Ndau of south-eastern Zimbabwe in particular, kept their distance from a person who had leprosy (*maperembudzi*). Views on how a leprosy patient was handled were summarised by one traditional leader (TL1) who submitted thus:

> Before the advent of clinics and hospitals, we used to have frequent cases of *maperembudzi* in our communities. This was a disease which could be transmitted very easily from one person to another. As a prevention measure we would isolate the infected person. A hut could be built some distance from the homestead and this person could be nursed from there. We made sure that the person does not come in contact with anyone for some reasonable period. Even conjugal rights were denied of that patient. Food was provided to him/her under very strict observances lest the one caring for the patient got infected too.

The above submissions were re-echoed by one ward councillor (WC3), who stated thus:

> As we were growing up, our elders used to tell us stories about *michhachha* (makeshift huts) built at the fringes of the homestead where people with contagious ailments like *maperembudzi* were kept for the period of the ailment. The person was quarantined and all other people were supposed to keep distance (social/physical distancing) from the infected. While the infected person was quarantined, his/her family members would ensure that s/he gets the family support such as provision of food, bathing and clothing. Those who could come closer to the patient needed to be careful not to get infected too by putting on protective clothing.

A female culturist academic (A2) who was interviewed also intimated:

> From the past people have had pandemics that warranted them to keep a distance from the infected. Although the keeping of distance was not known by 'social distancing' then, it is quite true that pandemics and epidemics of this nature abounded. Given that social/physical distancing has been there not only in the COVID-19 context but during other pandemics/epidemics in the past, building on what the people already know from their past experiences with pandemics or epidemics could increase the uptake of social distancing by locals as one of the containment measures against COVID-19.

### *Manyembana* (chicken pox)

Research participants understood *manyembana* (chicken pox) as skin boils (*maronda anobuda mvura mumuiri weshe*). The participants indicated that in severe circumstances, the disease had disastrous consequences such as crippling the patient, death and was said to be highly infectious. This was summed up by one traditional leader (TL4) who stated thus:

> *Manyembana* is no longer common but was a highly infectious disease that also made the patient to be quarantined. The patient was put in a hut away from the homestead and people would take turns to go and see the patient. Body contact was highly prohibited. The patient's food was placed at the entrance of the hut and the patient would serve himself/ herself. With full knowledge of their conditions, the quarantined patients would accept the treatment from family members. They could not begrudge them for they fully understood that coming in contact with the family members the infection would spread to others. They had to endure for the period until the ailment was completely healed.

The excerpts above are, indeed, illustrative of how the concept of separation/ quarantine was instituted among the Ndau rural communities when an individual was infected by a contagion. The above cited infectious diseases were as contagious as is COVID-19, meaning that measures that were instituted for these diseases can be applied to any infectious disease. Social/physical distancing is, therefore, not new when it comes to COVID-19 discourse.

### *Biripiri* (measles)

*Biripiri* (measles) was yet another ailment that called for caution and alertness when it afflicted an individual. Participants were unanimous that *biripiri* (in Ndau language), *was* (my use of the past tense is prompted by the fact that with immunisation most of these ailments are on the curb, though instances of them occurring are possible but with less severity as was in the past before immunisation), an infectious disease which warranted the infected person to be isolated from others. Most of the participants' views can be summarised by what one traditional leader (TL4) said:

> When a person was infected by *biripiri* one was given accommodation where others could not be in contact with him/her. Ordinarily, *biripiri* was very common among the young. When a child was infected, s/he was separated from the others. S/he was put in a hut (*muchhachha*) at the margins of the homestead. During the quarantine period, parents of the child were asked to refrain from sexual intimacy, for doing so would risk the child's life. In fact, *biripiri* had become a rite of passage for one was supposed to pass through it. If a child grew up into adulthood without having been hit by *biripiri*, the parents became worried. If one was infected by the ailment and recovered, one's immunity would have been boosted and would not be prone to other attendant ailments.

Additionally, another participant, an elderly ward councillor (WC3) had this to say:

> *Biripiri* is/was an ailment that could also affect the mature people, not only the young. It was a disease that one had to suffer from, especially when still young. When a person passed his/her teens without having been affected by the disease, people were sure that it would one day affect him in adulthood. At adulthood, the ailment could be more severe and would need rituals to be performed such as making confessions, commonly known as *kudura* in Ndau language. That a person affected by *biripiri* was quarantined in a hut away from the homestead was accepted at a family level, by everyone; both the patient and the family members were inducted to accept this reality.

### *Mphezi* (scabies)

This contagious disease was equally indicated to be one of the ailments that need no skin contact lest it spreads that way. One academic (A1) expressed that:

> As we were growing up in the villages, we were urged to stay away from friends who would have been infected by scabies, lest we too would get infected. Though it was difficult to separate oneself from an infected friend, we were told frightening stories that would force us not to be close to the affected friend. It did not make sense to us then but am now seeing the logic behind. It was meant to reduce the spread of the disease amongst friends. The affected friend was kept under close supervision by the parents so that s/he did not infect others in the community. This was another form of physical distancing, in my view.

The above excerpt illustrates that the separation approach was a painful experience. It hurts both the infected and his/her friends by physically marooning them, thereby emotionally make them miss each other. Mantineo (2021:29) sums up the emotional effect of social distancing by admitting that the dominant feelings of it are "sorrow, grief, and loneliness..." Although the net effect of this exclusion was meant to keep the pandemic/epidemic within manageable limits, it was psychologically numbing as evident in the excerpts above. In some cases, social distancing resulted in some stigma and labelling as A2 revealed that being afflicted by the epidemics was scorned at "*une maperembudzi*", a phrase not readily acceptable to the victim just like it was/is to say "*une* AIDS' (He/she has AIDS).

## The Ndau way of greeting as a safety net against COVID-19

Apart from the forced social distancing imposed by the cited diseases, the Ndau people, who are the participants of this study, have a unique way of greeting. Among indigenous Ndau people shaking of hands and hugging each other, especially between people of a different sex are not only discouraged but castigated as indecorous behaviour (though such taboos are under siege from globalisation and acculturation). The elderly interviewees' views were summarised by one traditional leader (TL5), a village headman. He had this to say:

> We are told that handshaking and hugging are some of the ways through which the virus is spread. As for some of us, who are the real custodians of our culture, handshaking and hugging are not very common because for us there is no respect in doing this. We greet each other with dignity, clapping our hands while sitting down especially when greeting the village head or chief. Reasonable distance is kept between the village head/chief and the subjects. For instance, sons and daughters-in-law keep a distance when greeting their fathers and mothers-in-law. Although we are witnessing changes in how greeting is done these days, in these contexts of COVID-19, our beliefs and practices reign supreme.

Probed further, the interviewee indicated the kind of greeting that happens between a mother-in-law and her son-in-law. The son-in-law takes a respectful body position clapping hands while the mother-in-law literally sits down clapping hands too, with the two literally not looking at each other face to face. This, according to the interviewee, is a sign of respect and a high demonstration of *untu* (humaneness, humility, meekness and gratitude). Chances that COVID-19 may be transmitted here are minimal for there is reasonable physical distance between the son-in-law and mother-in-law. The practice, which could be on the verge of extinction in the Fourth Revolution, can become handy if all people in the COVID-19 context treat each other in the manner the Ndau son-in-law and mother-in-law relate to one another. This traditional behavioural practice can be turned into a public health safety net.

## Social distancing and *Ubuntu* among the Ndau

On whether social distancing does not violate the principles of *ubuntu,* one traditional leader (TL3) summarised the interviewees' views as follows:

> There is a serious dilemma that we face when we are asked not to be in contact with our dear infected kinspeople. While we are aware of the consequences of the contact, it remains inhuman for us to separate ourselves from the sick. Firstly, it is extremely difficult for the caring person. Secondly, it has serious psychological effects on the patient. One feels rejected or rather discriminated against. Our *ubuntu* values teach us to care and love the infected. This care and love come in the form of closeness to the patient, talking to him/her, re-assuring her/him that this is just a passing phase. This is what this highly infectious disease thrives on. We are, therefore, left wondering what to do, keep ourselves away and not being infected or be close enough to the infected to be infected too?

The same pessimism was shared by another interviewee who talked about the way funeral proceedings of the victims of the pandemic are carried out. She (A2) had this to say:

> We are deeply concerned about the way our departing ones are being buried. We no longer observe burial rites for a person who has died of COVID-19 related complications that include: having the corpse in the house a night before burial, no body bathing, no body reviewing and many other associated funeral rites. A person, in some instances, is laid to rest by health and funeral agents who are not even related, strangers to the deceased. This has serious consequences for the deceased and the deceased's close relatives. This flouts our beliefs and values on death and funeral rites. That sense of communitarianism is no longer there. The 'I am because of others' is seriously challenged.

A female traditional healer, who was part of the key informant interviewees among the traditional leaders, had this to say:

> Oooh! To die and your children failing to touch your body is the most painful thing to happen in one's life. This is unacceptable in our culture as Ndau people. I will turn in my grave and definitely punish them for abandoning me. I must die in the hands of my children. My funeral rites must be observed fully.

During fieldwork, I observed that most funerals held in the rural areas compromised a lot on observing WHO and the Ministry of Health and Child Care (MoHCC) guidelines on funerals. Health officials, (who usually are members of the bereaved communities), who were supposed to enforce these stipulations, were held back by socio-cultural beliefs and values. As such COVID-19 containment measures like proper face masking, social distancing, handwashing using soap on clean running water and not coming too close to a COVID-19 corpse were relaxed, risking many lives. The health officials found it very difficult, in the rural areas, to coerce members of the communities they were too accustomed to, to abstain from carrying out the funeral rites. Instead, the officials tended to ignore the flouting of the COVID-19 regulations during mourning and burial.

## Discussion

Participants in the interviews were clear that social distancing was not necessarily new but a practice that was there from time immemorial, especially among the Ndau people. They indicated that the epidemics and pandemics were dealt with by putting in place the socio-cultural beliefs and practices (which I can refer to the Ndau people's indigenous knowledge systems) commensurate with the people's socio-cultural milieu. This puts traditional communities on a vantage position when it comes to the COVID-19 pandemic containment measures. Unfortunately, this vantage position is not utilised for the benefit of the communities confronted by what Okyere-Manu (2021) identified as 'the lion attacking the village'. Ndhlovu-Gatsheni is instructive when he argues thus:

> The ironic part is that even among Africans-who have a long history and experience of grappling with epidemics and pandemics, largely because of the negative impact of modern global power dynamics, which invented and reproduced the Global South as the geography of poverty-there is reluctance to tap into this history, experience, and knowledge about responding to the COVID-19 pandemic.
>
> (2020:370)

This argument emanates from the realisation that there is a tendency to look for answers to problems from outside the context of the problem. For instance, when the COVID-19 pandemic hit the world the most logical thing was to look for contextual responses. Rather, what happened is that WHO came up with a one-size-fits-all approach where the Global North and the Global South were, all of a sudden and surprisingly, symmetric. The assumption made was that all nations were *tabula rasa* when it comes to the pandemic. Little did the Global North know, that pandemics of this nature were not necessarily new to the Global South, as Ndhlovu-Gatsheni (2020:372) points out that "the COVID-19 has plunged the world into an unfamiliar territory though it is not so unfamiliar to the Global South, where a majority of people live in what Fanon (1968) termed the 'zone of nonbeing'". Admittedly, there is need for a global solution to a global problem but we need not lose sight of the heterogeneity that characterises continents and countries. Zeleza (2020) cautions that we need an African solution to a global problem.

Given the foregoing, the thesis I am advancing is that instead of coming up with a one- size-fits-all approach to the COVID-19 pandemic, WHO and ministries of health in various nations were supposed to prioritise flattening the curve taking into cognisance countries potentialities and capabilities. For example, when Madagascar tried to institute its local expertise to curb the spread of the virus, it received unwarranted criticisms from WHO and its allies. This inferiorisation and othering of other people's knowledge systems is tantamount to epistemic violence and genocide. As participants indicated, ailments such as measles, leprosy, and chicken pox warranted physical distancing. Instead of bringing social distancing as a new measure, WHO and its agents should have advocated for the utilisation of the local people's past experiences with pandemics/epidemics of a similar nature and use the experiences as building blocks towards finding solutions to the COVID-19 challenge. This is what developmental scholars believe in when they talk of the B4 model (Building the Build Back Better model) (Nhamo & Chikodzi 2021). The call is for the Global North to realise that circumstances differ. An anonymous writer says "If New York never sleeps because the lights are always on and there's always somewhere to be, Lagos never sleeps because there's no power and it's much too hot indoors", which brings us the stark reality that while other communities are luxurious and spacious, others, even if they want to, simply do not have the space to be that luxurious. Taking their existential circumstances when dealing with challenges is fundamental.

It has also been evident from the participants that while social distancing is recommended at funerals, it is not just practical in some socio-cultural contexts. The psychological pain that the bereaved have to go through when the loved departed one is never given the full burial rites as per custom is just unbearable. The idea of a victim of COVID-19 coming straight from a funeral parlour to the grave where trained health officials take over the proceedings is hard to accept. This is why COVID-19 funerals are very difficult to manage in the rural communities as observed during fieldwork. Deopa and Fortunato (2020) concur when they argue that while the health measures enacted have been, on the average homogenous across all cultures, compliance to these rules varied widely within the local context. The fear to anger the spiritual world forced some people to flout COVID-19 funeral stipulations. Imaging a mother dying not in her children's hands (literally) is treated as an anathema that may result in *kutanda botso* (appeasing the avenging mother's spirit). People find themselves in a *cul de sac,* either to follow health officials' guidelines and anger their ancestors or to flout the funeral regulations. Okyere-Manu (2021) poignantly says that this raises an ethical dilemma for us as Africans. We are to either choose life affirming practices or ignore the public health call.

An anonymous writer in the Correspondent of 27 March 2020 submits that social distancing will not work for Africans. For the anonymous writer, social distancing is not just alien to Africans, it is impossible for social and economic reasons too. We have witnessed how families' livelihoods have been affected by national lockdowns in the Third World countries. While social distancing is the catchword for WHO, WHO is forgetting (consciously or unconsciously) that there are many parts of the world where this single solution is contextually inadequate or even dangerous. I call to mind here fundamental questions that Okyere-Manu (2021) raises. She queries:

> Some of these choices are relatively rudimentary – choosing not to have an evening event with friends to share meat, music and conversation is simple enough. But what happens to that same choice when a baby is born? A young couple gets married? A young intelligent member of our neighbourhood graduates?

While the above excerpt may be looked at casually, the cited events call for the serious need to demonstrate *ubuntu*. Okyere-Manu points to the serious dilemma most people find in social distancing no wonder people flout it as it contradicts the people's sense of *ubuntu*. Sambala *et al.* (2019) attribute the rise of ethical problems to disproportionate interventions and intrusive public health measures. According to Sambala *et al.* (2019), interconnections, interdependence and interrelationships are the pillars of *ubuntu*. Social distancing defeats interrelationality and sociality. African people have to contend with dictates and teachings from African indigenous religions and the scientific pronouncements made about pandemics. The dichotomous variations between science and religions are at play, and because Africans, who are "notoriously religious" (Mbiti 1969: 1) revere and venerate ancestors, they fear angering their spiritual world. They would rather jeopardize their lives than angering the ancestors. This explains why they continue, against science recommendations, to attend and carry funeral rites that risk their lives in COVID-19 funeral contexts. They choose religion instead of science.

## Linking the past, present and the future: lessons from the Sankofa bird

The foregoing arguments are a culmination of what used to happen, what is happening and what we need to do. Using the Sankofa perspective, I submit that while the behaviour of WHO and health ministries of many governments, particularly in Southern Africa is acceptable, treating countries as homogenous who need a homogenous solution to a global problem stifles rooms for creativity, ingenuity and innovation. Southern African governments must not "cut and paste" (Mocamo 2020: 1) European responses to the COVID-19 pandemic. The clarion call is "let us go back to the past, take that which is useful and blend it with that which is at our disposal for sustainable solutions to existential challenges such as the COVID-19 pandemic" (Mocamo 2020: 1). This chapter is by no means a total rejection of modern measures by health experts but a plea for the need to tap from the known into the unknown, from a people's indigenous knowledge into science. Social distancing that used to be there in pandemics and epidemics mentioned by participants needs not to be ignored. I argue that we need to build from the known to the unknown. This has an advantage in that uptake of measures may be increased for a people's socio-cultural milieu would have been taken into consideration in the search for COVID-19 containment measures. In other words, let us learn from the Sankofa bird.

On how the past experiences can be the building blocks on flattening the curve, the creation of community-based task forces headed by traditional leadership to educate the public on the need to balance Western and local interventions to increase the uptake of WHO recommendations is more urgent than ever. This is where traditional chiefs, kraal heads and headmen become handy. These traditional leaders derive respect and trust from their members. This is a competitive advantage in that they are more likely to be hearkened to when they actively participate in COVID-19 containment measures education campaigns. Dziva argues:

> As custodians and enforcers of traditional customs and values, endogenous leaders are widely relied on and respected in rural communities such that their encouragements, orders and coercive interventions can positively combat the deadly coronavirus. With the fear for punishment in the form of cursing or being ostracized, ruralites often listen to and abide by traditional leaders' calls and pleas to stay at home, practice personal hygiene and observe social distancing. Based on these cutting edge advantages, chiefs and their decentralized structures can play a key role in community mobilization, raising awareness, dispelling pandemic rumours and myths, vaccine utilization and pushing for compromises where measures are incompatible with local traditions, cultural values and norms.
>
> (2020:509)

Failing to utilize this abundant resource at its disposal, the Zimbabwean government is failing the whole nation. If ever there was a time to seriously harness a people's socio-cultural capital, it is now. Traditional leaders must not only be found convenient during elections but also during health crisis such as COVID-19.

## Conclusion

This chapter has discussed social distancing from a Ndau religious indigenous knowledge systems, where the argument is that there is scope to tap from past experiences. It has concluded that social distancing is a safety valve that communities in south-eastern Zimbabwe utilised to reduce the impact of epidemics and pandemics and that it is, therefore, not a new strategy in the context of COVID-19. The containment measure has come in Eurocentric packages, ignoring what local communities used to do in the past. This one-size-fits-all approach has been rejected in this chapter. The chapter has suggested the B4 model where eventualities such as COVID-19 hits, there is need to build on build back better (BBBB) where the thrust is to tap on what communities used in curbing previous epidemics and pandemics and improve where need be. The chapter has also accounted for the lack of compliance when it comes to social distancing during funerals. Principles of *ubuntu* are not amenable to social distancing, particularly during religious burial rites. This dilemma needs to be untangled by robust education platforms where the locals are educated on the need to deal with COVID-19 in a culturally responsive context. Traditional mechanisms such as traditional leadership's agency must be used in the education of the locals, an education that is not too divorced from the socio-cultural milieu of the locals. Such an education would reduce confrontation and resistance in the fight against COVID-19.

## References

Aslam, F. 2020. COVID-19 and the importance of social distancing. www.preprints. org. Accessed 28 October 2020.

Bowen, G. 2009. Document analysis as a qualitative research method. *Qualitative Research Journal*, 9(2), 27–40. https://doi.org/10.3316/QRJ0902027.

Cabral, A. 1973. *A Return to the Source: Selected Speeches by Amilcar Cabral.* New York: NYU Press.

Deopa, N. and Fotunato, P. 2020. Coronagraben: Culture and social distancing in times of COVID-19. UNCTAD Research Paper No. 49. https://unctad.org/system/files/official-document/ser-rp-2020d8_en.pdf. Accessed 10 March 2021.

Dziva, C. 2020. The potential and challenges for traditional leadership in combating the COVID-19 pandemic in rural communities of Zimbabwe. *African Journal of Governance and Development,* 9(2), 509–523.

Fanon, F. 1968. *The Wretched of the Earth.* Cambridge: Grove Press.

Jaja, I.F., Umunna, M. and Jaja, C.J.I. 2020. Social distancing: How religion, culture and burial ceremony undermine the effort to curb COVID-29 in South Africa. *Emerging Microbes and Infections,* 9(1), 1077–1079.

Macamo, E. 2020. *The Normality of Risk: African and European Responses to COVID-19.*https://www.coronatimes.net/normality-risk-africa-european-responses/ Accessed 8 March 2021.

Mantineo, A. 2021. I have a dream: Restarting, but going where? In Pierluigi Consorti (ed.). *Law, Religion and COVID-19 Emergency.* Pisa: DiReSoM, 29–34.

Mbiti, J.S. 1969. *African Religions and Philosophy.* Blantyre: Heinemann.

Ministry of Health and Child Care. 2020a. Coronavirus (COVID-19) Update Statement. 14 April 2020.

Ministry of Health and Child Care. 2020b. Coronavirus (COVID-19) Update: Zimbabwe, 19 June 2020.

Ministry of Health and Child Care. 2020c. Zimbabwe COVID-19 SitRep: Update: Zimbabwe, 6 September 2020. http://www.mohcc.gov.zw/index.php?option=com_phocadownload&view=cate gory&id=15&Itemid=742. Accessed 28 September 2020.

Ministry of Health and Child Care. 2020d. Stay at home # stay safe # defeat COVID-19, 8 April 2020. http://www.mohcc.gov.zw/index.php?option=com_content&view=cat egory&layout=blog&id=103&Itemid=743. Accessed 28 September 2020.

Ndlovu-Gatsheni, S.J. 2020. Geopolitics of power and knowledge in COVID-19 pandemic: Decolonial reflections on a global crisis. *Journal of Developing Societies*, 36(4), 366–389.

Nhamo, G. and Chikodzi, D. 2021. *Cyclones in Southern Africa Volume 1: Interfacing the catastrophic impact of cyclone Idai with SDGs in Zimbabwe*. Switzerland: Springer.

Okyere-Manu, B. 2021. Coronavirus: The Lion is attacking the village. https://beatriceokyere.com/post/coronavirus-the-lion-is-attacking-the-village. Accessed 4 February 2021.

Prem, K., Liu, Y., Russell, T.W., Kucharski, A.J., Eggo, R.M., Davies, N., Flasche, S., Clifford, S., Pearson, C.A., Munday, J.D. and Abbott, S. 2020. The effect of control strategies to reduce social mixing on outcomes of the COVID-19 epidemic in Wuhan, China: A modelling study. *The Lancet Public Health*, 5(5), e261–e270. Published online 2020 Mar 25. doi: 10.1016/S2468-2667(20)30073-6

Reluga, T.C. 2010. Game theory of social distancing in response to an epidemic. *PLoS Computational Biology*, 6(5), 1–9.

Sambala, E.Z., Cooper, S. and Manderson, L. 2019. *Ubuntu* as a framework for ethical decision making in Africa: Responding to epidemics. *Ethics and Behavior*, 30(1), 1–13.

Slater, J. 2019. Sankofa-the need to turn back to move forward: Addressing reconstruction challenges that face Africa and South Africa today. *Studia Historiae Ecclesiasticae*, 45(1), 1–24.

Travis, D. 2016. Desk research: The what, why, and how. *User Focus*. https://www.userfocus.co.uk.

World Health Organization (WHO). 2020. *Coronavirus disease (COVID-19) outbreak situation*. https://www.who.int/emergencies/diseases/novel-coronavirus-2019?gclid=EAIaIQobChMIv5yAiOfY6wIVpoBQBh2LEwgEEAAYASAAEgLk u_D_BwE. Accessed 10 October 2020.

Zeleza, P.T. 2020. The coronavirus: The political economy of the pathogen. *Elephant*. 1–23. https://www.theelephant.info/long-reads/2020/03/25/the-coronavirus-the-political-economy-of-a-pathogen/ Accessed 5 March 2021.

# 4 Coping with the coronavirus (COVID-19)

## Resources from Ndau indigenous religion

*Macloud Sipeyiye*

### Introduction

The global pandemic of the coronavirus (COVID-19) has shaken the world in a devastating way. This is so tragic to Africa in particular, given that the continent had not yet completely ridden the tide of the HIV and AIDS. Indeed, Africa has not tasted the luxury of rest. Dube (2003:85) presents metaphorically the unfortunate story of Africa where she says,

> Only yesterday did we leave the delivery room, smiling with a new born baby: a free and independent Africa...And just as we began to smile, watching this child lift its foot to take its first step as an independent being...bang! Another oppressor struck Africa: HIV/AIDS!

Africa had almost begun to take stock of her success over HIV and AIDS when her space is intruded yet again by a ruthless novel coronavirus (COVID-19) that has compelled governments across the world to put their countries or parts thereof on lockdown where people are encouraged to remain indoors to stop the spread of the disease in the absence of a vaccine. On a positive note though, the contagious disease has not been as virulent with Africa as it has been with the global north, a feat that has found no clear explanation from health scientists, at least for now. One of the opinions that have been thrown around is that the continent is under-reporting the pandemic's statistical information owing to her incapacity to roll out massive testing to ascertain the levels of infection due, largely to poverty and lack of political will. Miller *et al.* (2020:1) opine that the impact of the disease is different in different countries. They attribute these differences to differences in cultural norms, mitigation efforts, and health infrastructure. The government of Zimbabwe in line with global trends put the country under an initial 21-day lockdown from 30 March 2020. The lockdown has since seen two two-week extensions that were followed by an indefinite extension with a fortnight review intervals announced on 16 May 2020. The government has also come up with a litany of statutory instruments that are intended to enforce the lockdown regulations.

DOI: 10.4324/9781003241096-4

Religions have been taken unawares by this unprecedented development forcing them to search deeper into their resources in order to remain relevant to their followers. It is a fact that these religions will emerge from this phase renewed. The most disturbing trait of the COVID-19 pandemic is that its major route of transmission, that is contact, is the mainstay of religious practices. Indigenous religions of Africa, for example, have been aptly described as religions that are based on relationships (Taringa 2014, Dube 2009, 2006, Cox 2007, Mbiti 1969). It is this social dimension; these relationships that COVID-19 pandemic has subjected to a big test of the times. The question that I seek to answer in this chapter is: What preventive and containment strategies can the Ndau indigenous religio-cultural resources proffer in mitigating COVID-19 pandemic? To achieve this objective, I explore strengths and challenges of the Ndau indigenous beliefs and practices in the context of the standard COVID-19 health measures and protocols. Given the diversity within African religio-cultures, my focus is primarily on Ndau indigenous religion of Zimbabwe. I use "religio-cultures" here for the simple reason that "religion and culture are so intertwined throughout Africa that it is impossible to speak of one without the other" (Thomas 2015:7).

## Theoretical framework

In this chapter, I employ spiritual capital theory. Ganiel (2009) tells us that at times the terms "religious capital" and "spiritual capital" are often conflated and seem to mean the same while at other times scholars draw distinctions between them. Çarkoğlu (2008) distinguishes the two differentiating between them by stressing that religious capital produces exclusivist 'bonding' identities within a group or individuals, while spiritual capital is a 'bridging' resource between groups or individuals that inspires people to act to help others beyond their immediate comfort zone. He distinguishes them by drawing an analogous relationship with Putnam's (2000) bonding and bridging social capital. Putnam defines social capital in terms of networks of relationships within (bonding social capital) and between (bridging social capital) groups and individuals. This denotes that the theory has its roots in the development of the concept of 'social capital'. Çarkoğlu's view is in tandem with the understanding that spirituality goes beyond the the usual limits of organised religion, which makes it less binding but more amenable to human transformation. Spiritual capital concretizes a family-like atmosphere that provides spiritual strength and bonding that generates social capital (Haynes 2007). Thus, spiritual capital is an important source for social capital. The theory was utilised in this article to enable an appreciation of how the Ndau invoke their spiritual capital enshrined in their notion of collective existence to provide a framework for solidarity and active compassion.

## Methodology

The chapter is an empirical qualitative phenomenological study that seeks to access the meaning embedded in the religious activities of the Ndau in the context of COVID-19 through audio and chat messages shared via WhatsApp. WhatsApp is a social media micro blogging site that is reasonably cheaper particularly to populations residing in rural areas compared to other social media platforms such as Facebook, Tweeter, Instagram and many others. I also employed telephone interviews with some key informants who had no access to WhatsApp. I found these methods to be compliant with the WHO COVID-19 recommended means of communication in the spirit of social or physical distancing. I purposefully sampled adult male and female participants on the basis of my knowledge of the population to provide the best information to address the purpose of the research. I did not include the actual sample size deliberately, opting to rely on the principle of theoretical saturation, that is, the point when new data no longer brought additional insights to the research question (Mack *et al.* 2005). The rationale for choosing the Ndau is based on my cultural setting; I am Ndau myself. Mack *et al.* (2005) stress that in qualitative research, researchers who possess a solid base of cultural awareness stand a better chance of gaining the confidence of the communities under study. This is particularly important for this research where data were retrieved via social media platforms that have the propensity to increase informant fears and suspicions. I was cautious also of the fact that familiarity with the researched community may lead to biases in data gathered. To guard against biases, I committed myself faithfully to the phenomenology of religion's methodological principle of *epoche* that calls for the bracketing of preconceived ideas about the phenomena researched (Chitando *et al.* 2013). Second, my interest on the Ndau is also driven by the fact that Ndau culture is transboundary, one of the characteristics that pose challenges to mitigatory efforts against COVID-19. It is therefore interesting to find out how the Ndau, in their geo-political and cultural locatedness mobilize their religio-cultural resources to respond to the dreaded COVID-19 pandemic.

## What is coronavirus (COVID-19)?

Coronaviruses are a large family of viruses which may cause illness in animals or humans. In humans, several coronaviruses are known to cause respiratory infections ranging from the common cold to more severe diseases such as Middle East Respiratory Syndrome (MERS) and Severe Acute Respiratory Syndrome (SARS). The most recently discovered coronavirus causes coronavirus disease that later came to be known as COVID-19. So, COVID-19 is the communicable or infectious disease caused by the recently discovered coronavirus. This new virus and disease were unknown before the outbreak began in Wuhan, Hubei Province, China in December 2019, hence the 19 to indicate year of discovery (Miller *et al.* 2020, WHO 2020). COVID-19 often causes fear and uncertainty to people since the disease is new and there are no scientifically known treatment or vaccine.

## Symptoms and modes of transmission of COVID-19

Symptoms of COVID-19 are similar to other types of illness such as flu that people usually do not take seriously, thus not detected or seek treatment before critical time (MoHCC 2020). The most common symptoms of COVID-19 are fever, difficulty in breathing and dry cough. Some patients may have aches and pains, tiredness, nasal congestion, runny nose, sore throat or diarrhoea. These symptoms are usually mild and begin gradually. Some people are asymptomatic; they become infected, but do not develop any symptoms and do not feel unwell. Such people have a strong immune system that successfully fights the coronavirus. Those people transmit the virus to others unknowingly. Their status can only be detected through testing. Most people, about 80%, recover from the disease without needing special attention (WHO 2020). Anyone can be infected with COVID-19, but older people and those with underlying medical conditions such as asthma, high blood pressure, heart problems or diabetes are more likely to develop serious illness. Children and young people can be infected and develop serious illness. Although serious illness in young people is less likely, they can spread the disease to others. COVID-19 is primarily transmitted through contact with respiratory droplets from infected persons and by contact with contaminated objects and surfaces.

## Global response to coronavirus

It is important to outline what the World Health Organization (WHO) recommends as ways of curtailing the spread of coronavirus since these recommendations will provide a platform for assessing the Ndau indigenous religion's competence or lack of it against coronavirus. WHO has come up with a raft of behaviour change strategies that have drastically changed the social landscape in an unprecedented way that they have been befittingly labelled the 'new normal'. Below are some of the strategies that nation-states' ministries of health, following the WHO guidelines, are campaigning for:

- People should avoid contact with anyone, especially if they have cold or flu-like symptoms by practising physical distancing of at least one metre.
- Cover mouth and nose when coughing or sneezing into your elbow or use a tissue and discard it into a bin with lid straight away.
- Avoid touching eyes, nose and mouth.
- Wash hands with water and soap regularly for at least 20 seconds.

- Self-isolate for 14 days if you have come from a country with case or have been in proximity to those with COVID-19.
- Use a mask when feeding or caring for the sick.
- Avoid travelling to countries, cities or local areas where COVID-19 is spreading.

## A brief social history of the Ndau people of south-eastern Zimbabwe

The present day Ndau people live in the vast region that comprises the south-eastern parts of Zimbabwe, specifically Chimanimani and Chipinge Districts of Manicaland Province, sprawling into the central and western parts of Mozambique (Dube 2017). The Chipinge district has seven Ndau chiefdoms, namely Garahwa, Gwenzi, Mpungu, Mahenye, Mapungwana, Musikavanhu, and Mutema while the Chimanimani area is home to five Ndau chiefdoms that include Chikukwa, Ndima, Mutambara, Muusha, and Ngorima (Sithole 2018). Most of the Ndau chiefs' jurisdictions stride the international border for example, the first six Chipinge and the first two Chimanimani chiefs above in the same manner that their Mozambican counterparts do, a typical example being chief Macuiana (Portuguese).

Herbst (1989) cited by Konyana (2018:52), avers that the Ndau community is quite expanse and always refers to some group of people separated by the colonial borderline between Zimbabwe and Mozambique. He further posits that before the partition of Africa, eastern Zimbabwe and south-western Mozambique were part of the precolonial Zimbabwe Plateau that was occupied by the Shona people of various ethnic languages, including the Ndau. Beach (1980:34) says that the Ndau is linked together by the bonds of intermarriages between families of different totems, the distinct Ndau dialect and the cultural beliefs and practices which they have always shared. Patricio (2011, 2010) and MacGonagle (2007) have shown that for many centuries, the Ndau have remained undisturbed by the border. They have maintained close links and are united in all spheres of social, economic and political lives to the extent that they are identified as one large community that extends from one country to the other across the international boundary. Patricio (2011:678) succinctly expresses this situation as follows:

> So the Ndau of Mozambique continue to cross the border like they did in the past and go to Zimbabwe to visit their family, to consult healers and traditional authorities, to go to school and to take part in ceremonies. It seems these people do not feel the impact of the international boundary demarcation in the daily lives-not in colonial times, not even today.

Konyana's (2018:55) observation aptly summarises the situation of the Ndau when he says that, "[T]he Ndau people have had uninterrupted *de facto* dual citizenship status of being Zimbabweans as well as being Mozambicans."

### The name *Ndau*

Sithole (2018:5) notes the obscurity of the history and etymology of the term Ndau as an ethnic label. There are various theories propounded to disentangle this Gordian knot. One of the theories suffices for the purpose of this chapter. The theory contends that the term was originally used as "an exclamation of deference" by Ndau speakers (Sithole ibid). The theory avers that the term was conferred on the Ndau by outsiders that include traders in acknowledgement of the hospitality, friendliness and respectfulness of the local people. Sithole (2018:5) aptly expresses it as follows:

> Ndau people follow 'unique' customs especially greeting forms as well as a generally respectful conduct. The Ndaus are believed to be a culturally 'down-to-earth' people governed by high standards of morality, humility and excellence. This is encapsulated in the phrase 'Ndauwe' which implies that 'We salute you!' This is an expression of friendliness and utmost humility. The essence of being Ndau was communicated through showing respect to elders and visitors (Kuhlonipha). It appears that the Ndau identity predicates itself on common behavioural and sociocultural values such as humility and morality...

MacGonagle (2007:548) concurs with Sithole where she says that 'Ndau', "was a nickname used by others in the 19th century to describe the people who said, 'Ndau-wee. Ndau-wee" as their customary unassuming greeting when they entered a homestead or received any strangers in their homesteads. This chapter focused on three chiefdoms in Chipinge, chiefs Mapungwana, Musikavanhu, and Gwenzi. These areas were chosen on the basis of the authors' familiarity with the places which enabled them to get informant consent without hassles.

### Ndau family institution

The Ndau notion of the *mphuri* (family) is an all-embracing phenomenon expressed through a web of relationships that goes beyond the living beings. It is rather a cosmic totality that includes the living, the living-dead, the unborn, the flora and the fauna, and the rest of other inanimate elements comprising the environment (Sipeyiye 2020). The Ndau *mphuri* is best described as referring to the whole clan. According to Rusinga and Maposa (2010:47), members of African families strive as far as possible to stay together in the same community, especially in rural areas. This is also true of the Ndau who cherish greatly the value of unity and communal existence. This interconnectedness is best explained by the Ndau concept of *Ukama* (kinship/relatedness) that Murove (2009) refers to as 'communal ethic'. *Ukama* (kinship/relatedness) expresses the interconnectedness and interdependence of the human and non-human within their environment. Konyana

(2018:57) maintains that *Ukama* is the concept which touches on the family relatedness and communal belonging which has kept the Ndau family much the same as it was before colonisation. The Ndau family is patriarchal. The most senior male member, in most cases the grandfather (*baba akuru*) is the revered head of the extended or connected family. He is the family leader whose major role is to advise the family on all matters of life and more importantly to connect the family with its ancestral spirits or the spirit elders (*midzimu*). Pfukwa (2001) cited by Konyana (2018:57), holds that the Ndau refer the family grandfather as "the great one" (*Musharukwa*) in reference to his central role as the family advisor and rapporteur between the living and the living-dead. Rusinga and Maposa (2010:18) posit that the Ndau people in general value blood relatedness to the extent that most of them strive to remain attached to their extended family members despite relocation and migration in pursuit of greener pastures. Gelfand (1973:105) explains that "the urge to live together is not something that took its effect, or was imposed, only with the beginning of colonization. It is traditional and the connection is that it is a survival strategy imperative of the culture." This suggests that the communal ethic of *ukama* inspires the Ndau to live close to each other and share everything, their blessings and sorrows.

## Ndau beliefs and practices

At the core of the Ndau indigenous beliefs and cultural practices is the belief in ancestral spirits or spirit elders or guardian spirits (*midzimu*) that are connected with the spirit world (Pfukwa 2001). The spirit world is fashioned in a way that reflects how the society is structured. In the Ndau chiefdoms, the chief, is at the top. He is approached through a mediator and only in cases of emergency is he addressed directly. Requests to the chief go through a process known as *kushuma* (protocols), the role that junior members in the spirit world perform. *Musikavanthu* (Creator of human beings) or *Marure* (The Creator) is at the apex of the hierarchy of the spiritual world followed by the royal ancestral spirits down to the level of the family in a way that mirrors the hierarchy of power present in the Ndau society. *Musikavanthu* or *Marure* is not perturbed by the petitions of the people; rather the family and territorial spirits are the busiest of the constituents of the spirit world. Among the Ndau, as in most African societies, ancestral spirits are the kingpin of the society. They influence the activities and lives of the living descendants of their community. The notion of ancestral spirits expresses the common African idea of the increased power of the dead in their role as the guardians of the land and the people (Schoffeelers 1979). The Ndau believe that ancestral spirits are at their best when they have been accorded proper funeral rites by their living descendants, which include decent burial and traditional ceremonies in their honour. As a result, the Ndau always make sure that they occasionally hold ceremonies to appease their ancestors at all the times. This feature of the Ndau belief system compels them to come together and share in all their problems and difficulties because they ought to constantly consult the *midzimu* together for solutions to social problems including appeasement, if need be, of the angered spirit elders (Konyana 2018).

## Indigenous communities and Coronavirus (COVID-19)

The United Nations Department of Economic and Social Affairs (2020) notes that the coronavirus poses a grave health threat to indigenous communities worldwide. This is so because even before the outbreak of the pandemic, most indigenous communities already faced challenges of food insecurity, poor communication technologies, poor access to healthcare, high rates of diseases, lack of access to essential services, sanitation and other key preventive measures such as clean water, soap, and disinfectants. Cotacachi and Grigera (2020) concur when they say that standard health protocols for hand washing and disinfection are difficult to follow in such a situation. In some cases, indigenous people face stigma and discrimination even when they are able to access healthcare services. It has also been observed that indigenous peoples' lifestyles are a source of their resilience, and can also pose a threat in preventing communicable diseases in general and coronavirus in particular (United Nations Department of Economic and Social Affairs 2020). Regular traditional gatherings for religio-cultural ceremonies to mark special events, and multi-generational housing are the hall mark of indigenous communities that put indigenous peoples and their families especially the elderly at risk of contracting coronavirus. Cotacachi and Grigera (2020) express it aptly when they say that "implementing isolation and social distancing protocols is challenging when family and community structures are intrinsically collective and strongly socially cohesive." The situation of indigenous women, who are often the main providers of food and nutrition to their families, is even graver. To this effect, calls have been made to make sure that "immediate health responses to address the worldwide emergency should be differentiated and prioritise indigenous peoples as a high risk epidemiological population" (Cotacachi and Grigera 2020). Regardless, it has also been observed that indigenous communities are seeking their own solutions to combat the threat of COVID-19 pandemic. They are taking action and employing their indigenous knowledge and practices such as voluntary isolation and sealing off their territories as well as preventive measures in their own language (United Nations Department of Economic and Social Affairs 2020).

## Ndau indigenous responses to COVID-19: challenges and promises

In this section, I present and analyse findings on the Ndau indigenous responses to coronavirus. I took cognisance of areas that need reflection for improvement and those that provide potential sites for improved responses to the pandemic. My key respondents were coded to ensure confidentiality. I used numbers instead of their real names so that they remain anonymous. Many respondents shared a common puzzle about the coronavirus pandemic. They have never met anyone suffering from the disease. The handling and management of the disease emphasise individual rights and privacy at the expense of the community. Respondent 1 has this to say:

> *Atisati tachiziya kuti tizoona kuti marwarire akhona akadini. Atisati tamboona wachirwara. Chichi chokuzwira mumphepo kuti munthu wabatwa ndicho unokotsora, kufemera mudenga nekuvhara miro. Hezvinonga zvekunyepa kee, pane wakambozvionawo ere? Azvina kutodzana nezvemagandanga epaWhatsApp ayani ere?* (We have not yet known the disease for us to establish the pattern of sickness. We have never seen anyone suffering from it. We just hear about it in the news where it is said that a person who has contracted it, coughs, has short breathing and congestion of the nose. It may appear as lies, has anyone ever seen this? Is it not the same with those stories about terrorists that once appeared on WhatsApp?)

Respondent 3 echoed the same sentiments metaphorically when they said:

> *Kana mhondoro ikafungidzirwa kuti iri kuhamba muntharaunda vaisa vanoungana vototorosa matsiko kuti vabate gwinyiso kuti ndizvo ere kana kuti idede. Zvinoita kuti vave nekuzwisisa kwakakwana kuitira kuti dantho reshe ravachatora mukuteera nekurwisa chikara ringe rine unyanzvi negwinyiso rekuti vanonyisa* (If the community suspects a threat of a prancing lion in their neighbourhood, men come together and study trails to ascertain whether it is really a lion or that it is just a baboon. It ensures certainty so that any move they take in tracking and attacking it be informed by dexterity, tact and a strong conviction that they would emerge victorious).

The views of the two respondents above show that indigenous communities' responses to the challenge of coronavirus are often thwarted by lack of knowledge of the identity of the invisible enemy that they are supposed to combat. This situation has a tendency of making the COVID-19 a distant myth that has remote chances of being part of their lived experiences. This is also compounded by the fact that the disease has a foreign origin and could therefore remain a foreign disease. This scenario negatively impacts on the uptake of preventive measures. For example, one respondent was subjected to a humiliating experience on her way to the family nutritional garden when a group of locals jeered at her just for masking. The group shouted at her, "*Kwai chati chaauno ere, kusiri kuda zviro!*" (Has it (coronavirus) ever been recorded here or you just want things!) She was blamed for allegedly being overzealous and she felt stigmatized and discriminated against just for her caution consciousness. Mobilizing cultural resources may be a challenge if the nature of the disease is unknown. This is in line with Konyana (2014:125) who avers that the Ndau believe that all illnesses and diseases can be overcome for as long as the source of the illness is identified.

As observed above, the Ndau indigenous religio-culture is about collective existence based on a strong web of relationships, which has a high likelihood of posing a great challenge to the practice of self-isolating and social or physical distancing. Respondents admitted that the coronavirus pandemic has indeed caused panic across the world and disturbed lifestyles, and the Ndau have also been affected. Respondent 4 maintains that:

> *Kubvira kudhaya nakudhaya vaNdau tine ukama hunotambarara kubatanidza vanthu vakawanda vari jinga remuZimbabwe neMozambique. Midiro yedu nechianthu chedu cheshe zvinotibatanidza. Anyari matenda nemarufu emene tinotoonera nekubatira pamwepo ngekuti tine mazwisisiro ekuti denda rinothya kuwandirwa. Zviro zvinorema kuti veukama vakorere kuhanira zviitiko zvakadai. Hino dika tika remukuhlana unoronzwa uyu ratishatira.* (Since time immemorial the Ndau have shared closely knit kinship that spread over the Zimbabwean side of the border and beyond into Mozambique. Our social and religio-cultural ceremonies and other practices bring us together. Even cases of illness and deaths are events that bring out the best of our oneness as they bring us together because we believe that illnesses fear solidarity of purpose. It is very difficult for the kin to fail to attend such important occasions. Now the threat of coronavirus that is talked about has been a big problem for us).

The views of the respondent above confirm Patricio (2011), MacGonagle (2007) and Konyana's (2018) findings that the Ndau have for a long time maintained close links and are united in all spheres of social, economic and political life to the extent that they are identified as one large community that strides the international border. In short, the vast region is home to the Ndau. The lockdown regulations of staying home, self-isolating and social distancing have proved unworkable as they run against the self-consciousness of the Ndau. This is in line with Cotacachi and Grigera (2020) who aver that implementing isolation and social distancing protocols is challenging when community structures are intrinsically collective and strongly socially cohesive. Among the Ndau the elderly, the age group that is vulnerable to COVID-19, are the indispensable pillars of authority and heads of the extended families and therefore difficult to isolate even when the virus causes serious threats to their lives. The collective existence has also inspired returnees from epicentres of coronavirus to skip the quarantine camps and take refuge in the comfort of the family. There are numerous reasons for this practice, but the motivating factor behind the Ndau is the warm reception proffered by the family institution, the danger of spreading the disease not-withstanding. One respondent stressed that *veukama hwake vanomuika kuti asaenda kunoronzwayo kwavanofanira kungwarirwa* (relatives hide their kin so that they do not go to the places that they are supposed to be kept).

In cases of illness and death rituals such as *doro rekufa* ceremony (traditional beer to mourn the dead) and *tsvisa* (home bringing ceremony) that bring the members of the Ndau kinship web together, the respondents agree that the *nyanga* (traditional healer) plays a central role, to establish the cause of illness and to provide guidance on process of conducting the rituals, respectively. Besides, these ceremonies bringing a number of people together, the practices of the *nyanga* equally have high chances of exposing their consulting patients and themselves to the virus. Respondent 2 explains that:

> *Pakuhamba panobviswa songo remunoshuma ndiro mubati wemushando. Songo iri rinoashidzwa kuna nyamakumbi unozogumisa kuna chiremba. Chiremba ndiro raanoshuma ndiro kumagwasha anomuitira mushando. Pari pakutsvake chakarya munthu, wabatwa ngehakata unobatiswa mphete yakaotsirirwa ngetunzi kutenda ndaa. Hino mukuashidzana ashidzanamwo mukuhlana unopinda ndimwo.* (When consulting a traditional healer, a consulting team produces a token, that is, a gesture to officially announce their mission. The token follows protocols from the assistant of the healer to the traditional healer. The traditional healer uses the same token to communicate the presence and mission of the visitors to the spiritual powers that they use in their trade. In the case of finding a culprit over death, the guilt is obliged to accept responsibility by receiving a token possessed by the death-causing spirit. The method of transferring the spirit onto the token is through a breath or cough).

Dube (2006:142) observes almost the same divination procedure in the Setswana culture where,

> the diviner-healer begins by handing the divining set to the concerned person, to blow his or her breath on the set, and in so doing write his or her story on the set, which is then read communally by the diviner-healer, the consulting patient, and the accompanying relatives.

The divining set and the token money have the risk of transmitting the virus to the *nyanga* and its clients. According to WHO guidelines, the traditional healer is at risk of contracting and transmitting the virus. They should avoid prescribing any medicines and putting people and oneself at risk. This is echoed by a ZINATHA official who urged,

> Traditional healers and prophets to stop lying that they can cure coronavirus. Instead of exposing themselves while performing their prangs,

they should stay indoors and observe the 21 day nationwide lockdown decree, while praying to god and ancestors to help us discover a cure for this disease.

(Mafirakureva 2020)

These messages, noble as they are, run against the worldview of the Ndau where the traditional healer is the fulcrum of their indigenous health delivery system (Konyana 2018). Ironically, the same official confirms that, "traditional healers have herbs that can boost the immune system and we urge people to eat traditional foods, lots of fruits, and drink warm water..." (Mafirakureva 2020).

However, challenges notwithstanding, Ndau religio-cultural beliefs and practices possess rich sites for mobilising formidable responses to COVID-19 pandemic. As Chitando (2007a:50) observed, "African Traditional Religions swing into action whenever life-threatening forces besiege individuals, families or the community. They demonstrate a sense of urgency." The Ndau are not an exception. They are on record for their tact in transforming dehumanizing experiences into a community-serving heritage. Hlatywayo (2017) posits that the Ndau were successful in transforming the oppressive Nguni ear-piercing practice for men meant to express their subject status into a rite of passage for Ndau men. They also transformed the Nguni dance, *muchongoyo*, into their own cultural heritage. The Ndau invoke their spiritual capital enshrined in their notion of collective existence that provides a framework for solidarity and active compassion. Respondent 2 holds that there is nothing new about most WHO guidelines. For example, with regard to social or physical distancing, they had this to say:

*VaNdau avazi kumbovheya vashandisa njira yekuchingamidzana veiqhebu-rana nyara kana kukwambatirana. Zvakazouya kubudikidza ngechikora. Vanthu veichingamidzana veukama zviya vanonga vakataraukirana, um-weni akaqochocha iyo umweni apo. Vaisa ndivo vanoqochocha madzimai anogwadama kana kuita chibondokoto. Pari pokuti vanthu vasangana panjira vanotherukirana, votekesana, vaisa veichaya paditi ngenyara. Madzimai anoembera asi veichingamidza vaisa vanonga veidzasa madhoyo nekuembera. Kazhinjitu amutoningirani muhope.* (The Ndau have never used handshakes and hugs in their greeting protocols. All this came with the school system. When relatives are exchanging greetings, men squat and women touch the ground with their folded knees, allowing a respectable space between them. If people meet along the path, they both step aside on either side of the path and exchange greetings. In a man to man greetings, either man beat their chests with their right hand in rhythmic manner as they exchange greetings. In a man to woman situation, the man claps their hands while women cross their cupped palms as they clap in rhythmic manner lowering their knees in the process. Usually, the interactants avoid looking into each other's face).

MacGonagle (2007:56) concurs when she maintains that each clan had its own particular greeting that involved a customary clapping of hands and these salutations have changed little over time. When men clap they place their palms together so that their fingers are in front. Women cross their palms as they clap...While speaking to the king, they clapped their hands, in the customary manner of greeting...Rather than clapping, in some areas today women perform a courteous lowering of their body when they encounter men." According to the respondent, it is worth noting that offering a handshake to a chief, whether at a ritual occasion or just ordinary social life, is punishable by a fine. It is believed to be undermining the authority of the chief.

One respondent explained the avoidance of handshakes in a separate cultural setting of Ndau funeral wakes. They say that:

*Mukugara kwevaNdau, parufu apasaibatanwa mazicho. Zviro zvaitoita chihlamariso pakutanga zveitobva ngekune imweni mihlobo. Vaiuya kookhuza vaitoguma veichaya chiriro, vari pamuzi patamikiwa paya vodairawo chiriro chiya. Vanokhuza ava vaichigara pashi vakati taraukei kwaakuchibvunza mahambire ezvakaita. Vana vadoko nevabva zero avasaikwedera padhuze, vaitozwi vaende kumizi yehama dziri padhuze kusina rufu. Vasharuka ndivo vainingirana nezveshe zvinoitikapo. Zvinonga zvaiitirwa kuti vana vadoko vasaziya kufa kwemunthu.* (In the Ndau culture, handshakes were unknown at funerals. This was a surprising practice at first coming from other ethnic groups. Members of the community who came to express their condolences were often led by women wailing at the top of their voices, which was reciprocated by the bereaved at the homestead. Instead of offering handshakes, they would sit down apart, express their heartfelt condolences for the loss and finally, made an inquiry into the cause of the death. Children, including adolescents were not welcome at a funeral. Those from the bereaved family would be sent to homes of relatives in the neighbourhood away from death. Adults would handle everything that was involved. I think it was done to avoid exposing children to death and dying).

The Ndau customary greetings and conduct at funerals imply that implementing social distancing through avoidance of handshake and hugs in line with the COVID-19 preventive measures, is never a problem. In fact, it is a revival of their culture and its elevation to an international scene. To the Ndau, some of the WHO and health experts' recommended methods of greetings such as using the elbow or feet are cumbersome compared to their cultural way that had for long maintained avoidance of contact. Again, the call to limit numbers at funerals dovetails with the indigenous Ndau conduct of funeral. The Ndau customary greetings and funeral protocols are cultural resources that can be exploited to reinforce responses to the COVID-19 pandemic. Thus, I agree with Cotacachi and Grigera (2020) who hold, "that COVID-19 disproportionately affects indigenous peoples. This presents a major health challenge requiring immediate responses that account for indigenous peoples' diverse cultural and linguistic contexts." Once the health guidelines are repackaged in local cultural resources, indigenous communities are bound to find them convenient to their health and well-being.

Self-isolation and quarantine among the Ndau are not a new phenomenon. Respondent 3 says:

> *Kune matenda anoti wamarwara unotogariswa mumbatso mwako wega. Kana zvoonyanyisa zviya mutenda unoakirwa kamuchacha kake ega ngekubanze kwechianze. Zvakaita biriripiri, mai vemwana ndivo vega vanotenderwa kumuona nekumupa chikafu ngekuti rinoera. Rikadarikirwa mwanawo unofa. Mai nababa vanotoenda pachizilo munguwa yakonayo. Kwozotiwo reshe dendanje, kana ratora nguwa yakareba zvisisna shwiro, mutenda unobekwa mumuchacha kubanze kwemuzi kwakasitika zvekuti kuvazhinji kunonga kweizwi wakambohamba. Asi panonga pane nyanga nevashomani veukama vasingafungidzirwi uroyi, vanonga veimuhloya nekuona kuti wakangwaririka.* (There are some diseases that cause the ·patient to be quarantined to their own house. When the situation deteriorates, the patient is moved to a makeshift shelter often constructed at the margins of the homestead. For example, measles, the mother of the patient is the only person allowed to nurse them because there are a number of taboos involved. If the patient is exposed to the general public they are bound to die. Parents of the patient suspend sexual intercourse for that period for it has adverse effect on the patient. Generally, any prolonged illness warrants isolation from the public. The public is told that the person had gone on a journey. A traditional healer and a few selected elderly members of the family who are not suspected of witchcraft, monitor the proceedings to ensure uninterrupted care).

Konyana (2014) concurs when he points out that,

> the *nyanga* consulted before and during the construction of the *muchacha* becomes the administrator of the ill person's delicate welfare. They advise the council of family elders on how to prepare the patient's food while they are solely responsible for the preparation of the daily doses of traditional medicines. At the *muchacha* visitors are strictly vetted and approved by the *nyanga*.

The Ndau quarantine system utilizes their spiritual capital that inspires the social and cultural structures of the family that do not remove the patient from the company and love of the family. Çarkoğlu (2008) posits that spiritual capital is a bridging resource between groups or individuals that inspires people to act to help others beyond their immediate comfort zone.

In Zimbabwe, quarantine centres for COVID-19 patients have been criticised for a number of reasons including overcrowding, lack of food and lack of constant monitoring from health personnel to the extent that the critics have dubbed them incubatory sites for the disease (Frey 2020). Integrating indigenous quarantine systems into the health care delivery system holds a potential for improved responses to the COVID-19 pandemic.

Responding to the question on the competence of traditional healers in dealing with coronavirus, respondent 1 maintains that:

> *Kune matenda akawanda angahluya nyanga, asi azvironzi kuti apana nachimwe chevanokona kuita ndiwo matendawo. Kubvira kudhaya nyanga ndidzo dzaidetsera vanthu pamahlupeko anochekuita nezvehlonzi yevanthu. Ukazwa zvinobhuyiwa ngedenda remukuhlana riri zvakada kutodzana nemaitiro eamweni matenda akadai ngekukotsora, chifuwa nekuzarirwa. Zveshe zvitenda izvi nyanga dzinodetsera. Kunyari nechemazuwa ano chiya anditi dzine madetserero adzo anonyaradza kupanda kwemwiri.* (There are so many types of diseases that may challenge the competence of traditional healers, but that does not mean that they cannot do anything about them. Since time immemorial, traditional healers have rendered services for any health challenges. If you listen to what is said about coronavirus, it has symptoms that are almost similar to other types of diseases such as flu, chest pains and asthma. A traditional healer assists in all these types of diseases. Even with HIV and AIDS traditional healers have fared well in providing palliative herbal concoctions).

The sentiments of the respondent means that traditional healers have the confidence of indigenous communities in matters of health. This means that they are an indispensable constituency that has to be included in any efforts that are meant to come up with preventive and containment strategies for any health crisis. It is for this reason that there are calls for a multi-sectorial approach to coronavirus that involves biomedical practitioners, public health practitioners and traditional healers. This is a practical approach that takes cognisance of the indigenous communities' worldviews that prioritize their traditional pharmacology for any ailment. What is pertinent at the moment is not to discourage traditional healers, but to roll out programmes that educate them on the best practices that are COVID-19 compliant when conducting their business just like what was done in Zimbabwe with HIV and AIDS.

Besides dealing with direct effects of COVID-19, Ndau spiritual capital addresses indirect challenges that have a lasting effect on efforts to contain the health crisis. For instance, the threat of coronavirus comes fast on the heels of the devastating trails of cyclone Idai in early 2019. The natural disaster has had adverse effects on the Ndau communities' yields thereby compromising to some extent, the Ndau responses to food insecurity. The

COVID-19 pandemic takes advantage of such compromised socio-economic safety nets. However, the spiritual capital of the Ndau that informs their collective existence provides a framework for solidarity and active compassion that abhors indifference to the challenges of fellow human beings. Behaving otherwise, ultimately denies one's own humanity. A lot of sharing of food stuffs and ideas on dealing with respiratory diseases is common as families show great determination to pull through in the likelihood of an outbreak. The Ndau collective existence inspires compassion that invariably "translates into activism for the human rights of the infected and the affected" (I am indebted to Chitando (2007a:60) for the phrase).

Muyambo (2018:108) maintains that chiefs, as traditional leaders in Ndau communities are the custodians of the communities' culture and includes the values, beliefs, practices and norms of the community. In times of social stresses that overwhelm the family institution, the Ndau stick hopes on the judgement of their leaders and established safety nets designed to deal with disasters and stress (MacGonagle 2007:53, 67). The pivotal role of the traditional leaders that include the chiefs, headmen and village heads is crucial in managing stressful social stresses as they become a rallying point for order and common good in the community. The Ndau are not comfortable with abandoning their ritual practices for fear of offending the spirit elders be it at family or community level. Traditional leaders also help disseminate and oversee the implementation of government policies on health in their areas of jurisdiction. The chiefs' pronouncement is not resisted because they are believed to speak on behalf of the territorial spirits; spirits of the deceased tribal rulers mostly from the lineage of the chiefs in a particular village (Hlatywayo 2017). Respondent 2 describes how their community once conducted a ritual of *kusuka mapadza* (washing hoes) guided by WHO COVID-19 guidelines. *Kusuka mapedza* is a ritual that is conducted to break the mourning period following the death of a member of the family of the tribal rulers:

> *Takaenda kwamambo tiri muzvigaba zviiri zvevanthu vasikadariki ma-kumi marongomuna takasunga miromo chero ngechawaonawo zvako chinoita inyari mitsoto. Munthu weshe wakageza nyara pachigubhu giya ngesipo. Mutape vakazotanga ngekuchumaira ngendaa yedenda remuku-hlana ririyo veibhuya ngenjira dzekuri vhikeya. Zvigaba zviiri zvaiyapo zvakachizoita majana ekupinda mumunda. Kwaichizwi muchigabamwo, umwe naumwe waipuwa kandima kekushanda kasakanyauranje takata-ranuka. Chigaba chekutanga chapedza chotobuda chogeza nyara kwaa-kutoqonde kanyi. Chimweni chopindawo.* (We went to the chief's home in two small groups of people not exceeding forty when combined wearing face masks of any kind even rags. Everyone washed their hands with soap and running water from a chigubhu-giya (a leg-operated system involving a five-litre container of water balancing on a rake).The traditional leader then addressed people about COVID-19 explaining

recommended ways of preventing infection. The two groups then took turns to go into the field where each one was allocated a small portion to work on respecting social distance at all times. When the first group was done, they washed their hands once again and left for home. It was now time for the second group.

The narrative above shows that the Ndau ritual activities are not suspended in the context of COVID-19 but are performed following WHO and ministry of health's guidelines under the guidance of rituals leaders. It is important to note that in the case above, the chief's role is that of balancing the indigenous religious requirement and the modern health responses to a health crisis. The adopted *chigubhu-giya* system is a sustainable interventionist strategy meant to ensure that communities prioritise hand washing amidst the challenge of shortage of water in most rural communities. Hand washing with soap is the most effective and inexpensive way to prevent diarrhoea and acute respiratory infections. Dhoba (2016:4), claims that "turning hand washing with soap at all critical times into an ingrained habit saves more lives than any single vaccine or medical intervention." Many Ndau households have installed the *chigubhu-giya* system at their homes following the embracing of the system by village health workers and traditional leadership. Those who cannot afford soap have turned to *mutombera* (fermented by-product from soaked grain) and ash. One interviewee contends that *mutombera* is an effective indigenous alternative to any commercial detergents. As said before, the chief commands the respect and confidence of their people. In this regard, traditional leaders are a deserving constituency in virus prevention and containment measures programmes in indigenous communities. They ensure the embrace of existing preventive measures as well as new indigenous initiatives. Cotacachi and Grigera (2020) could not have said it better when they opine that, "indigenous organisations and traditional indigenous authorities have representative structures at the national, subnational, and community levels each of which plays a vital role in virus prevention and containment measures."

## Conclusion

In this chapter, I have shown, through the case of the Ndau people, how indigenous peoples' belief systems are both a source of their resilience and can also pose a threat in preventing and containing COVID-19 pandemic. This resonates well with the findings of Miller *et al.* (2020:1) that the impact of the disease is different in different countries. They attribute these differences to a number of factors including differences in cultural norms. It is pertinent that any declaration of war on a pandemic should take stock of local cultural resources with a view to appropriating those that can reinforce responses to the challenge and transforming the negative ones. It has also been observed that the Ndau have a penchant of reviewing their cultural resources with a view to making them relevant to their immediate existential concerns. The Ndau notion of communal or collective existence anchored on their spiritual capital that finds expression in the institution of the extended family, has for generations proved to be an invaluable resource for building resilience in dealing with social crises or stresses. As Haynes (2007) opines, spiritual capital concretizes a family-like atmosphere that provides spiritual strength and bonding that generates social capital. The Ndau indigenous spiritual capital allays fears as well as stigma, discrimination and stereotyping of the people infected and affected by any disease, coronavirus included. Taking a cue from the Ndau communal existence, there is need to reimagine the notion of communities that respect and empower all their members to focus on community-serving behaviours as opposed to the prioritization of individual whims. It is true that the coronavirus pandemic has taken religions by surprise, but it is equally true that it has availed an opportunity for indigenous religio-cultures to retrieve the best of their practices in seeking to prevent and contain the pandemic in partnership with medical and public health practitioners.

## References

Beach, D.N. 1980. *The Shona and Zimbabwe, 900–1850: An Outline of Shona History*. Gweru: Mambo Press.

Çarkoğlu, A. 2008. Social vs. spiritual capital in explaining philanthropic giving in a Muslim setting: The case of Turkey. In Day, Abby (ed.). *Religion and the Individual: Belief, Practice, Identity. Theology and Religion in Interdisciplinary Perspective*. London: Ashgate, pp. 111–126.

Chitando, E. 2007a. *Living with Hope: African Churches and HIV/AIDS 1*. Geneva: WCC Publications.

Chitando, E., Mapuranga, T.P. & Taringa, N.T. 2014. On top of which mountain does one stand to judge religion? Debates from a Zimbabwean context. *Journal for the Study of Religion* 27, 2, 115–136.

Constitution of Zimbabwe (amendment number 20). (2013). Harare: Government Printers.

Cotacachi, D. & Grigera, A. 2020. The 2020 Pandemic: The need for urgent, culturally appropriate responses for indigenous peoples. https://blogs.iadb.org/igualdad/en/covid-19-response-for-indigenous-peoples/. (Date Accessed: 16 June 2021)

Cox, J.L. 2007. *From Primitive to Indigenous: The Academic Study of Indigenous Religions*. Aldershot: Ashgate.

Dhoba, L. 2016. Mubaira Growth Point, a Place to be on the 25th of November 2016, *WASH Connector Newsletter*, October 2016, Issue 4.

Dube, E.E.N. 2017. *Getting married twice: the relationship between indigenous and Christian marriages among the Ndau of the Chimanimani area of Zimbabwe*, University of South Africa, Pretoria, http://hdl.handle.net/10500/23809. (Date Accessed: 5 March 2020)

Dube, M.W. 2009. 'I Am Because We Are': Giving Primacy to African Indigenous Values in HIV & AIDS Prevention. In M. F. Murove (ed.). *African Ethics: An Ontology of Comparative and Applied Ethics*. Durban: University of KwaZulu Natal Press, pp. 188–219.

Dube, M.W. 2003. Culture, gender and HIV and AIDS: Understanding and acting on the issues. In M.W. Dube (ed.). *HIV/AIDS and the Curriculum: Methods of Integrating HIV/AIDS in Theological Programmes*. Geneva: WCC Publications.

Dube, M.W. 2006. Adinkra! four hearts joined together: On becoming healing-teachers of Africa indigenous religion/s in HIV & AIDS prevention. In I.A. Phiri & S. Nadar (eds.). *African Women, Religion and Health: Essays in Honour of Mercy Amba Ewudziwa Oduyoye*. Maryknoll, NY: Orbis Books, pp. 131–156.

Frey, A. 2020. Quarantine Centres spreading COVID-19 in Zim. https://clubofmozambique.com/news/quarantine-centres-spreading-covid-19-in-zim-162465/

Ganiel, G. 2009. Spiritual capital and democratisation in Zimbabwe: A case study of a progressive charismatic congregation. *Democratization*, 16(6): 1172–1193.

Gelfand, M. 1973. *The Genuine Shona: Survival Values of an African Culture*. Gweru: Mambo Press.

Haynes, J. 2007. *Religion and Development: Conflict or Cooperation?* Basingstoke: Palgrave.

Hlatywayo, A. 2017. Indigenous knowledge, beliefs and practice on pregnancy and childbirth among the Ndau People of Zimbabwe. An unpublished DPhil Thesis submitted in the School of Religion, Philosophy and Classics (College of Humanities), UKZN.

Konyana. 2014. Euthanasia in Zimbabwe? Reflections on the management of terminally-ill persons and the dying in Ndau traditions of Chimanimani and Chipinge, South-East Zimbabwe. In D.O. Laguda (ed.). *Death and Life after Death in African Philosophy and Religion: A Multidisciplinary Engagement*. Harare: African Institute for Culture, Peace, Dialogue & Tolerance Studies, pp. 115–131.

Konyana, E. 2018. When culture and the law meet: An ethical analysis of the interplay between the Domestic Violence Act and the traditional beliefs and cultural practices of the Ndau people in Zimbabwe, DPhil Thesis submitted to the School Philosophy and Classics, UKZN.

MacGonagle, E. 2007. *Crafting Identity in Zimbabwe and Mozambique*. Rochester: University of Rochester Press.

Mack, N., Woodsong, C., MacQueen, K.M., Guest, G. & Namely, E. 2005. *Qualitative Research Methods: A Data Collector's Field Guide: Family Health International (FHI)*, USA.

Mafirakureva, G. 2020. Be wary of fake COVID-19 healers, *Southern Eye*, Friday 10 April 2020.

Mbiti, J.S. 1969. *African Religions and Philosophy*. Oxford: Heinemann.

Miller, A., Reandelar, M.J., Fasciglione, K., Roumenova, V., Li, Y. & Otazu, G.H. 2020. *Correlation between universal BCG vaccination policy and reduced morbidity and mortality for COVID-19: An epidemiological study*, CC-BY-ND 4.0 International License. https://doi.org/10.1101/2020.03.24.20042937

The Ministry of Health and Child Care, Zimbabwe. 2020. *Key Messages Brief on COVID-19*.

Murove, M.F. 2009. An African environmental ethic based on the concepts of *Ukama* and *Ubuntu*. In M.F. Murove (ed.). *African Ethics: An Ontology of Comparative and Applied Ethics*. Durban: University of KwaZulu Natal Press.

Muyambo, T. 2018. Indigenous Knowledge Systems of the Ndau People of Manicaland Province of Zimbabwe: A case study of *bota reshupa*. Unpublished Ph.D Thesis, School of Religion, Philosophy and Classics of the University of KwaZulu-Natal, South Africa.

Patricio, M. 2011. Ndau identity in Mozambique-Zimbabwe Borderland. *International Organization,* 43(94): 673–692.

Pfukwa, C. 2001. Unwritten ethics and moral values: The human face of Chimurenga II. In M.T. Vambe (ed.). *Orality and Cultural Identities in Zimbabwe.* Gweru: Mambo Press.

Putnam, R.D. 2000. *Bowling Alone: the Collapse and Revival of American Community.* New York: Simon and Shuster.

Rusinga, O. & Maposa, R.S. 2010. Traditional religion and natural resources: A reflection on the significance of indigenous knowledge systems on the utilisation of natural resources among the Ndau People in South-eastern Zimbabwe. *Journal of Ecology and the Natural Environment,* 2(9): 201–206.

Sipeyiye, M. 2020. Rethinking environmental sustainability through Ndau notion of communal existence. In N. Penxa-Matholeni, G.K. Boateng & M. Manyonganise (eds.). *Mother Earth, Mother Africa & African Indigenous Religions.* Stellenbosch: AFRICAN SUN MeDIA.

Sithole, E. 2018. Identity consciousness among the Ndau people in Zimbabwe: Unravelling mysteries, misconceptions and justifications, *African Identities,* DOI: 10.1080/14725843.2018.147314.

Taringa, N.T. 2014. *Towards and African-Christian environmental ethic.* Bamberg: University of Bamberg Press.

Thomas, E. Douglas. 2015. *African traditional religion in the modern world* (2nd ed.). Jefferson, NC: McFarland & Company, Inc, Publishers.

United Nations. 2020. The Impact of COVID-19 on Indigenous peoples, United Nations Department of Economic and Social Affairs policy Brief #70

WHO. 2020. COVID-19 for Religious leaders of Faith-based organisations and communities of faith https://www.who.int/publications-detail/practical -considerations-and- recommendations-for-religious-leaders-and- faith-based-communities-in-the-context-of-covid-19 (29 July 2020).

# 5 Living with COVID-19 in Zimbabwe

## A religious and scientific healing response

*Bernard Pindukai Humbe*

## Introduction

Over the past two decades, the world has been struck by serious health crisis. Of note is COVID-19 which was declared a public health concern by the World Health Organization on 11 March 2020. The global disease highlights the interplay between religion and science in a contemporary society. This chapter explores Zimbabwe's scientific and religious responses as explanatory models to the Coronavirus crisis. It must be emphasised from the onset that there are numerous diverse characterisations of the terms "religion and science". This chapter gives the intended meaning of these terms in Zimbabwe, without necessarily assuming all of the meanings and connotations that are attached to them outside the context of the discourse of COVID-19 pandemic. Science is a derivative word from the Latin *scientia*, which means knowledge. Bhagat (2018) posits that science is systematic knowledge based on facts, observations and experimentations. Science seems to provide the only reliable path to knowledge since many people view science as objective, universal, rational, and based on solid observational evidence (Barbour, 1968:3).

Scientific tactics to COVID-19 pandemic encompass an amalgamation of mutually experiential and interpretive fundamentals. The experiential element in COVID-19 discourse comprises observations and tests, while the interpretive component includes the concepts, laws, and theories, which constitutes the theoretical side of science (Barbour, 1966:138). A scientific procedure on COVID-19 research would start with observation of cases, from which tentative hypothesis would be formulated, whose implications would be tested experimentally. These experiments would lead to the construction of a more complete theory, which in turn would suggest new experiments resulting in modifications and extension of the theory, which may also suggest a paradigm shift.

As suggested by the topic of this chapter, I also looked at the response of religion to the Coronavirus crisis. Unlike science, a major obstacle to investigating the role of religion in COVID-19 management is its contentiousness though it is a critical existential phenomenon which is as old as

DOI: 10.4324/9781003241096-5

humanity itself. In view of the religious plurality in the world today, several approaches ranging from various disciplines such as theology, ethics, philosophy, sociology and psychology have been employed to define religion. However out of the numerous definitions proffered by scholars of religion, I affirm an operational definition which Young (2005:4) advances when he claims that 'Religion is human transformation in response to the perceived ultimacy'. Basing on three key terms in the definition, which are *human, transformation* and *ultimacy*, the following are some deductions that can be made:

First, **Religion** is a phenomenon that solidifies a human community. The indigenous Zimbabweans exist and behave as an existential community. Second, the concept **human** implies that in religion, the observer will find a particular understanding of what it means to be peculiarly human. So, one finds several essential characteristics of Zimbabwean personality. Third, the term, **transformation**, carries with it the dynamic inner quality of religion. Accordingly, this helps the researcher to understand that every facet of life among the indigenous Zimbabwean people is religious, be it in terms of their thoughts, feelings, interests, aspirations or actions. Therefore, the religious aspect of anything or something about the human life is only realised if there is transformation, that is, the integral change from one state to another. This religious transformation sets a target towards which the transformation is directed. This insight was clearly posited by Mbiti (1969:4) when he advanced the now classical niche that an African is 'notoriously religious'. Fourthly, in terms of the notion of **ultimacy**, the indigenous people perceive themselves to be at the centre of their lives which defines what holistic and wholistic life is all about in the Zimbabwean community. Now, in African indigenous cosmology, *Mwari* (God) and or *vadzimu* (ancestors) are regarded to be the *causal nexus* (centrality) of indigenous people and well-being in Zimbabwe (Maposa and Humbe, 2012).

Religion has the capacity to influence the way individual/groups conduct themselves, interact with others and interpret certain phenomena in this case COVID-19. By implication, religion can influence health and well-being of people. Characteristic features of religion are that it is subjective in its experiential component, emotional, and based on faith, traditions or authorities. This is the reason why in the modern world of biomedicine it is mistakenly understood as parochial.

In this study, focus is paid on two religious traditions namely Christianity and African Traditional Religion (ATR) which I take as religions of healing. At the most obvious level, the two provide adherents with a soteriological belief system, hope, protection and escape from sickness, misfortune, and death (Porterfield, 2005:vii). Christian religious tradition in Zimbabwe is expressed in so many ways through its varied denominations, sects and cults. The same is with African Traditional Religion, which has been understood to be diverse due to differences in language, cultural belief systems and practices in various regions. So collectively, this may justify the idea of having Christianities and African Traditional Religions respectively thriving on the Zimbabwean religious landscape. However, for convenience sake, I make reference to Christianity and African Traditional Religion in singular forms. Religiously, the indigenous people of Zimbabwe's response to COVID-19 is manifestly expressed through their beliefs, practices, ceremonies, rituals, festivals, symbols, objects, sacred places, morals, religious leaders and the revered practitioners (Mbiti (1969:4).

The chapter shows that in Zimbabwe, the pandemic has emerged at a time when life is unbearable due to political and socio-economic crises since the year 2000. It is against this backdrop that the coming of this pandemic to Zimbabwe provides the indigenous people an opportunity for human reflection on transcendent life since it is a challenge to science and human wisdom. The problem emanates from the nature of this disease, especially the obscurity of its origins, compounded by the fact that it is incurable. This study then explains why religious and scientific knowledge systems should coexist productively to tackle challenges such as the COVID-19 pandemic.

## Conceptual framework

Any academic discipline is characterised by its own methods, its own content and its own terminology. Conceptual discourse on COVID-19 places its emphasis on the irrefutable prevalence of the disease in Zimbabwe. To describe something in this manner is to say that there is very little or virtually nothing one can do about it in face of a gruesome phenomenon. More often than not, language on Coronavirus seems to be having a paralysing rather than an energizing effect on people. Among other concepts, the majority of Zimbabweans use 'pandemic'. There are other terms which are used in conjunction with pandemic like 'crisis, 'agonising', and 'devastating'. For a pandemic to occur, there must be an epidemic (Isiko, 2020:78). So, the following is a clarification of the concept epidemic which the study calls epidemiology.

## Epidemiological paradigm of COVID-19

Etymologically, the term, 'epidemiology' is derived from three Greek words: *epi* = 'upon', *demos* = people and *logos* = study of. Literally translated, the word epidemiology means the study of what is upon the people. Bartlett and Judge (1997:331) think that epidemiology is the study of disease in populations. The term is used to mean any disease that kills many people quickly in an unpleasant and arbitrary way regardless of age, gender, religion, race, nationality and/or health status of the victims (Isiko, 2020:78). Specifically, this study perceives epidemiology as denoting the prevalence and spread of the Coronavirus disease in the Zimbabwean population and the factors that influence or determine the spread of this disease. So, epidemiology is the study of health-event, health-characteristic, or health-determinant patterns within the Zimbabwean societies from a scientific and religio-cultural perspective. Having a good conceptualisation of the virus and the science of epidemics is handy in explicating the decisions that are being made by the government, public health officials and local scientists. There are three main concerns for medical and public health professionals: the uncertainty of the virus, the severity of infections and the rapidity of spread the virus. Though it is rendered to the periphery, in this study a religio-cultural epidemiological approach is the cornerstone methodology of COVID-19 public health research. It helps to articulate the relationship between science and religion regarding the mourning, grief and burial of COVID-19 related funerals.

## Pandemic

When an epidemic is experienced in several parts of the world at a given time, it is then categorised as a pandemic. Therefore, a pandemic is defined as an epidemic occurring worldwide, or over a very wide area, crossing international boundaries and usually affecting a large number of people (Isiko, 2020:78). By 11th March 2020, the World Health Organization (WHO) declared COVID-19 a pandemic because it had spread to over 110 countries and territories around the world. Whereas there exists numerous medical works on pandemics by the governments, Non-Governmental Organisations (NGOs) and scientists, composition of treatises about pandemics has, over the centuries, been a concern of religious scholars, interpreting the occurrence of diseases according to pious traditions, as well as guiding society on proper conduct during pandemics. The sudden occurrence of pandemics has often been traumatizing for societies all over the globe with the initial search for answers more often associated to religion (Isiko, 2020:78). It explains why in the Zimbabwean context, the ordinary people postulate COVID-19 as a mysterious disease which has caused serious suffering. The notion of pandemic in this study presents the cruel and tragic facet of COVID-19, a serious disease of which individuals suffer and die alone, a situation of intense distress.

## Methodology

This was a qualitative study that used phenomenology of religion. During the inquiry, procedures of *epoche*, empathetic interpolation and eidetic intuition were adopted to study varied symbolic expressions of that which people appropriately respond to as being of unrestricted value of them. Accordingly, the reality of COVID -19 could only be understood and made sense for by exploring indigenous Africans' lived experience of religion and the meaning that such people have attributed to it through their experience.

   A purposive sampling frame was used to select 15 key informants to serve a specific purpose of finding the scientific and religious response to the problem of COVID-19 in Zimbabwe. They were aged between 20 and 65. The study was carried out from March 2020 to February 2021.The participants were adequately informed about the research, comprehended the information and had the power and freedom of choice to allow them to decide whether to participate or decline Arifin (2018:30). Information from the participants was coaxed through observations (both participant and non-participant) and interviews. Due to lockdowns and quarantines, face-to face interviews were complimented by telephoning, messaging and WhatsApp voice notes. The key informants were identified considering their demographic characteristics (e.g., gender or age), sociocultural factors (e.g. religious affiliation, marital status, ethnicity, education, or area of residence) or occupation characteristics (e.g. religious experts, working, retired, or unemployed). What the participants had is what Bourdieu (1986:105) calls 'cultural competence' to understand the religious narrative of COVID–19 in Zimbabwe. Cultural competence included the 'forms of skill and knowledge which enabled participants to make sense' of the intersection between religion and health in their daily life. Anonymity and confidentiality were well-kept by not revealing names and the identities of participants in the data collection, analysis and reporting of the study findings. In addition to observations and interviews, I also did a review of secondary data which included media reports and online sources of information.

## Flattening the curve: mitigatory measures to harness COVID-19

In the context of this study, the scientific perspective is the one adopted by the Government of Zimbabwe. Since the inception of COVID-19 in Zimbabwe, the Government has demonstrated practically that when it comes to health matters especially health pandemics, the scientific route is the only recommended practice to harness the situation. The Government through the Ministry of Health and Child Care (MoHCC) has become the mouthpiece and implementer of WHO guidelines and measures on COVID-19. Dr Agnes Mahomva, who is the National COVID-19 Response Chief Coordinator, vehemently stated that the Government has played the essential role in leading and coordinating the national response by ensuring that scientific comprehensive measures are outlined and protocols are met in all sectors. So strong community ownership of the response was very critical, taking action without waiting to be caught by the Government, for example, by the police to enforce the set rules and measures. Sharing of fake and misleading messages and information by individuals and communities about COVID-19 pandemic that would jeopardise the Zimbabwean national response was discouraged. Some of the messages shared on social media had caused a lot suffering to the general populace. In addition, the Government maintained that surveillance and testing were key elements to the country's national response.

Though science had prescribed ways to flatten the curve, another dimension from some Christian circles emphasised introspection as the heart of survival from this pandemic. Some Christian adherents expounded that in the context of suffering brought by the COVID-19 pandemic, the Holy Spirit was "protecting" the holy ones. One participant bluntly declared that "introspection is a precondition for a religious healing of the coronavirus". In its foundational meaning, Christian healing is about repentance and forgiveness of sin. Linkages between repentance and healing to end suffering derive from Old Testament stories about the blessings of health, fertility, respect, and prosperity that accompanied God's forgiveness of Israel's sins after He called her to repent. God chastised Israel for her sins and turned her toward repentance with punishments of sickness, barrenness, disgrace, and misery. Thus, affirmation of a connection between sickness and sin lies at the root of Christian healing (Porterfield, 2005). In other instances, as reflected by Porterfield (2005), Christians discerned surrounding forces of evil and sin as causal agents of disease and suffering. The gospel writers understood the healings performed by Jesus along these lines, describing them as acts that defeated evil spirits (Porterfield, 2005). This might serve to imply that God is in control of the situation and ultimately, He is the solution to the pandemic if and only if people pray to Him.

The Government reiterated the importance of being guided by science in everything people do in their daily life as well as in treatment guidelines and protocols. For example, the need to follow science-based processes of introducing new medicine ensured that all patients were protected from unsafe practices. Strengthening of the national response to COVID-19 was done through deployment of vaccines. Vaccines are simply an additional prevention measure meant to compliment what the Government was already doing. Deployment of vaccines was done in line with WHO and African Union guidelines. Using the national vaccine framework, Health Care workers administered the vaccine working together with the Medicine Control Authority of Zimbabwe and local scientists throughout the deployment period and after the deployment. On 18 February 2021, General Retired Dr Constantino Chiwenga the Vice President and Minister of Health and Child Care became the first person to be inoculated with Sinopharm vaccine from China.

However, vaccination in Zimbabwe has been associated with confusing information such that the initial response was characterized by complacency in embracing the vaccination drive. Respondents admitted that they had accepted information which was propagated by some Church leaders who encouraged their members from taking the vaccines. On 19 January 2021, Ndoro reported in iHarare News that popular Zimbabwean prophet Emmanuel Makandiwa of the United Family International Church (UFIC) claimed that the DNA of Africans had also been tampered with for the search of the COVID-19 vaccine. Makandiwa's sentiments on COVID-19 vaccine were heavily criticised specially by those who embrace science as a response to the pandemic. The critics argued that due to his massive following, Makandiwa's words had the potential to undermine public health as his followers always take his words to be gospel. The Government also responded on the national broadcaster Zimbabwe Broadcasting Corporation (ZBC) by urging the public to ignore such conspiracy theories from religious leaders. Given this scenario, unpredictable and chaotic, atypical situations begin to proliferate, bringing along a sense of unreality in the face of an overwhelming experience in times of pandemic (Oliveira-Cardoso et al., 2020). The State's subsequent reaction to defiant religious leaders was a demonstration of its ultimate authority despite the legal guarantees to religious freedom and expression. The reality on the ground was that religious opinions on the pandemic were not only unwelcome but also posed a great danger to public health and, therefore, the need for religious restraint. So, the implication was that scientific knowledge, but not religious ideologies, was the key to combat the pandemic (Isiko, 2020). On 25 July, *The Herald* captured Makandiwa addressing his followers on a live broadcast Sunday, backtracking on the conspiracy theory of the vaccination drive urging his followers to get vaccinated (https://www.herald.co.zw).

## Conspiracy theory and COVID-19

The challenge with Zimbabwean bio-medical delivery system is that a significant percentage of frontline workers were found to have a poor attitude towards COVID-19 (Isiko, 2020:79). This is because of serious shortage of Personal Protective Equipment (PPE), unavailability of drugs in the hospitals, etc. On 25 March the Zimbabwean Nurses Association went on strike because of a lack of PPEs, unreliable water supplies and the need for a COVID-19 allowance. A healthy official reiterated that "the situation in the hospitals is pathetic, our own hospitals are now death traps". She went on to emphasise that when she tested positive, she refused to be admitted into a hospital. She argued that "it was rare for Coronavirus patients to come alive from hospital". From the responses she gave, it could be noted that some health officials had moral distress. According to Wallace (2020) moral distress is "the physical or emotional suffering that is experienced when constraints (internal or external) prevent one from following the course of action that one believes is right". Moral distress is a significant issue facing critical care providers in hospitals and is associated with burnout, where the health staff experience emotional exhaustion and depersonalization, or even dehumanization, of the patients in their care. Some participants allegedly claimed that when a COVID-19 patient is admitted, some health officials avoid the patient to limit risk of exposure. The pain endured by the patients and ultimately their deaths may cause grief for the health officials.

In addition, lack of scientific research carried out in Zimbabwe on COVID-19 has exacerbated intensified establishment of fear in Zimbabwe. The national broadcaster, ZBC Television, reported in the first week of February 2021 that the Government was yet to start working on COVID-19 research. This means that since the emergence of the pandemic what the

Government was regarding as official information on COVID-19 was imported from other countries especially South Africa. Two possible threats were feared: loss of a family member and loss of a sense of control over events, triggering experiences of helplessness (Oliveira-Cardoso et al., 2020).

## Importance of religious and cultural epidemiology

Knowing the importance of the spiritual component in health and well-being of indigenous Africans, an online publication (www.aa.com.tr) reported that the President of Zimbabwe, Emmerson Mnangagwa declared 15 June 2020 as Presidential Day of Prayer and Fasting to seek divine intervention in tackling the Coronavirus outbreak. He urged Zimbabweans to come together, pray, fast and continue to observe precautions necessary to prevent the virus spread. The Head of State urged Zimbabweans to join him for a virtual Church service from 10am to 12pm local time which was broadcast live on ZBC and other social media platforms. In January 2021, The First Lady Amai Auxillia Mnangagwa called women of Zimbabwe to join a ten-day series of prayer and fasting to seek for divine intervention in face of the deadly pandemic scourging, a request which was welcomed by most churches. She also has implored the nation to join her in seven days of prayer and fasting from 28 June to July 4 to pray for Zimbabwe in the face of a spike in COVID-19 cases and other ailments. Some interviewees criticised these prayer calls from the First Family arguing that it was a sign of desperation after having noted that scientific approach locally is struggling and unconvincing to a highly Zimbabwean distressed and suffering populace. A certain respondent maintained that there is no need to panic and portray a discorded policy framework in the Government's fight against COVID-19. The leaders should stick to science. Differing from the above views, one pastor thought that there was nothing wrong in calling for national prayers to contain COVID-19. He argued that what the President and the First Lady had done demonstrates that the country's leadership is using a multi-pronged approach to quell this calamity. However, it should be noted that Zimbabwe houses various religious traditions. So, the multi-pronged approach should reflect inclusivity in religious recognition as a response tool to COVID-19 pandemic. This reignites the long-standing debate whether Zimbabwe is a Christian state or not, a view which is dislodged by the provisions of the country's constitution. Mentioning only Christianity on the part of spiritual interposition is connoted bearing in mind that it is a religious tradition with origins from the West. At national and international levels, maybe, it was a shrewd move to appease the Western world which has been the author of western science being subscribed to by the Government to combat COVID-19.

The Church in Zimbabwe has been proactive to end suffering through instigation of prayers. One cleric cited the Zimbabwe Catholic Bishops' Conference which has been supportive of national prayers, viewing the disruptions occasioned by coronavirus as a novel way for the church in the country to rediscover itself. He said the Church was encouraging congregants to pray for each other as families in both sickness and death. Another participant pointed out that the Roman Catholic Diocese of Masvingo did Novena Prayers asking God through the intercession of various saints to have the pandemic come to an end. Catholics were also encouraged to donate PPEs, sanitizers, soap, buckets to be given to the poor and disabled. Prayers for healing of COVID-19 patients helped in relief of suffering and enhanced ability to cope with coronavirus ailments. For example, part of Christianity's appeal as a means of coping with suffering is the idea that suffering is not meaningless but part of a cosmic vision of redemption (Porterfield, 2005).

The above approach was also associated with African Traditional Religion as adherents seek for a religious response to end suffering caused by COVID-19. They highlighted that there is an affirmation of the existence of Mwari (Shona Supreme God) in the religion's approach to harness the pandemic. The designations *Mwari* (God), *Musikavanhu* (Creator of people), *Samasimba* (The Omnipotent one) among others are replete with meanings, showing what the indigenous Shona people think of Him including health matters. Between *Mwari* and humanity are ancestral spirits who serve as conveyor belts. The Ancestors are the founders of the "Shona community". Chavhunduka (2001:4) argues that ancestors occupy a central position in our African religion largely because of their ownership of land and to their relationship to God. They are referred to as *varipasi* (those below) and dwell in a spirit world called *nyikadzimu*. They are guardian spirits who are influential in people's lives (Bourdillon, 1976:263). The Shona people are in the presence of their ancestral spirits wherever they are and whatever they do. The sacred practitioners interviewed clarified how suffering caused by COVID-19 is understood in indigenous communities through aphorisms like *vadzimutiringe,* (ancestors take care of us) *vadzimu vatirasa* (ancestors have forsaken us) and *vadzimu vadambura mbereko* (ancestors have broken their back sling). These maxims serve to confirm the gravity of suffering being experienced by the indigenous of Zimbabwe. The ancestral spirits perform various positive roles provided the living relatives honour them regularly through libations. Some of their functions are; protection of their progenies from danger, misfortunes, natural disasters and deadly diseases pandemic.

Through interviews and observations in rural areas, the study discovered that in exploring the ATR's response to COVID-19 pandemic, rituals for the Shona begin, control and end all the affairs of life suffering. Using Idowu's view of categorization of rituals, they were typical of preventive rituals (Idowu, 1994:125). The COVID-19 preventive rituals in the rural communities are either public or private. They are often a precautionary measure to ward off evil or misfortunes which cause suffering. So, supplications and incantations are continuously done especially at family level seeking for ancestral protection from the scourging disease.

On healing of COVID-19 related symptoms to alleviate the pain endured by victims and caregivers, traditional healers pointed out that ATR was very pragmatic in its approach when dealing with disease pandemics. They cited traditional herbs like Zumbani (*Lippia javanica*), Mufandichimuka (*Myrothamnus flabellifolius*), Chifumuro (*Dicoma anomala*), Rimiremombe (*Sonchus oleraceus*), among other herbs as being very effective when used to manage the coronavirus. This is in agreement with what Tribert Chishanyu (online) said:

> Traditional medicine practice is older... than science and it is accepted by the majority of Zimbabweans," he said. "If modern scientists are given opportunities to try whenever there is an emergency disease (outbreak), why can't we do the same to traditional medicine practice? We are treating symptoms related to COVID-19, so by (some) chance we may be able to treat COVID-19 (https://www.voanews.com/science-health/coronavirus-outbreak/zimbabwes-government-says-herbal-treatment-ok-covid-19).

During the study it was observed that the majority of Zimbabweans both in the rural and urban areas are using traditional home remedies to treat symptoms of COVID-19. They used the traditional methods like *kufukira* (steaming) which involved inhaling steam covered with a blanket. Before the emergence of coronavirus, ATR has been always prescribing *kufukira* to exorcise evil spirits and to cure respiratory diseases. One participant had this to say: "Since I used traditional and the so-called conventional medicine prescribed by medical doctors, I wonder if what I did constitutes a syncretic approach, *ndainatira nekunamata* (I steamed and prayed)". Although no confirmed medical assurance has been issued by government medical experts, most Zimbabweans used a traditional herb called *Zumbani* as medicine to treat COVID-19 symptoms. Some respondents thought that it is important for Zimbabweans to thank ancestors for providing desperate citizens with *Zumbani* which has saved lives of millions in this pandemic. Ndoro (2021) argues that what makes this herb unique is that since immemorial past it has been understood to have some mystic powers. Because of its spiritual properties it is used in pre-burial, burial and post burial rites. It is a ritualistic plant which wards off keep evil spirits. In contemporary Zimbabwe, people showing signs of mental disorder, madness, or hysterical outbursts are required by traditional healers to wash their bodies with leaf infusions.

According to Ncube (2021), in a press statement, Health and Child Care Minister, Vice President Constantino Chiwenga commented on the use of *Zumbani* to treat COVID-19, saying:

> Some Traditional Doctors were said to be claiming that their patients recovered after administering herbs. Yes, it is possible that some

traditional medicines can be used to treat COVID-19. However, there is a need for scientific researches to be done to ascertain their efficacy. The Ministry of Health and Child Care actually operationalized the Traditional Medicines Department, which is pre-occupied with research in this area (https://iharare.com/vice-president-chiwenga-speaks-on-the-use-of-zumbani-and-moringa-to-treat-covid-19).

It is important to note that taking time to finalize researches on the efficacy of some of the traditional herbs in managing the coronavirus is fuelling suffering in Zimbabwe for its health delivery system has collapsed.

## Dying, death and burial of COVID-19 victims

Coronavirus disease has severely affected death and burial rites. During lockdowns, the government banned citizens to gather for funerals only allowing a limited number of not more than 30 people as a way of reducing transmission. In January 2021 the government also put restrictions on movement of COVID-19 related deaths, saying police would only clear body movements for burial straight from a funeral parlour/hospital mortuary to the burial site. Breaking these stipulated injunctions have resulted in those who subscribe to scientific interventions in curbing COVID-19 to reason that traditional ways of handling funerals have become super spreaders of the virus. On 2 July, *The Herald* reported that eight people died after attending a COVID-19 death funeral. Mourners had converged at the deceased's homestead in their numbers. Traditional mourning practices included close contact with the deceased's body including folding, bathing and viewing. This meant that there was a prolonged period of contact of mourners with the corpse. These attendees could then establish new chains of transmission, leading to an unchecked transmission of the virus Rammohan et al. (2012:1).

In most cases, during bereavements, the funeral wake, it was observed that the homes were never disinfected, no practice of social distancing, no sanitization, no masking up of faces, people hand shaking, hugging and body viewing. In line of this situation, Sachiti (2021) in *The Herald*, cited the Community Working Group on Health Executive Director Mr Itai Rusike suggesting that

> family members, relatives and friends should consider other options to mourn and pay their respects to the departed instead of physically attending the funeral, avoid touching of hands and embracing as a way of consoling the mourners. They should keep their masks on when singing or dancing at the funerals.

Confronted by this unprecedented situation, some participants suggested use of information technology in attending funeral sessions. A certain COVID-19 survivor had this to say:

without a proper plan of action, I still think use of information technology for funeral is a good option. Better to err on caution than risk lives in the name of gatherings for funeral service. But as a survivor, the risk is not worth it.

However, the majority of Zimbabweans do not have information technology gadgets and those who own them cannot afford high speed bundles for Internet. Failure of observing the traditional death and burial rites has contributed to disenfranchised grief. It occurs when families are unable to grieve in traditional practices of funeral services or being unable to attend a loved one's burial (Wallace, 2020). For the Shona people of Zimbabwe, funeral gatherings are meant to show one's sense of belongingness.

Misery in communities which have COVID-19 deaths has been nursed by stigmatization. Response from a woman who attended a funeral of a relative who died of COVID-19 opined that after the funeral, she experienced stigmatization though she had tested negative. The pathogen's invisibility and dangerousness are two additives that enhance persecutory anxiety (Oliveira-Cardoso et al., 2020).Thus according Oliveira-Cardoso et al. (2020) the mourner ceases to be an object perceived as vulnerable, someone who needs support and protection and becomes stigmatized as a potential vector of transmission, a threatening and persecutory object, which further amplifies feelings of loneliness and discouragement.

**Psycho-social support in religious healing: family power**

The lockdown restrictions have rendered people to be intensely affected by grief. The African person is defined as a member of a family, and so is never alone either in self-concept or in the perception of others. The life of a person is wholly dependent on the family and its symbiotic functions of biological lineage, communal nurture, and moral formation (Paris, 1995:101). A COVID-19 survivor, emotionally charged saying "When I was quarantined, I felt lonely, disconnected and isolated from my family and friends" Most of the people in Zimbabwe like elsewhere in the world, are suffering from an ambiguous grief. This is because the COVID-19 deaths occur without the opportunity to say good-bye, engage in traditional rituals and obtain closure, making unresolved feelings commonplace. The rapidness of dying, death and burial changes since the emergence of this pandemic has caused many people to be left with a real sense of unease.

A certain man narrated that when he fell sick his COVID tests were positive. His wife was the caregiver but a few days after his recovery the wife succumbed to COVID-19. So he was feeling guilty blaming himself that he had caused the death of his wife. This is supported by Wallace (2020) who thinks that when an individual has not followed the social or mandated "rules" to limit exposure and becomes infected or spreads illness to others, feelings of blame, anger, and sadness, among others, will be entwined with their experience of losing their family members (Wallace, 2020). The respondent said the Church was giving him comfort in the notion that there may be a greater purpose in the loss of his loved wife.

## Unification of a divided people

With the arrival of coronavirus, religion has been associated with the construction and maintenance of social peace. At the core of their social practice, believers have built families out of strangers, and the extraordinary success of religion in human affairs can be attributed, in part, to this social feat. Believers understood the formation of close communities as manifestations of the Divine power. This has become handy in coping up with the adverse effects of the pandemic especially accepting the reality of death of a family member and processing the pain of grief.

When looking at the response of religion in managing COVID-19 pandemic in Zimbabwe, one is not compelled to pay too much attention to religious membership as an indicator of religion. What is on the ground is existence of home religion where people have just become independent religious people. The idea of independence comes to exonerate the person from being involved in various religious expectations. For example, in some instances, Christians were involved in steaming with *Zumbani*, sniffing snuff, sprinkling snuff, libations, while traditionalists would also listen to Biblical verses cited on coming to end of the world. Mostly all these ritualistic practices were done at home. The home has become the sacred place for unchurched believers. In most cases, women operate as home frontline workers in taking care of the COVID-19 patients hence they have endured more suffering compared to other members of the family.

## Final reflections of the study

Findings of this study opened up new ways of thinking about indigenous people's response to a pandemic like COVID-19 in terms of religious experience and practice. Basically, the study showed how competing regimes of knowledge in Zimbabwe were unveiled and how a combination of these is used in the discourse of coronavirus (Botha, 2008:153). This is viewed side by side with scientific approach which provides healing as a biological process thereby leading to better comprehension of how religious experience and practice can stimulate bodily strength and vitality. Using religion as a coping strategy appeals to the brain of the affected people. Relief from stress can affect all of the systems and functions of the body, from heart rate, blood pressure, digestion, and immunity to improvements in the exercise of thought, speech, and memory.

The two religious traditions used in this study equipped people with skills to offer psycho-social support when dealing with daily coronavirus-related challenges and other mundane concerns. The coronavirus crisis made many people believe that to be a health worker means to receive a divine calling to help people whose life is threatened by COVID-19. The study also noted that women were the most vulnerable people in COVID-19 era. The role they played in caring for the sick exposed them to COVID-19 hence they fulfilled a divine mission of *musha mukadzi* (a woman is the pillar of an indigenous home).

Because of coronavirus, the following is generally what the participants agreed to be severely affecting dying, death and burial rites:

- Those in quarantine die alone without the company of relatives
- No relatives to perform folding rites
- No relatives to perform bathing rites
- No hand shaking and embracing
- No body viewing
- Sometimes interment of the deceased is done by strangers.
- In some cases the deceased are buried on alien lands without the presence of their relatives.

On death and burial practices, one participant clarified saying African traditional practices overshadow Christianity. She emphasised even in Christian circles, there is no Christian burial but African burial of a Christian. However, COVID-19 has contributed towards omission of some of the important rites during burial procedures. Instead of using sayings such as *tamuradzika* (we have laid her/him, and *tamuchengeta* (we have kept he/her) participants have resorted to the aphorism *tamurasha* (we have disposed her/him. In this context, the process of burial does not become the means of ensuring a smooth transition from the living membership of the family to a membership as an ancestral spirit (Humbe, 2020). The failure to perform the prescribed dying, death and burial rituals makes the living relatives to suffer from serious grief. Participants were in agreement that science does not address the emotional effects that COVID-19 impacts on the victims and those who live in fear of contracting it. On this note some respondents admitted that they appeal to religion during these convalescing moments of grief.

Synecdochisation played an important role in the characterisation of religious healing for COVID-19 in Zimbabwe. Through synecdochisation, only a particular aspect was generalised to be the essence of managing COVID-19. For example, mostly the healing aspect at national level was administered with the use of science only. This was predominantly propagated by modernised people in their interpretation of religious and cultural healing practices in Zimbabwe as retrogressive especially in a pandemic situation. That characterisation was proliferated in print and electronic media for public consumption. This resulted in an undervaluation of religion since the Government's COVID-19 response framework subscribed to a scientific approach. This undervaluation of religious congregations, reliance on faith healing and performance of rituals constituted the main strategy to morally justify condemnation of religious healing (Martí, 2015). There is no doubt that in the processes to understand the efficacy of science to fight against COVID-19, overvaluation also appears. For example, this is noted in the Government's position that it is guided by science in whatever it does. However, there are situations which need religion, especially in understanding the religio-cultural epidemiology of the indigenous people. Because of the undervaluation of religion and overvaluation of science, in a public forum, religion took a backstage in its response to COVID-19 pandemic. This is well expressed by Isiko (2020:93) in the following words "Religious institutions' attitude of passivity, inactivity, distance or mute indifference in the face of such a monumental catastrophe was driven by thinking that it was an absolute responsibility of the state".

## Conclusion

There are several approaches used to deal with a health pandemic. This study detected two which are: public health approach and individual health approach. The government of Zimbabwe is using the public health approach which mainly subscribes to science. High state intervention also signifies a political response to the pandemic. But the majority of Zimbabweans have resorted to use the individual approach using home-made remedies to alleviate COVID-19 symptoms. This one has been widely embraced because it takes cognisance of one's religio-cultural values. However, the conflicting visions and interpretations of COVID-19 in Zimbabwe have created a certain ambiguity in the country's health sector, as well as in other aspects of national thought and life. In this COVID-19 era, interest in the salutary effects of religious belief and practice far exceeds interest in its pathological aspects. To reduce Zimbabwe's medical development to a scientific exercise in rational planning without fully recognizing its religious and cultural dimensions is to tell an incomplete story (Porterfield, 2005:12).

## References

Arifin S.R.M. (2018) Ethical Considerations in Qualitative Study, *International Journal of Care Scholars*, 1(2), 30–33.

Barbour G.I. (1968) *Science and Religion: New Perspectives on Dialogue*, New York: Harper and Row Publishers.

Bartlett P.C. and Judge L.J. (1997) The Role of Epidemiology in Public Health, *Revue scientifique et technique (International Office of Epizootics)* 16(2), 331–336.

Bhagat R.P. (2018) *Introduction to Science,* https://www.researchgate.net/publication/32932111.

Botha N. (2008) HIV/AIDS Discourse and the Quest for a Rebirth in Africa: A Theological Perspective, in Adogame A., Gerloff R. and Hock K. (eds), *Christianity in Africa and the African Diaspora The Appropriation of a Scattered Heritage*, London: Continuum.

Bourdieu P. (1986) Forms of Capital, in Richardson J.G. (ed), *Handbook of Theory and Research for the Sociology of Education*, London: Greenwood Press.

Bourdillon M. (1976) *The Shona People: Ethnography of the Contemporary Shona, with Special Reference to their Religion*, Gweru: Mambo Press.

Chavhunduka G (2001) *Dialogue among Civilisations, the Africa Traditional Religion To-Day*, Harare: Crossover Communication.

Idowu E.B. (1994) *Oludumare, God in Yoruba Belief*, New York: Wazobia.

Isiko A.P. (2020) Religious construction of disease: An exploratory appraisal of religious responses to the COVID-19 pandemic in *Uganda, Journal of African Studies and Development*, 12(3), pp. 77–96.

Maposa R.S. and Humbe B.P. (2012) *Indigenous Religion and HIV And Aids Management in Zimbabwe: An African Perspective*, LAP Lambert Academic.

Martí J. (2015) Representing African Reality through Knotty Terms; *Cahiers d'Études Africaines*, 55, pp. 85–105; Cahier 217, EHESS Stable.

Mbiti J.S. (1969) *African Religions and Philosophy*, Blantyre: Heinemann.

Oliveira-Cardoso E.A., Silva B.C.A., Santos J.H., Lotério L.S., Accoroni A.G., and Santos M.A. (2020) *The Effect of Suppressing Funeral Rituals during the COVID-19 Pandemic on Bereaved Families. Revista Latino-Americana de Enfermagem*, 28, p. e3361 (Accessed on 10/08/21).

Paris P.J. (1995) *The Spirituality of African Peoples: The Search for A Common Moral Discourse*, Minneapolis: Fortress Press.

Porterfield A. (2005) *Healing in the History of Christianity*, Oxford: Oxford University Press.

Rammohan A., Ramachandran P. and Rela M. (2021) Bereavement management during COVID-19 Pandemic: One size may not fit all! *Journal of Global Health*, 11, p. 03009.

Wallace C.L., Wladkowski S.P., Gibson A. and White P. (2020) Grief During the COVID-19 Pandemic: Considerations for Palliative Care Providers, *Journal of Pain and Symptom Management*, 60(1), 1–14.

Young W.A. (2005) *The World's Religions. An Introduction*, Pretoria: University of South Africa.

**Internet Sources**

Ankara, 11 June 2020, "Zimbabwe Leader Calls for Prayer to Tackle Coronavirus", *https://www.aa.com.tr › africa › zimbabwe-leader-calls-*, Accessed on 11/03/21.

*The Herald*, 25 July 2021, "Makandiwa Endorses Vaccination Drive", *https://www. herald.co.zw*, Accessed on 10/08/21.

Mavhunga C, 07 April 2021, "Zimbabwe's Government Says Herbal Treatment OK for COVID-19", *https://www.voanews.com/science-health/coronavirus-outbreak/zimbabwes-government-says-herbal-treatment-ok-covid-19*, Accessed on 06/03/21.

Ncube L.A. (2021) "Vice President Chiwenga Speaks on the Use of Zumbani and Moringa to Treat Covid-19", *https://iharare.com/vice-president-chiwenga-speaks-on-the-use-of-zumbani-and-moringa-to-treat-covid-19*, Accessed on 07/03/21.

Ndoro T.E (2021) "Health Benefits of Zumbani and All You Need to Know about the Plant", *https://iharare.com/health-benefits-and-all-you-need-to-know-about-zumbani*, Accessed on 06/03/21.

Ndoro T.E. (2021) "Zimbabwean Prophet Makandiwa Blames Vaccines for Africa's Poverty, Underachievement", https://iharare.com/watch-zimbabwean-prophet-makandiwa-blames-vaccines-for-africas-poverty-underachievement, Accessed on 20/03/21.

Sachiti R. (2021) "Zimbabwe: Covid-19 Community Deaths Increase—Funerals, Defiance", *The Herald,* https://www.allafrica.com, Accessed on 10/08/21.

# 6 Religion, law and COVID-19 in South Africa

*Helena Van Coller and Idowu A. Akinloye*

## Introduction

This chapter appraises the state regulatory response in containing the spread of the new coronavirus disease (COVID-19) in light of the constitutionally guaranteed right to freedom of religion[1] in South Africa. The increased complaints (Chothia, 2020b; Pillay, 2020; Tsotetsi, 2020) and lawsuits[2] challenging the impact of the regulatory measures on the flourishing of religious freedom in South Africa heighten the need for the appraisal. According to the World Health Organization (WHO, 2020a), the COVID-19 is a deadly virus that was first identified in Wuhan, China in December 2019. It is said that the virus causes a contagious respiratory disease that spreads through physical contact. On 30 January 2020, the WHO declared the outbreak of the virus as a public health emergency of international concern, and on 11 March 2020 characterized it as a pandemic (WHO, 2020b). As of 2 June 2021, 172,159,531 infected cases have been reported worldwide and 3,696,931 reported deaths (Worldometer, 2021)

For almost a year of its existence, no scientifically proven cure or efficacious treatment was found to heal anyone who contracted the virus. Even now that some vaccines said to be of probable cure to the spread of the virus have been discovered in some countries like in the United States and the United Kingdom, as at early February 2021, South Africa has not started vaccinating (Mwai, 2021). Accordingly, following the advice from health specialists, the South African government, like most other countries, came up with radical measures to reduce the rate of transmission, impact and deaths arising from the virus. Some of these measures are backed by regulations (hereafter, "lockdown regulations") with an attendant effect of fine and imprisonment for their violation (Chothia, 2020a).

An apparent effect of the lockdown regulations is that they restrict the constitutionally guaranteed human rights, including the rights to freedom of movement, freedom of association, freedom of religion and the right to human dignity, among others. Possibly due to the widely held view of South Africans' religiosity, the restriction touching on religious freedom appears to have elicited much public debate. Whilst some members of the public

DOI: 10.4324/9781003241096-6

welcome the regulations and legal restrictions (Swain, 2020a), others took serious exceptions to some of the regulatory measures, particularly the provisions of the lockdown regulations that ban religious gatherings. Similarly, the South African courts have delivered conflicting rulings in a number of lawsuits that challenged the legality and constitutionality of the ban of religious gathering in an attempt to curb the spread and the numbers of death arising from the virus. The lockdown regulations and their effects on all spheres of human rights may not be effectively evaluated given the limited scope of this chapter and the specific focus of this book. Against the backdrop of the above, this chapter, by using a doctrinal research approach through analysis of literature, statutes and case examples, will evaluate the state regulations enacted to curb the spread of the COVID-19 in South Africa vis-à-vis the constitutional provisions protecting freedom of religion in the country. The primary essence of the evaluation is to determine the constitutional justification of the regulations.

The chapter is structured as follows. After the introduction, it briefly examines the constitutional framework for the protection of the right to freedom of religion in South Africa. Thereafter, some of the provisions of the lockdown regulations that impact on freedom of religion are highlighted. This is followed by an examination of the responses of the religious groups to the regulations. In this section, the opinions of public commentators as well the court rulings were analysed to determine the justification of the regulatory measures in light of the constitutional limitation to human rights, and thereafter, the summary is made and the conclusion is drawn. From the analysis made, the chapter observes that legislative wise, South Africa was clearly not prepared for the pandemic because the government had to hurriedly enact regulations without adequate consultations or planning. It argues that although parts of the regulations that provide for the total or partial ban of religious gatherings in the wake of the outbreak of the COVID-19 may have increased the suffering and violates the rights of most South Africans, they are permissible limitations of religious freedom.

## Legal framework for freedom of religion in South Africa

Freedom of religion is a recognised human right that means different things to different people. This is perhaps because the scope of what it entails varies between states, religions, individuals and legal instruments (Evans, 2001; Sullivan *et al.*, 2015). What appears to gain consensus, however, is that freedom of religion would imply a state's duty to refrain from interfering in an individual or community's pursuit of a chosen religious belief; a right to choose and change one's religion without force and coercion, including the freedom to manifest and practise the religion individually or in fellowship with other believers. The importance of the protection of freedom of religion as a fundamental human right has been widely acknowledged as crucial for the development of an individual's self-definition and the promotion of democratic pluralism within society. It is regarded by some as 'the most sacred of all freedoms (Robertson, 1991; Ouashigah, 2014).

South Africa has given constitutional recognition to the protection of the right. Section 15(1) of the South African Constitution 1996 (the Constitution) provides: "Everyone has the right to freedom of conscience, religion, thought, belief and opinion." Chaskalson P, in *S v Lawrence* (1997) described the scope of this provision as the

> right to entertain such religious beliefs as a person chooses, the right to declare such religious beliefs openly and without fear of hindrance or reprisal, and the right to manifest religious belief by worship and practice or by teaching and dissemination.
> (Van der Schyff, 2003; Govindjee, 2016)

It is submitted that the full ambit of this right can only be ascertained when section 15 of the Constitution is read conjunctively with sections 9(3),[3] 31,[4] and 185[5] of the Constitution (Constitution of the Republic of South Africa, 1996). The combination of the above provisions protects individual and group religious autonomy, equality of all religions, and non-discrimination on the basis of religion. It further protects the rights to belong to any religion; change one's religion; *manifest and propagate* one's religion either in public or in private or either alone or in community with others.

The right which is majorly violated by the lockdown regulations is the right to *manifest one's belief* in community with others—religious gathering that is guaranteed in terms of sections 17 and 18 of the Constitution (Constitution of the Republic of South Africa, 1996). This right is at the heart of the freedom of religion because it underscores the collective group or institutional right to freedom of religion. Dinstein rightly argues, "Freedom of religion, as an individual right, may be nullified unless complemented by a collective human right of the religious group to construct the infrastructure making possible the full enjoyment of that freedom by individuals" (Dinstein, 1992; Govindjee, 2016).

Freedom of religion is, however, not absolute in the Constitution. The state may be obliged in certain cases to limit a fundamental right including the right to freedom of religion. But in terms of section 36 of the Constitution, where the state is to limit any of the constitutionally guaranteed rights, such limitation must be reasonable and justifiable in an open and democratic society based on human dignity, equality, and freedom. Usually, to determine the validity of a limitation, the court will delve into a limitation analysis involving "… the balancing of means and ends." This will involve an analysis of all relevant considerations

> to determine the proportionality between the extent of the limitation of the right considering the nature and importance of the infringed right, on the one hand, and the purpose, importance and effect of the

infringing provision, taking into account the availability of less restrictive means available to achieve that purpose.

(Minister of Home Affairs v NICRO, 2005)

As noted previously, some of the provisions of the lockdown regulations
limit the freedom of religion. The next section will highlight some of these
provisions.

## The lockdown regulations

After the COVID-19 hit the shores of South Africa, and following the ex-
ponential spread and the fear of the numbers of death it may cause in the
country, Dr Mmaphaka Tau on 15 March 2020, in his capacity as Head of
the South African National Disaster Management Centre and in terms of
section 23(1) of the Disaster Management Act 57 of 2002 (DMA) categorised the pandemic as a national disaster.[6] Subsequently, the Minister of
Cooperative Governance and Traditional Affairs (COGTA), in terms of
section 27 of DMA promulgated Regulations (lockdown regulations) that
imposed lockdowns in different spheres and sectors in South Africa. In
terms of the regulations, lockdowns are stratified into alert level 1 to alert
level 5, with alert level 5 as the strictest. To date, a number of regulations
have been made. The first regulations – Regulation 11B94 (hereafter, the
Level 5 Regulations) took effect on 26 March 2020 and it governed the
level 5 lockdown. The second regulations (hereafter, the Level 4 Regulations) came into force on 1 May 2020 to govern alert level 4 lockdown. The
third regulation (hereafter, the Level 3 Regulations) came into force on
1 June 2020, and it relates to alert level 3. A number of other regulations
have further been made, but their provisions are largely the same with
those already mentioned.

Section 11B (i) and (ii) of the Level 5 Regulation and section 24 (1) of the
Level 4 Regulations provides that any place or premises normally open to
the public where religious and cultural or similar activities take place are to
be closed during the period of the lockdowns. Curfews were also placed between 8pm and 5am in terms of the two regulations. Section 18 of the Level
4 Regulations specifically permits attendance at funerals during the time of
the lockdown, but limits the attendance to 50 people and specifically states
that "no night vigil shall be held".[7] It also further requires that "all safety
measures are strictly adhered to".

The above provisions mean that worship places like churches, synagogues
and mosques were closed for worships during the day and at night in alert
Levels 4 and 5 Regulations. It further means that individuals may also not
invite any other person to their home for prayer, worship, cell group meetings, to anoint the sick with oil or pray for healing for them, etc. However,
in the alert Level 3 Regulations, the ban on religious gatherings was lifted
subject to adherence to some protective protocols.

The regulations were further relaxed in 2021 and people started to become lax about observance of COVID-19 hygiene protocols. In May 2021, nine people who form part of a small Uniting Reformed Church in Vredendal, in the Western Cape, succumbed to COVID-19 complications. The church reopened when COVID-19 restrictions were eased, but with infections rising it has closed its doors again (Masweneng, 2021).

March and April 2021 saw coronavirus infections continue to rise in South Africa, which has prompted the South African government in the beginning of May 2021 to consider introducing additional measures in order to stave off a third wave. The original Alert level 2 was in place from 18 August to 20 September 2020. A new adjusted Alert level 2 was put in place from 31 May 2021.[8] In terms of the movement of persons, the regulations introduced a closing time for all venues hosting faith-based, or religious gatherings to 22H00. All faith-based or religious gatherings are permitted but limited to 100 persons or less for indoor venues and 250 persons or less for outdoor venues. If the venue is too small to hold the prescribed number of persons observing a distance of at least one and a half metres from each other, then not more than 50% of the capacity of the venue may be used, subject to strict adherence to all health protocols and social distancing measures.

Attendance of a funeral is further limited to 100 persons and not more than 50% of the capacity of the venue may be used, subject to strict adherence to all health protocols and all persons maintaining a distance of one and a half metres from each other. The regulations also prohibit night vigils and after-funeral gatherings, including "after-tears" gatherings. During a funeral, a person must wear a face mask and adhere to all health protocols and social distancing measures. The duration of a funeral is restricted to a maximum of two hours.

## Responses to the regulations

Various groups have reacted differently to the lockdown regulations. For instance, immediately after the alert Level 5 Regulations that introduced "the strictest lockdowns" was announced, most religious organisations appear to accept it as a laudable step by the state to guard the inhabitants of the country against the virus. But some people considered the total and a blanket ban on religious gathering as unreasonable and unconstitutional given that funerals with a maximum of 50 persons were allowed. The state and those who welcome the ban on religious gatherings justify the ban on a number of grounds. First, it is argued that the ban was imposed on all religions; it therefore passes the constitutional test of non-discrimination. Second, there were no effective measures to manage the risk or to prevent the spread of the infection and the possible numbers of death that may occur at the outbreak of the virus in the country. The ban is thus to allow the state to build up an extensive public health response for the anticipated surge of infections (Swain, 2020a). Third, the ban followed similar measures adopted by other countries. Furthermore, the purpose of the ban was to curb the spread of the virus in order to save lives. Akin to this is that the ban is to allow citizens to access the constitutionally entrenched rights to health care and an environment that is not harmful.

Those that oppose the ban on religious gathering have also predicated their position on a number of grounds, which include first, given that a person's faith and the manifestation thereof is central to their dignity as a human being, the blanket ban of any form of religious gathering (except for a limited waiver for funerals) is unfair and prejudicial to religious adherents. It also violates their essential humanity (Barmania and Reiss, 2020; Swain, 2020a). Further, given the religiosity of most South Africans, to think that people's spiritual needs are not paramount at a time like this is unreasonable, especially that many are isolated, lonely, and may have lost loved ones or jobs, and are fearful of what the future holds. In fact, for a great many people being a part of a religious body at a time like this is a source of healing, a mode of alleviating suffering and their only lifeline. Some religionists have further argued that the ban had created, anxiety, fear and mental suffering and "spiritual depression" on their adherents (Kowalczyk *et al.*, 2020; Pillay, 2020). Furthermore, throughout history, the religious community has typically been at the forefront of the response to the ravages of disease. Apart from offering fervent and continual prayers for the government and those suffering in the communities, it also offers practical service, spiritual counsel and support (Swain, 2020a). Shutting down religious gathering in a country where faith is deeply woven into the fabric of the society is arbitrary and irrational (Swain, 2020b). Also very related is that some religionists believe the current pandemic is a punishment from God due to the human sinfulness, and it is in worship places that many will seek the face of God for forgiveness and get divine healing (Ozalp, 2020). Thus, the blanket ban on religious activities overlooks the unique contribution of the religious community (Chothia, 2020). Second, it is posited that there are various comparable diseases plaguing the country like tuberculosis, influenza, and so on, for which no worship centre is closed, restricting all religious gatherings at this time is therefore an overreaction. Thirdly, it is argued that if the lockdown could be relaxed for funerals to be held, taxi and grocery stores to operate, it is unreasonable not to allow worship places to open subject to taking precautionary measures to avoid the infection (Chothia, 2020b; Pillay, 2020).

Furthermore, the legality and constitutionality of the lockdown regulations banning religious activities have been challenged in the court, and some are still reportedly about to go to court (Mokhoali, 2021; SABC, 2021; Shange, 2021). But so far, the courts have not been consistent in their rulings on this issue. The remainder of this section will summarise the facts and rulings of two case examples: *Mohamed v The President of the Republic of South Africa (Mohamed)*[9] and *De Beer v The Minister of Cooperative Governance and Traditional Affairs (De Beer)*.[10]

*Mohamed case*

The applicants are Imams and worshippers at a mosque managed by the third applicant. The applicants asked the court to, among other things, declare the provision of the lockdown regulations, which provides for a blanket ban on religious gatherings as overbroad, excessive and unconstitutional to the extent that it fails to allow congregational worship; to allow "an exception" to be made for them to gather and worship under certain conditions; that the respondent be ordered to amend the regulations to permit movement of persons between their residence and places of worship on such reasonable conditions as the court deems appropriate; and that the third applicant be allowed to conduct each of the five daily prayers for a congregation limited to 20 people each under certain strict sanitary precautions.

In the presentation of their case, the applicants submitted that they accepted that the lockdown regulations were rational and a permissible response to the COVID-19 pandemic, they nevertheless argued that their religious obligations are suffering serious and egregious inroads by the lockdown. They posited that it is obligatory for them to perform the five daily prayers in congregation and at mosque even in the face of the COVID-19 pandemic. Accordingly, they claim that the lockdown regulations violate their constitutional rights to freedom of movement, freedom of religion, freedom of association (including religious association) and the right to dignity. Their argument is that if the government could frame some exceptions to the present rule such as for funerals and for taxis to carry 75% of their usual passenger load, they should be able to do so for purposes of congregational worship as well.

In response, the respondent posited that indeed the lockdown regulations imposed severe restrictions on every person's constitutional rights and particularly those regarding movement and association. However, those limitations are both reasonable and necessary given the suffering and threat that COVID-19 poses to human life, dignity and access to healthcare. The respondent submitted that the regulations encompass a serious limitation of rights, but are justified to protect the rights to life, access to healthcare, an environment that is not harmful to one's health and wellbeing, and the right to dignity that are entrenched in the Constitution.

In her ruling, Neukircher J held that the application is about whether the state's refusal to craft an exemption permit to allow for congregational religious worship, is reasonable and justifiable in terms of the provision of the Constitution. In her limitation analysis in terms of section 36 of the Constitution, the court held that for the lockdown regulations to constitute a constitutional limitation, the government needs not to show that they will invariably achieve their objections of stemming the COVID-19 pandemic, it is sufficient if they show that the lockdown regulations are a rational measure designed to achieve that end. She held that the restriction was neither unreasonable nor unjustifiable on the basis that the blanket ban was not selective, discriminatory or against a particular religion. She further held that the current pandemic calls for every citizen "in the name of the greater good" and in the spirit of *Ubuntu* to make sacrifices to their fundamental rights.

This approach seemed sensible, especially given the fact that a church gathering in Kwasizabantu in KwaZulu-Natal in December 2020, which was attended by more than 2,000 people, resulted in at least 48 COVID-19 infections in the province (Nombembe, 2020). At the same time, the Roman Catholic Diocese of Mariannhill, west of Durban, has confirmed that nine nuns, who belonged to Daughters of Saint Francis in Port Shepstone, Mariannhill Diocese that have succumbed to COVID-19. All the affected nuns had attended a church function in the past two weeks (Mhlongo, 2020).

### De Beer case

The applicants in this case claimed, among other things, that the declaration of the national state of disaster and all the lockdown regulations promulgated to curb the spread of COVID-19 are unconstitutional, unlawful and invalid; that all the gatherings be declared lawful alternatively be allowed subject to certain condition. It is apposite to state that at the time the ruling in this case was delivered on 2 June 2020, the latter relief has, to an extent, been overtaken by events since the alert Level 3 Regulations that came into force on 1 June 2020 allows religious gatherings, subject to certain conditions. The applicants did not challenge the categorisation of the pandemic as a national disaster; rather they attacked the rationality or constitutionality of the regulations. This is unlike in the *Mohamed* case where the claimants accepted that the regulations were rational and a constitutionally permissible response to the COVID-19, but only asked for an exception. To justify their claim, the applicants in this case contended that the state's response to the pandemic was irrational and constitute an overreaction. They further contended that in terms of section 59(1) and (4) of the DMA. They were unlawful because the minister did not obtain the approval of the National Council of Provinces prior to the promulgation of the regulations. But this argument was rejected by the court on the ground that the provision is inapplicable in the instant case. In its ruling, the court emphasised that where the power to make a specific regulation is exercised as in the instant case, the regulation made must be rationally related to the purpose for which the power was conferred (this is called the rationality test). The question the court asked was: is there a rational connection between the intervention and the purpose for which it was taken? In construing the rationality test, the court submits that "it is not to determine whether some means will achieve the purpose better than others, but only whether the means employed are rationally related to the purpose for which the power was conferred." To the court, if the means employed to achieve the purpose are disconnected and irrational, then they will be unconstitutional and not permissible limitation in terms of section 36 of the Constitution.

The court used some illustrations to evaluate the rationality of the regulations. For instance, it reasoned that the provisions of the regulations that prohibited religious leaders and people (who are willing to take prescribed precautions) to leave their homes to visit and support their loved ones on a deathbed, but allowed them to attend the funeral of the loved one who is departed who needs no support is not rational. The court also observed that a total blanket ban on gathering that implicates the observance of religious vigil for the dead but allows 50 people for a funeral is also not rational. In summary, the court highlighted that the lockdown regulations, including the alert Level 3 Regulations, are replete with instances of sheer irrationality. On the final analysis, the court held that although the Minister's declaration of a national state of disaster in terms of the DMA in response to pandemic is rational, the lockdown regulations do not satisfy the rationality test. Also, their limitations to the Bill of Rights are not justifiable in an open and democratic society based on human dignity, equality and freedom. The court therefore declared them unconstitutional and invalid. The government has rejected this judgment and indicated its intention to appeal it (Rabkin, 2020).

## Findings and conclusion

Although the court attempted to distinguish the facts of *Mohamed* from the *De Beer* on the ground that the applicants in the former accepted the rationality of the lockdown regulations which the latter did not accept, the questions for determination in the two cases are essentially the same. The questions bother on the constitutionality of the lockdown regulations. We are of the view that the decision in *Mohamed* represents the true position of the law. The fact is that no right is absolute. The restriction placed on religious gathering is legitimately permissible given the circumstances of the current pandemic and the fact that people can be exposed to risk in large gatherings. The COVID-19 pandemic presents a "deep health crisis" to the country and the effort to curtail the same in the way the government has done will be legitimate. Although the South African approaches in dealing with the pandemic might have been at the expense of the livelihood of the people, they are based on saving lives and preserving livelihoods.

As for the *De Beer* judgment, it lacked cogency and appears not to deal thoroughly enough with the issues. Some other commentators have similarly argued that the judgment of *De Beer* may not be able to stand the scrutiny of the higher court if it is appealed (Comins, 2020; Shange, 2020). Notwithstanding this view, *Mohamed* and *De Beer* cases, as well as other cases that have challenged the validity of the lockdown regulation raise some important issues and positive outcomes.

First, the increased number of lawsuits relating to religious ban reiterates the widely held view that religious institutions are forces to reckon with in state governance in South Africa and most African countries (Agbiji, 2015; Mbiti, 1990). It further reinforces the assertion that freedom of religion is one of the most controversial of all human rights and a potent source of social conflict (Cheadle *et al.*, 2002), and therefore, it should be well managed.

Second, the cases reveal some vacuum and lacunae in the extant legislation that deal with the management of a pandemic in the country, which perhaps had not been subject of court or public scrutiny prior to the outbreak of this present pandemic. The court in *De Beer* observed this point when it stated "there is no existing legislation and contingency arrangement to adequately manage COVID-19." The implication of such vacuum is that state government would have to promulgate new regulations in a hurry and this may create a tendency of making the state to promulgate arbitrary rules or rules may lead to "unintended" interference with the guaranteed human rights. And this may further open the gate of litigation against the state. For instance, in the *De Beer* case, the court and the respondent (the state) confirmed that there were many concurrent similar cases challenging the lockdown regulations in other jurisdictions of the court. Akin to this is that the state should not in the name of a pandemic assume that it can limit human rights. The state should always prioritize the realisation and protection of human rights at all times.

In conclusion, the increased number of lawsuits is a signal to the government that citizens could go to court to challenge the limitations of their rights or seek clarity on the rationale behind the lockdown regulations and their constitutionality. This is a sign of a flourishing democracy where the people keep the state in check, even during a national state of disaster. Accordingly, the state must be conscious that **in a constitutional democracy like South Africa, any legislation by the government must be rational and must justifiably limit the rights of citizens.** Even though the decision of the *De Beer* is likely to be successfully appealed, the judgment, at least emphasises the fundamental principle that every exercise of state power, whether legislative or executive cannot be arbitrarily conducted; it must be subject to the constitution and give respect to the bill of rights. Put differently, in the exercise of public power or performance of a public function, there is the need for state apparatus to self scrutinize in order to ensure the legality and constitutional compliance thereof. Furthermore, South African religious institutions have been widely recognised as major civil institutions that play a role in the provision of social services to complement the state effort (Goodchild, 2016; Koegelenberg, 2001). Even despite the limitation that was placed on religious gatherings during this time, religious communities have reportedly played, and are still playing an important role in alleviating the effects of the pandemic on the citizens. For example, the religious communities were at the forefront of alleviating the suffering of citizens in the face of illness and mobilizing resources (Swain, 2020a) – spiritual, monetary and psychological to support the needy, as well as calming an already restless society (Barmania and Reiss, 2020; Maromo, 2020; Nzwili, 2020; Swain, 2020a). Accordingly, for religious communities to continue to play a role in the provision of social services, it is expedient that the state respect and protect their institutional religious rights; such rights should be limited only in exceptional circumstances, as illustrated by *Mohamed*.

## Notes

1 Religion in this context refers to any particular system of faith and worship, such as Christianity, Islam, Buddhism, African traditional religion, and so on.
2 *De Beer v The Minister of Cooperative Governance and Traditional Affairs* (Case No: 21542/2020. Judgment delivered on 2 June 2020); *Moela v Habib*(Case No. 2020/9215, Judgment delivered on 23 March 2020); *Khosa v Minister of Defence and Military Veterans and of Police* (Case No. 21512/2020, Judgment delivered on 15 May 2020); *Mohamedv The President of the Republic of South Africa* (Case No: 2140/20 Judgment delivered on 30 April 2020).
3 Section 9(3) provides: "The state may not unfairly discriminate directly or indirectly against anyone on one or more grounds, including race, gender, sex, pregnancy, marital status, ethnic or social origin, colour, sexual orientation, age, disability, *religion,* conscience, belief, culture, language and birth." Emphasis added.
4 Section 31(1) provides: "Persons belonging to a cultural, *religious* or linguistic community may not be denied the right, with other members of that community—(a) to enjoy their culture, practise their religion and use their language; and (b) to form, join and maintain cultural, religious and linguistic associations and other organs of civil society.
5 Section 185(1) provides for the functions of the Commission for the Promotion and Protection of the Rights of Cultural, Religious and Linguistic Communities to among others things, "promote respect for the rights of cultural, *religious* and linguistic communities." Emphasis added.
6 The Classification of a National Disaster published in government Notice No. 43096 of 15 March 2020.
7 The night vigil is a religious and cultural practices usually observed by the family of the deceased to honor the deceased.
8 Gazette 43620 of 17 August 2020) as amended by Gazette 44642 of 30 May 2021.
9 Case No: 2140/20; *Khosa v Minister of Defence and Military Veterans and of Police* (Case No. 21512/2020). The case was decided by Fabricius J on 15 May 2020.
10 Case No: 21542/2020.

## References

Agbiji, O.M. and I. Swart. (2015) 'Religion and Social Transformation in Africa: A Critical and Appreciative Perspective' *Scriptura*, 114(1), pp. 1–20.
Barmania, S. and M.J. Reiss. (2020) 'Health Promotion Perspectives on the COVID-19 Pandemic: The Importance of Religion' *Global Health Promotion*, 28(1), pp. 15–22.
Cheadle, M.H., D.M. Davis and N.R.L. Hayson. (2002) *South African Constitutional Law: The Bill of Rights.* Durban: Butterworths.

Chothia, A. (2020a) 'Police Raid Mosque, Arrest Men for Gathering during Ramadan' *The South African*, 25 April. Available at: https://www.thesouthafrican.com/
news/police-arrest-men-mosque-lockdown-video/ (Accessed: 28 April 2020).

Chothia, A. (2020b) 'Reformed Churches Ask for One Gathering on Sundays During Lockdown' *The South African*, 28 April. Available at: https://www.thesoutha-
frican.com/news/reformed-churches-gathering-during-lockdown/ (Accessed: 30
April 2020).

Comins, L. (2020) 'Mixed Views on Lockdown Judgment' *The Mercury*, 4 June.
Available at: http://themercury.newspaperdirect.com/epaper/showarticle.aspx-
?article=1764b401-6a7e-430b-99256d9a1eace631&key=tufNkZaqqzutAhv2E%-
2bU90g%3d%3d&issue=64032020060400000000001001 (Accessed: 3 July 2020).

Constitution of the Republic of South Africa, 1996.

Dinstein, Y. (1992) 'Freedom of Religion and Religious Minorities', in Dinstein, Y.
(ed). *The Protection of Minorities and Human Rights*. Netherlands. Springer.

Evans, C. (2001) *Freedom of Religion under the European Convention on Human
Rights*. Oxford: Oxford University Press.

Goodchild, E. (2016) *Best Corporate Governance Practices: Financial Accountability
of Selected Churches in the Free State Province* (LLM thesis, University of the
Free State).

Govindjee, A. (2016) 'Freedom of Religion, Belief and Opinion', in Govindjee, A
(ed). *Introduction to Human Rights Law*. 2 ed. Durban: LexisNexis.

Koegelenberg, R.A. (2001) 'Social Development Partnership between Religious
Communities and the State: Perspectives from the National Religious Association for Social Development' *Journal of Theology for Southern Africa*, 110, pp.
97–109.

Kowalczyk, O., K. Roszkowski, X. Montane, W. Pawliszak, B. Tylkowski and A.
Bajek (2020) 'Religion and Faith Perception in a Pandemic of COVID-19' *Journal
of Religion and Health* 59, 2671–2677.

Maromo, J. (2020) 'Religious Leaders Asked to 'Practise Charity', Help the Poor
during Covid-19 Lockdown' *IOL*, 15 April. Available at: https://www.iol.co.za/
news/politics/religious-leaders-asked-to-practise-charity-help-the-poor-during-
covid-19-lockdown-46721704 (Accessed: 30 April 2020).

Masweneng, K. (2021) 'Nine Congregants Die as Covid-19 Sweeps Through Vredendal Church' *Times Live,* 1 June 2021. Available at: https://www.timeslive.
co.za/news/south-africa/2021-06-01-nine-congregants-die-as-covid-19-sweeps-
through-vredendal-church/ (Accessed: 4 June 2021).

Mbiti, J.S. (1990) *African Religious and Philosophy*. Portsmouth: Heinemann.

Mhlongo, F. (2020) 'Ninth Death Reported at Durban's Roman Catholic Diocese
amid COVID-19' *SABC News,* 21 December. Available at: https://www.sabcnews.
com/sabcnews/ninth-death-reported-at-durbans-roman-catholic-diocese-amid-
covid-19/ (Accessed: 4 June 2021).

Mokhoali, V. (2021) 'SANCF Takes Govt to Court Over Decision to Ban Religious Gatherings' *Eyewitness News*, 11 January, Available at: https://ewn.
co.za/2021/01/16/sancf-takes-govt-to-court-over-decision-to-ban-religious-
gatherings (Accessed: 30 January 2021).

Mwai, P. (2021) 'Coronavirus: When Will South Africa Start Vaccinating?' *BBC News*,
10 February. Available at: https://www.bbc.com/news/world-africa-55675806 (Accessed: 13 March 2021).

Nombembe, P. (2020) 'Church Gathering Ignites 48 Covid-19 Cases as Virus Spreads in KZN' *Times Live*, 12 December. Available at: https://www.timeslive. co.za/news/south-africa/2020-12-20-church-gathering-ignites-48-covid-19-cases-as-virus-spreads-in-kzn/ (Accessed: 4 June 2021).

Nzwili, F. (2020) 'African Church Leaders Work to Curb Domestic Abuse During Lockdown' *CNS News*, 19 May. Available at: https://www.catholicnews.com/services/englishnews/2020/african-church-leaders-work-to-curb-domestic-abuse-during-lockdown.cfm (Accessed: 30 June 2020).

Ozalp, M. (2020) 'How Coronavirus Challenges Muslims' Faith and Changes their Lives' *The Conversation* 2 April. Available at: https://theconversation.com/how-coronavirus-challenges-muslims-faith-and-changes-their-lives-133925 (Accessed: 30 April 2020).

Pillay, K. (2020) 'Muslim Groups Plead with President to Relax Regulations for Daily Prayers' *Mercury News*, 6 April. Available at: https://www.iol.co.za/mercury/news/muslim-groups-plead-with-president-to-relax-regulations-for-daily-prayers-46315332 (Accessed: 30 May 2020).

Quashigah, K. (2014) 'Religion and the Republican State in Africa: The Need for a Distanced Relationship' *African Human Rights Law Journal*, 14, pp. 78–92.

Rabkin, F. (2020) 'Dlamini-Zuma Seeks to Appeal the Judgment that Set Aside Lockdown Regulations' *Mail and Guardian*' 9 June. Available at: https://mg.co.za/politics/2020-06-09-dlamini-zuma-seeks-to-appeal-the-judgment-that-set-aside-lockdown-regulations/ (Accessed: 30 June 2020).

Robertson, M (ed) (1991) *Human Rights for South Africans*. Oxford: Oxford University Press.

SABC. (2021) 'Freedom of Religion SA Goes to Court to Demand Lifting of Religious Gatherings Ban' *SABC News*, 28 January. Available at: https://www.sabcnews.com/sabcnews/freedom-of-religion-sa-goes-to-court-to-demand-lifting-of-religious-gatherings-ban/ (Accessed: 30 January 2021).

Shange, N. (2020) 'Lockdown Judgment Should Have Been More Concise and Persuasive: Legal Experts' *Times Live*, 3 June https://www.timeslive.co.za/news/south-africa/2020-06-03-lockdown-judgment-should-have-been-more-concise-and-persuasive-legal-experts/ (Accessed: 30 June 2020).

Shange, N. (2021) 'Doors Might Be Open, But Church Council Wants Government Stopped from Ever Shutting them Again' *Times Live*, 2 February. Available at: https://www.timeslive.co.za/news/south-africa/2021-02-02-doors-might-be-open-but-church-council-wants-government-stopped-from-ever-shutting-them-again/ (Accessed: 30 February 2021).

Sullivan, W.F., E.S. Hurd, S. Mahmood and P.G. Danchin (eds), 2015. *Politics of Religious Freedom*. Chicago: University of Chicago Press.

Swain, M. (2020a) 'Lockdown Regulations: What about the Religious Community?' *FOR SA*, 14 May. Available at: https://forsa.org.za/lockdown-regulations-what-about-the-religious-community/ (Accessed: 30 June 2020).

Swain, M. (2020b) 'COVID-19 Lockdown: A Case for Limited Exemption for Religious Organisations' *FOR SA*, 16 April 2020. Available at: https://forsa.org.za/covid-19-lockdown-a-case-for-limited-exemption-for-religious-organisations/ (Accessed: 30 April 2020).

Tsotetsi, D. (2020) 'CHANGE Calls for Reopening of Religious Gatherings During Level 3 Lockdown' *SABC*, *News* 6 May. Available at: https://www.sabcnews.

com/sabcnews/change-calls-for-reopening-of-religious-gatherings-during-level-3-lockdown/ (Accessed: 30 May 2020).

Van der Schyff, G. (2003) 'Freedom of Religious Autonomy as an Element of the Right to Freedom of Religion', *Journal of South African Law*, 3, pp. 512–539.

WHO (2020a) 'Statement on the Second Meeting of the International Health Regulations (2005) Emergency Committee Regarding the Outbreak of Novel Coronavirus (2019-nCoV)'. Available at: https://www.who.int/news-room/detail/30-01-2020-statement-on-the-second-meeting-of-the-international-health-regulations-(2005)-emergency-committee-regarding-the-outbreak-of-novel-coronavirus-(2019-ncov) (Accessed: 30 April 2020).

WHO (2020b) 'WHO Director-General's Opening Remarks at the Media Briefing on COVID-19'. Available at: https://www.who.int/dg/speeches/detail/who-director-general-s-opening-remarks-at-the-media-briefing-on-covid-19---11-march-2020. (Accessed: 30 April 2020).

Worldometer. (2021) 'COVID-19 Coronavirus Pandemic' Available at: https://www.worldometers.info/coronavirus/? (Accessed: 2 June 2021). Nam voluptaqui officid que in corro consed quossi de quid quid explani mporerit oditent.

# 7 Tele-evangelism, tele-health and cyberbullying in the wake of the outbreak of COVID-19 in Zimbabwe

*Lucia Ponde-Mutsvedu and Sophia Chirongoma*

## Introduction

The outbreak of COVID-19 has indeed changed human interactions in the 21st century. Although how this epidemic actually originated remains unclear, it is apparent that the epidemic has impacted heavily on human communities and the global economic systems have been torn asunder. What is even more worrisome is that COVID-19 is still in its prime stages with a very high probability of ongoing for an unforeseeable period of time. As noted by Okon (2011), like any other global epidemics, COVID-19 necessitates that humanity be equipped with the dos and don'ts in order to stem the tide of the epidemic. In an endeavour to contain the epidemic, global health institutions such as the World Health Organization (WHO) have disseminated information and guidelines on how to practice physical and social distancing as measures to minimize chances of spreading the coronavirus. Focusing particularly on the African context with particular reference to the Karanga-Shona people in Zimbabwe, this chapter reflects on some of the efforts that have been put into place in order to observe these stipulated measures. The use of Information and Communication Technology (ICT) to bridge the social gap created by these measures will also be deliberated upon. The challenges posed by observing the stipulated guidelines in light of the African understanding of being in community is the focus of discussion in this chapter. Hence, the discussion centres on how the use of Tele-evangelism, Tele-health and other virtual means of making contact impact heavily on the African ethos of living in a community. In this undertaking, the chapter also seeks to weave another strand on the tapestry of "Online religion" in Africa as already deliberated upon by other scholars, particularly Goliama (2010), Asamoah-Gyadu (2015) as well as Sibanda and Hove (2018). This pre-existing literature interrogates the pros and cons of online religion in our contemporary times. In unison with these scholars, this chapter focuses particularly on the Karanga-Shona and how their worldview has been radically reshaped by the stipulated guidelines necessitated by the COVID-19 epidemic.

DOI: 10.4324/9781003241096-7

## Methodology and theoretical framework

This chapter draws insights from Bronfenbrenner's ecological model and the African ethic of *Ubuntu/Unhu* as guiding theories. Adopting the ecological model in this chapter helps to illustrate the impact of self-quarantine, social and physical distancing as opposed to the tradition of communal interactions which has been embedded in the African communities since time immemorial (Swearer & Susan, 2011). Life as presented in the African culture is indeed communal (Mabvurira, 2018). Clearly, the stipulated measures guiding human contact in the wake of COVID-19 are contrary to the African social interactions especially in the family, communal and religious circles. These measures also present major barriers for political gatherings which thrive in numbers.

Bronfenbrenner's ecological theory is anchored on examining how human interactions are linked to one's environment. Initially, his theory was mainly applied when studying the development of children. However, the theory has also been used to analyse the interconnectedness of human relationships in general. Hence, Bronfenbrenner's theory emphasizes on the importance of analysing the interconnections in human communities. This makes this theory relevant in this discussion because it helps to unpack how the "new normal" in the wake of the COVID-19 epidemic disrupts the web of connections within the African communities. The family, school, peers and the social environment play pivotal roles in maintaining the positive vibe to someone who is suffering either emotionally or physically. This is how the ecological model becomes relevant because the experiences of those suffering from ailments related to the coronavirus are inextricably linked to the conditions that the environment is throwing at them. Gaining such information can only help the affected and infected in trying to come to terms with the present situation in a contextualised framework; the social environment.

The ecological theory endorses the interconnectedness amongst families and the environment while the spirit of *Ubuntu/Unhu* echoes the notion of communitarianism. In this regard, the *Ubuntu/Unhu* philosophy upholds the importance of the community over the notion of an individual. According to Kimmerle (2006), *Ubuntu* emphasizes on 'we' in contrast with 'I'. Similarly, Mugumbate and Nyangura (2013:83) define the principle of *Ubuntu* as "being human through other people." The conclusion reached in this chapter is that the spirit of "Ubuntu" rides on the collective notion. The relationship between the individual and the social environment plays a pivotal role in human relationships. Human beings thrive on each other's encouragement, physical and social contact. Contrary to this, the COVID-19 epidemic has brought about the need to self-quarantine, especially in the event that one has tested positive for the coronavirus. This entails being isolated in an enclosed space, with absolutely no contact even with all those whom one holds so dear. In this chapter, we argue that as African indigenous people who thrive on communal interactions, being required to self-isolate in times of illness due to COVID-19 related ailments might leave a permanent void not only on the patient but more so, on those closely related to the patient. This is because they will be agonizing with the harsh reality of the fact that they have been deprived of their duty to care for their loved one in their most crucial time of need. In concurrence with Goliama (2010), we also contend that the stipulated guidelines on maintaining social distance, which underscores that people should neither exchange handshakes nor hugs is totally contrary to the indigenous African concept of *Ubuntu/Unhu* and being in community. Hence, our chapter resonates with Asamoah-Gyadu (2015) in underlining the fact that the use of tele-evangelism, tele-health services and other non-direct physical space sharing as necessitated by online platforms are inconsistent with the spirit of *Ubuntu/Unhu*.

## Proliferation of information and communication technology (ICT)

The proliferation of Information and Communication Technology (ICT) has brought about vast advantages in the face of the COVID-19 epidemic. For example, ICT enables individuals to listen to the word of God in the comfort of their own homes by turning on the television, radio or other social media platforms such as WhatsApp, Facebook or Instagram. People are attending church services via Facebook live streaming and they have continued to receive spiritual upliftment. In another vein, families have been maintaining regular communication channels through the use of WhatsApp video calls, Zoom Conferencing and Hangouts. The use of ICT is therefore facilitating constant communication which helps to maintain family and social ties. Consequently, using the virtual platform as a mode of communication is helping to foment the spirit of *Ubuntu/Unhu*. The idea of interacting with a loved one during a video call or video conference gives both parties comfort and solace. Making connections via the virtual space helps to maintain relationships and to bring loved ones together, especially those who are separated through time and space.

## Tele-evangelism

As noted by Biernatzki (1991), tele-evangelism refers to the process of conveying the Bible message to the people via various forms of media. Similarly, Hoover and Clark (2002) describe tele-evangelism as the mainstreaming of religious activities and messages via the television or a radio. In other words, tele-evangelism focuses on uniting the men and women of God through inspired Bible messages via media. In the contemporary context, the use of television, twitter and Facebook can never be underestimated (Sibanda and Hove, 2018). Globally, tele-evangelism has been in use since time immemorial. Tele-evangelism as highlighted by Okon (2011) is anchored on the importance of the pastor or the sharer of the word, the type of message to be delivered and the audience (those receiving the word). According to Okon

(2011), televisions are a sure way of conveying Bible based messages to millions of people across the world. In a similar light, Thomas and Lee (2012) aver that the media has been the mainstay of the people's faith in the contemporary world. It has been used as a vehicle to transmit the gospel to the whole world. In this pandemic era, people need to stay abreast with the word of God which keeps encouraging them to hold onto their faith as they go through the trying times. The spirit and the body cannot be separated; thus, it is of great importance for the people of God to maintain a certain grain of faith through the word. Live streaming on Facebook pages, videos and WhatsApp audio also help to disseminate religious messages to the bulk of African communities who either do not have access to or they cannot afford to pay for the DSTV subscription due to financial constraints.

Furthermore, the lockdown regulations in Zimbabwe which limits worshippers to only 50 people in a particular church service leaves the majority without the much needed spiritual caretaking. Consequently, the use of ICT is bridging the gap by bringing the word to different people in various parts of the world via the media. The use of media to share religious messages has sustained the spirituality of most people as they continue to fellowship together as families in their own homes. With just one click, the message is delivered instantly. This has actually helped to build relationships by cementing and increasing family interactions. In one of the audios sent via WhatsApp, a woman recorded a message articulating the goodness of COVID-19; she was rejoicing that due to the lockdown measures, she is now having an opportunity to spend more time with her husband and the children, something that was not possible before then. Others are also welcoming the lockdown restrictions because with limited opportunities for traveling, they are now able to save money as there are no transport costs to and from church. On the other hand, tele-evangelism also saves time, because people will not need to spend time travelling to the church building when the church service is being broadcast online.

In Zimbabwe, various churches and ministries are utilizing tele-evangelism to propagate the gospel especially as the lockdown restrictions have persisted for several months. For instance, the Prophetic Healing Deliverance Ministries (PHD Ministries) through its tele-evangelism arm, Yadhah TV which was originally founded in 2012 is currently making waves not only in Zimbabwe but globally. Likewise, Ezekiel TV, which was founded by Apostle Ezekiel Guti, the founder of ZAOGA (Zimbabwe Assemblies of God) is another powerful ministry. Another really popular tele-evangelism station is Emmanuel TV which was founded in 2006 by Prophet by T.B. Joshua, the Pastor of The Synagogue, Church of All Nations (SCOAN) based in Lagos, Nigeria. It is also the most subscribed Christian ministry channel on YouTube worldwide with well over 1,000,000 subscribers, as of January 2019 (https://www.scoan.org/, Accessed 20 October, 2020). Emmanuel TV has become a household ministry in most Zimbabwean homesteads particularly due to its prophetic, healing and deliverance ministry which appeals to the hearts of many amidst the uncertainties compounded by the COVID-19 epidemic. The Seventh Day Adventist Church (SDA) in Zimbabwe which is popularly known for holding annual camp-meetings in August has also been innovative by hosting various virtual camp-meetings spreading between the months of August and September, 2020.

## Tele-health

Wotton (2001) describes tele-health services as health care from a distance. Mars & Erasmus describe tele-health as the provision of health care over a distance through the use of ICT. The burden of caring for patients who have succumbed to the COVID-19 epidemic in various parts of Africa is real. For most African countries, the COVID-19 epidemic exacerbates the already over-stretched health care facilities (Mars, 2013). More so, as noted by Chirongoma (2016), these strained health care facilities are often staffed by very few medical professionals who were already sighing under the heavy yoke of long working hours, coupled with very poor remuneration, long before the outbreak of the COVID-19 epidemic. Against such a background, access to tele-health services in most parts of Africa becomes scarce due to limited resources and personnel (Mars & Erasmus, 2012). Wootton (2006) describes Africa as having the "digital divide" obstacle. Several segments of the African communities do not yet have access to efficient and reliable tele-communication networks due to poor infrastructure, which raises challenges in rolling out tele-health services. This is mainly because the health care service providers will be trying to guard against issues of liability, licensure and jurisdiction. However, the use of ICT remains a challenge to most Africans. As such, Wootton (2006) advocates for tele-health, since it breaks the barrier of geography and shortages of health personnel in Africa. In actual fact, the implementation of tele-health comes in handy during the current COVID-19 era, where self-isolation, social and physical distancing and quarantining are the order of the day.

Technology use such as Facebook, Twitter and WhatsApp may fail to reach some of the rural areas in Africa. Whilst mostly the elite are enjoying the broadband access, the bulk of the ordinary African populace regard such a facility as a luxury which they cannot afford. There is therefore need for improving the usage of telephones as this is the easier and faster channel of passing on the information in most African societies. In the 1st world, a wide range of medical consultations can be done either physically or virtually. Hence, most people in the 1st world countries have got the privilege of consulting their medical practitioners either in the comfort of their homes or offices. In this contemporary world, information dissemination is afforded to most people by the use of cell phones and video calling. WhatsApp has been the major transmission device in Africa. However, the downside is that in trying to relay some information, unauthenticated information is also transmitted along the way, without verification. Due to the fact that some African societies are rather detached from the outside world, this compromises their capacity to properly sift through and verify the authenticity of some life-giving and life-saving information. For instance, some elderly and rural-based folks are being bombarded with loads of misinformation regarding the genesis or the prevention measures for the COVID-19 epidemic. Others have been misled into believing that alcohol consumption will insulate them from contracting the coronavirus. The continuous help from the young generation to the older one is greatly appreciated as the older generation continue to navigate the ICT pool of information which may be too much to assimilate.

## Social media

Social media is indeed the most important and sustaining mode of communication in the contemporary world. Baruah (2015) postulates it as a means of communication amongst the new generation. As the modern technology has continued on a path of evolution, there is need for everyone to keep abreast with modern technology. Media on the other hand, runs a very high risk of being hijacked and used negatively by peddling lies and uncertified information. It is undisputedly known that the social media has spearheaded false information and some people solely rely on the social media for information sharing. Indeed, this tool can be misused. Technology is like a double-edged sword, on one end it gives connectivity, while on the other, it can be the source of emotional disturbances. Some videos and pictures can actually scare people, help them or cause them to live in fear while the same platforms can be the pillars of strength for some people. Very few people take time to verify information circulating on social media, which can provide pathways for spreading some of the very crude and unreliable information. Technology spearheads the sharing of essential information but at the same time it can facilitate the spreading of false information which can cause unnecessary panic and apathy.

## Cyberbullying/pornography

Zimbabwe, like most African countries, with high literacy, has a generally high rate of cell phone usage as well as access to computers and the internet (POTRAZ, 2014). That high level of access to ICT increases children's vulnerability to cyberbullying. This is particularly so during the current COVID-19 lockdown induced measures which have consequently precipitated the increased usage of computers and cell phones as children continue to do most of their school work online. In Zimbabwe, most private schools have engaged online lessons and that has given the young adults an opportunity to navigate and experiment online, while the parents are at work. Children, including those still in primary school are spending a considerable amount of time watching 'Netflix" as a pastime. Spending long hours on Facebook, Twitter and other social media platforms has also become the order of the day as children continue to study, research and keep in touch with friends and relatives. The flipside of ICT use is the fact that it has the propensity of becoming addictive. Through excessive ICT use, come some strands of violence and emotional abuse as screen time for both children and families is increased. Studies have shown that the more the screen time, the higher the abuse. The probability of coming across pornography is also high and with this volatile environment, parents are also not in the right space of monitoring what the children are doing at home. Concerns on the bread and butter issues are now on the increase, following closures of companies and businesses.

As the children navigate online, their parents are focusing on bread and butter issues and cyberbullying is indeed stemming in, thereby causing undue emotional strain. The younger generation is more susceptible to cyberbullying as they participate in various online activities without adequate monitoring from the adults. A study by Safaria (2016) found out that advancements of technology exacerbate cyberbullying. Apart from advances in technology, cyberbullying is also precipitated by the generational gap between parents and children, as parents are often behind when it comes to dealing with technology (Ordun, 2015). The ideology behind the use of ICT is that some programmes are not age appropriate, but who will be there to monitor what this young generation are watching? Who monitors these children so as to ensure that we continue to cultivate the right values, beliefs and norms amongst the young generation so as to maintain the African moral fabric? The caregivers' capacity to properly monitor children under their care continues to be compromised as the burdens imposed by the coronavirus weighs in heavily on them.

The generational gap and sometimes the constrained relationships between parents and children where there is no open dialogue often exposes the children to become victims of cyberbullying without their parent's knowledge. As the "Generations" advance for example from X, Y and Z, the later generations are likely to fall prey to cyberbullies because they spend more time on the internet than the antecedent generations. The more time they spend on the internet, the greater the risk to being cyberbullied. Technology indeed has compromised the spirit of *Ubuntu* among families. Instead of enhancing the inter-generational sharing and mentorship, it is instead causing a rift between parents and children as the children spend countless hours learning information from the media platforms rather than tapping from the older generations. The younger generation has a high affinity to technology and this predisposes them to mental health. Thus, the more they get exposed to technology, the greater the risk to numerous emotional problems and pornography.

## The "new normal" runs counter to the spirit of Ubuntu/Unhu

The COVID-19 pandemic seems to be hovering on earth for a bit longer than originally anticipated. Thus, it's of utmost importance to draw the dos and don'ts so as to enable human life to cope and be able to survive. The normalcy includes, wearing of masks, social distancing, elbow greeting, no embracing at funerals, hand washing and many others. All these are an antithesis of the *Ubuntu/Unhu* cultural values and norms. Suddenly adjusting to these new norms is especially daunting to the older generation who are steeped in their traditional values. Since time immemorial, the indigenous African greeting, particularly among the Shona people in Zimbabwe involves hand shaking. It is a way of showing respect and one cannot claim to have greeted an elderly person without exchanging a proper handshake. Similarly, at funerals, relatives, friends and neighbours are expected to gather at the homestead of the bereaved and to spend several nights there as a sign of solidarity and to comfort the bereaved. What then is prescribed to be the new normal is that we continue to unite and help each other in such predicaments, bearing in mind that we also have to exercise caution by observing social distancing.

The spirit of *Ubuntu/Unhu* emphasizes on communal interconnectedness and it frowns upon individualism. Hence, the prescribed measures to self-isolate in the event that one suspects that they have been exposed to the coronavirus or after having tested positive to the coronavirus runs contrary to the true spirit of *Ubuntu/Unhu*. No opportunity to look after a sick loved one, or being required to wear protective clothing such as gloves and masks when interacting with the loved ones smacks of the African interconnected web of relating. More so, being restricted from sharing utensils and other personal effects with a close family member who is either suspected of being infected or is actually infected with the coronavirus does not sound very pleasant in the African traditional context. The notion of the *Ubuntu/Unhu* ethos takes into cognisance the role of the environment, which in this case is the family. The microsystem (family, peers, and school) takes into cognisance the importance of the immediate environment which includes the family and peers. These interactions are very personal and in this environment, the family which is supposed to take care of each other is required to distance itself as a way of avoiding transmission. The African context has its own social dynamics which require a certain attitude and experience in order to evaluate other people's feelings and experiences. For instance, due to the intertwined nature of African social networks, it can cause a lot of emotional turmoil to realize that a blood sister or brother can be denied entrance into their sibling's homestead because the family is trying to guard against contracting or spreading the coronavirus. This new normalcy can actually strain social relationships as some family members might not see this from the same perspective. Both the behaviour of the infected and the affected and the impact of their dilemmas can be understood in their environmental context.

As noted by Bronfenbrenner, the environment plays an important role in bringing out the best in a human being. As such, the prescribed burial for corpses that would have died due to COVID-19 causes immense turmoil in those who were close to the deceased. The fact that in the early days of the COVID-19 related death, relatives of the deceased were not even allowed to physically attend the burial exacerbated their grief. This is made apparent by the comments made by one of the Zimbabwean women whose relative was among the first Zimbabweans to die of COVID-19 complications in April 2020. She expressed the grief and perplexity in the following words, "*Mukoma wangu kuvigwa muplastic sembwa here veduwe!*" [It is heart-wrenching that my brother was buried in a plastic bag, he was treated like a dog!] (Interview with an Anonymous Source). Another incident that drew massive social media attention occurred in Harare in June 2020 whereby a young Shona man hysterically protested at the graveyard after having been informed that his deceased grandmother's corpse was forbidden by the health restrictions to lie in state at their homestead because she had tested positive to the coronavirus. The widely circulated video clip which was recorded at the graveyard when the young man was making a scene whilst pleading for permission from the law enforcement agents to be allowed to accord his grandmother a "decent" burial made a social media sensation. Whilst on one hand some viewers heavily critiqued this young man for being insensible, others also sympathized with him by arguing that from a Shona cultural point of view, his protests were justified. These are some of the scenarios which are emitting the "Ubuntu spirit" and culturally, it's not easy for the Shona people who have their own values and beliefs to go through this kind of lamentation. The African notion of having loads of people at a funeral is regarded as "*kuchemwa kwakanaka*" [a powerful and moving send-off]. Normally, the Shona people perceive a huge crowd of mourners as a sign of the "power of love."

Clearly, the regulation that COVID-19 corpses are supposed to be buried within 24 hours has caused heartache beyond measure for most indigenous African people. This is mainly because most indigenous Africans are used to gathering at funerals, sometimes for more than three days which gives them an opportunity to perform their traditional ceremonies. Regrettably, due to COVID-19, they are being deprived of such opportunities, this leaves most bereaved people devastated and feeling lost. Not being able to actively participate in the burial rituals and being deprived of the opportunity to see a loved one being laid to rest leaves the bereaved with deep emotional wounds. This also presents a major barrier towards getting closure, particularly to those who were close to the deceased. The African communitarian spirit emphasizes the importance of family members and friends visiting each other in their homes and also in the hospital in the event that someone has fallen ill and has been admitted in hospital. This presents a platform for them to offer each other comfort and encouragement. Unfortunately, most of these social interactions have been ground to a halt by the restrictions imposed due to the COVID-19 social distancing measures.

Bronfenbrenner's mesosystem upholds the essence of relationships among the loved ones, which in this case are the parents, teachers and the children. Since the focus is on the relationships and interlinks between those that surround the individual, there is need to maintain a balance between health care and relationships. Failure to have such a balance may result in disequilibrium of the system. Drawing from Bronfenbrenner's ecosystem (indirect environment), a person can take it out on another person because of some unresolved issues in his or her life. For instance, if someone has contracted the disease, one may find himself/herself, lashing out on the very person who is genuinely trying to help them out. Just the news that one has tested positive for the coronavirus might take a huge toll on someone. The microsystem, (social and cultural values) and chronosystem (changes over time) play an important role in the shaping of human behaviour. The accumulation of values, beliefs and ideas can never be underestimated for it plays a major role in an adult's life. A change which might befall a family, like in the case of death, can take a huge toll on those who are left behind. A little change in the family structure can revolutionise everything in a family set up. There is therefore need for every family to learn how to resile in such an environment.

Gender relations are another aspect of human relationships that have been heavily impacted by the COVID-19 epidemic. Since the onset of the lockdown measures, the available global and regional statistics reveal a high rise of women and children abuse, and Zimbabwe is no exception. The pandemic did not only alter the people's social lives, but it has precipitated the rates of suicidal tendencies as caregivers lose either their jobs or sources of livelihoods. As the old adage goes, "an idle mind is the devil's workshop," consequently, in some instances, those who have lost their means of sustenance have resorted to crime and violence. Idle time has been increased and that places most people on the verge of committing crime as they struggle to fend for their families.

Furthermore, due to its oral transmission and in the absence of a well-established treatment or cure, there is stigma associated with COVID-19. Upon announcement by the health sector personnel that one has contracted the disease, those who are around you tend to distant themselves. Some of these announcements by the health sector exacerbates everything as most WhatsApp groups will disseminate prejudiced information like a veld fire, which exposes the infected individual to the vulnerability of stigma and discrimination.

There is also need for continuous conscientization especially for some conservative religious groups which adamantly defy the stipulated lockdown measures. A case in point is the unfortunate incident that led to the death of three male members of the Sungano Apostolic Church in Mutare, Zimbabwe during the early days of the lockdown phase in April 2020. As reported by several Zimbabwean newspapers, the Manicaland police spokesperson Inspector Tavhiringwa Kokohwa confirmed that the deceased trio were part of a ten member team that had gone to Murahwa Hill in Mutare to observe ten days of prayer and fasting in a cave. They lit a fire which gathered smoke inside the cave resulting in these three men choking to death. Those who lived to tell the tale are the ones who eventually reported the incident to the local police (Masekesa, 2020).

## Conclusion

The outbreak of COVID-19 has impacted heavily on human communities worldwide. Apart from very few advantages which entail increasing family time and drawing families together, the disadvantages however outweigh the advantages. In the indigenous African communities, for instance among the Shona, most of the social distancing regulations impinge on their deeply cherished norms and values. For most indigenous communities, particularly in Southern Africa, being required to desist from exchanging handshakes, hugging and being restrained from gathering in numbers at a funeral is tantamount to touching their raw nerves. The introduction of ICT has played a pivotal role in establishing a smooth and easy access to information, at churches, gatherings, and medical institutions as well as facilitating individual daily communication. Though it seems very hard to adapt to the new normal, the harsh reality of the matter is that if human communities wish to survive this catastrophe, difficult as it is, we simply have to learn to adjust to the new way of being in the world. Appreciating the gift of life and exercising responsible stewardship for our lives, our loved ones' lives and the lives of all those we interact with as we await the eventual harnessing of the epidemic should be our main goal. Now, more than ever, there is a pertinent need for information dissemination which is accurate, especially to those in the very remote areas who are still living either under the blanket of ignorance or those who are still in denial regarding the gravity of the challenges and threats presented by the novel coronavirus. Clearly, COVID-19 is a wakeup call to the human race, and the earlier we get it, the better. Being alert to these facts of life will help us to understand the nature of the problem and to take the requisite corrective action.

The African communal understanding is that people live for each other, hence, the African proverb, "it takes a village to raise a child." Simply put, relationship building and interconnectedness as emphasized in Bronfenbrenner's ecological model are the treasured right ingredients for positive human interactions in the African community. Whilst realistically upholding the spirit of *Ubuntu*, as African indigenous communities, we also need to acknowledge that the earlier we all learn how to adapt to this new normalcy the better, because it's going to be a long journey before most people can embrace reality. The concept of individualism has come in its full force through this very pandemic and so we need to adjust for our own good and for posterity's sake. The above discussion contributes to the current national and international drive to raise awareness in regard to COVID-19 and reduce the mortality rate especially in the spirit of the African community.

## References

Asamoah-Gyadu, J. K. (2015). ""We are on the internet": Contemporary Pentecostalism in Africa and the new culture of Online Religion" in *New Media and Religious Transformations in Africa* (eds) Rosalind I. J. Hackett and Benjamin F. Soares, Bloomington, Indiana: Indiana University Press, 157–170.

Baruah, S. (2012). Effectiveness of social media as a tool of communication and its potential for technology enabled connections: A micro-level study. *International Journal of Scientific and Research Publications,* 2(5), 1–10, May 2012 1 ISSN 2250–3153.

Biernatzki, W. E. (1991). Televagelism and the religious uses of television. *Communication Research Trends. Communication Research,* 11(1).

Chirongoma, S. (2016). "Exploring the impact of economic and socio-political development on people's health and well-being: A case study of the Karanga people in Masvingo, Zimbabwe" in *HTS Theological Studies Special Issue on Engaging Development: Contributions to a Critical Theological and Religious Debate* (eds) Afe Adogame and Ignatius Swart (Volume 72, Issue 3, pp. 1–9)

Goliama, C. M. (2010). *Where Are You Africa?: Church and Society in the Mobile Phone Age.* African Books Collective, 71–110.

Hoover, S., & Clark, L. (2002). *Practicing Religion in the Age of the Media: Explorations in Media, Religion, and Culture.* New York City: Columbia University Press.

Kimmerle, H. (2006). Ubuntu and Communalism in African philosophy and art. *Prophesies and Protest-Ubuntu in Glocal Management,* 79–91.

Mabvurira, V. (2018). Making sense of African thought in social work practice in Zimbabwe: Towards professional decolonisation. *International Social Work.*

Mars, M. (2013). Telemedicine and advances in urban and rural healthcare delivery in Africa. *Progress in Cardiovascular Diseases,* 326–335.

Mars, M., & Erasmus, L. (2012). Telemedicine can lower health care costs in Africa. *Innovate,* 32–33.

Masekesa, C. (2020). "Lockdown: 3 Apostolic church members suffocate to death" https://zimmorningpost.com/lockdown-3-apostolic-church-members-suffocate-to-death/ April 14, 2020

Mugumbate, J., & Nyanguru, A. (2013). Exploring African philosophy: The value of Ubuntu in social work. *African Journal of Social Work,* 3(1), 82–100.

Okon, G. (2011). Religion, media and politics in Africa. Teleevangelism and the socio-political mobilization of pentecostals in Port Harcourt metropolis: A KAP Survey. *Politics and Religion,* 5(1), 2–475.

Ordun, G. (2015). Millenial (Gen Y) Consumer behavior their shopping preferences and perceptual maps associated with brand loyalty. *Canadian Social Science,* 40–55.

Potraz, Z. (2014). *Information and Communication Technology (ICT) Household Survey 2014 Access by Households and Use by Individuals.* Harare. Zimbabwe: Zimbabwe National Statistics Agency (ZIMSTAT) and Postal and Telecommunications Regulatory Authority of Zimbabwe (POTRAZ).

Safaria, R. (2016). Prevalence and Impact of cyberbullying in a sample of Indonesian junior high school students. *The Turkish Online Journal of Educational Technology,* 15(1).

Sibanda, F., & Hove E.F. (2018). Unlocking the media and the politics of televangelism in Zimbabwe: A contemporary discourse in *Power in Contemporary Zimbabwe* (eds) E. Masitera and F. Sibanda. Routledge, 149–165.

Swearer, N., & Susan, M. (2011). Risk Factors for and Outcomes of Bullying and Victimization. *Educational Psychology Papers and Publications,* 132, 1–9.

The Synagogue, Church of All Nations (SCOAN). https://www.scoan.org/ Accessed 20 October, 2020.

Thomas, P., & Lee, P. (2012). *In Global and Local Televangelism: An Introduction. In Global and Local Televangelism* (pp. 1–17). London: Palgrave Macmillan.

# 8 The role of religion in response to COVID-19 pandemic challenges in Tanzania

*Paskas Wagana*

## Introduction

Corona Virus Disease (COVID-19) is a virus-related disease that affects the respiratory system (Amon, 2020; Kumar et al., 2020). It first appeared in the province of Wuhan, in China in December 2019. By mid-January, 2020, the COVID-19 cases were reported in many places in Asia including Thailand, Japan, South Korea, Vietnam, Nepal, Malaysia, Sri Lanka, Philippines and India (Kumar et al., 2020). In a short span of four months, the virus had already reached all the continents (Iroulo & Boateng, 2020). On 11 March 2020, COVID-19 was declared a pandemic by the World Health Organization (URT, 2020b; TCSDF, 2020). Such inconceivable bad news caused mayhem worldwide triggering panic, suspension of economic activities, disruption of healthcare services, inflating COVID cases, and heightening of COVID-19 related deaths.

In response to the outbreak, the World Health Organization recommended standard guidelines for prevention and management of COVID-19. The recommended measures include quarantining of infected or suspected patients, contact tracing, lockdowns, travel restrictions, border closures, wearing of masks, and physical distancing (WHO, 2020a, 2020b). These measures were readily adapted by countries in Asia and Europe where COVID-19 was initially extremely intense (Iroulo & Boateng, 2020) and later other countries also started using them.

In East Africa these standard guidelines were implemented in varied degrees. Some countries, Rwanda to be specific, enforced total shutdown. Other countries like Uganda and Kenya tried partial lockdown and partial curfews, respectively. Only Tanzania out rightly refuted the lockdown as a counterproductive measure to combat COVID-19. Instead, it decided to localize its response program by preserving all other WHO standard guidelines and implemented them in tandem with religion. Religion in this context is understood in its broadest sense as a belief to a supernatural agent.

Tanzania's unique approach to COVID-19 has raised many questions; often being belittled and downplayed as weak, ineffective, soft, disappointing and dangerous. But, in a way, it has worked. In the following sections the

DOI: 10.4324/9781003241096-8

outcome of this unique strategy for Tanzania is discussed by first briefing out the existence of COVID-19 in Tanzania, then efforts are made to interpret Tanzania's unique strategy in the light of the theory of governmentality and, finally, discussions on the role religious leaders, religious organizations and institutions played in supporting the Tanzanian government to implement preventive measures for COVID-19 are presented.

## COVID-19 pandemic and its effects in Tanzania

The first case of COVID-19 was reported in Tanzania on Monday 16 March 2020. And by mid-May 2020, over 500 people were already infected by the diseases and 21 people succumbed to death (URT, 2020b). Like many other countries in the world, the outbreak of COVID-19 found Tanzania virtually unprepared in terms of vaccine, medical infrastructure and treatment. The news caused public Punic; people started stockpiling food and medical supplies such as masks and hand sanitizers. This was followed by closure of education institutions (URT, 2020e). For just a short period of time normal life changed in Tanzania particularly in urban and semi-urban areas with many services being halted due to the fear of infection.

The initial response was to target affected people, isolate them, trace their contact friends and isolate them too. However, the exercise soon became complex because of the inflating number of cases. Hence, new methods of precautions were devised.

In response to counteract the devastating effects of COVID-19 pandemic, Tanzania established a special COVID-19 taskforce to implement strategies for management of the disease (URT, 2020b). Measures of precautions and containment were more enhanced and implemented: surveillance at airports, border crossings, and other points of entry were enhanced; public meetings and sporting events were strictly prohibited, and all international passenger flights were suspended. Stern measures were taken to encourage hand washing, house quarantining, and physical distancing. Several public and private hospitals were designated as isolation centers to accommodate people infected with coronavirus (WBG, 2020). Guideline to help healthcare workers to trace, make follow up and serve self-quarantined people in their homes and those in designated places of quarantine were issued (URT, 2020c).As the disease continued to spread, special guideline were issued on how hospitals should handle cases of COVID-19 by setting aside separate wards for specific COVID-19 treatment (URT, 2020d). Measures of prevention were adhered in all places which could attract a large number of people. Thus, places like retailer shops, hospitals, clinics, schools, markets and banks had to provide water and soap to their customers before they could offer them any service (Mpota, 2020). Generally speaking, Tanzania implemented a strong public campaign to prevent the infection of corona virus.

In addition to measures outlined in the national guidelines for COVID-19 prevention, the ministry of health in Tanzania encouraged the use of traditional medicine to arrest COVID-19 symptoms as the disease had, by then, neither cure nor vaccine (Mpota, 2020).This advice was warmly welcomed and easily adopted by the public as the practice of using local herbs for treatment of various diseases is widely in use in Tanzania. The government approval made it public and even more popular. The use of local herbs was further promoted by herbalists and other people who shared the procedures of blending the herbs to obtain appropriate dosages through the social media. Tanzania is extraordinarily reach in local herbs and is cheaply available in almost every place around the country. Lemon, ginger, chilly, pepper, neem tree leaves are boiled and mixed with honey to obtain a syrup for treatment. Sometimes same materials are boiled and patients incubate themselves from the steam produced thereof.

And above all these, community engagement was also envisaged as a significant strategy to promote COVID-19 public awareness. This is where religion found precedence and soft entry into the COVID-19 program in Tanzania. Religious leaders were motivated to continue offering special prayers to implore the merciful God to deliver His people from the fatality of Corona Virus (Mpota, 2020).

**Theory of governmentality**

The theory of Governmentality refers to the practice through which an agency such as the state, medical institution, and religion, is able to exercise control over a large population. The theory is associated with a French philosopher and psychologist, Michel Foucault (1926–1984). In his famous book *Discipline and Punish (1975)*, Foucault outlines how disciplinary power is far more efficient in disciplining people compared to coercive compliance. Therefore, modern states and non-state entities prefer to control their citizens, not by force, but though governmentality. That is, people are made to govern or comply with state or institutional policies by themselves even without the presence of the supervising central authority.

In other words, the central authority or institution acts as a reference center which imparts governing guidelines to its subjects and leaves them to implement those guidelines or policies by themselves. A classic example given by Foucault is the health system where patients are informed about their health statuses, treatment needed and the precautions an individual patient has to take. Afterwards, individuals are left free while responsibility is highly expected of them to govern their own bodies as directed by medical personnel.

This theory was originally written to describe the difference between sovereign and disciplinary powers. However, some of its features can be drafted to explain the scenario of COVID-19 management in Tanzania. Tanzania was the third country in East Africa to register the COVID-19 case following Rwanda and Kenya which recorded their cases much earlier. Unlike other East African countries which imposed outright coercion to implement restrictions, Tanzania chose the trajectory of engagement and cooperation with religion to implement its COVID-19 prevention guidelines. This approach was comparatively effective in motivating people to adhere to COVID-19 standard guidelines and practices for the prevention and control of COVID-19 in comparison to other measures used in different parts of East African region.

Rwanda was the first country in East Africa region to impose the lockdown. All movements were banned, employees were ordered to work from home, and borders were completely closed except for cargo and returning citizens, who had to undergo a forced two weeks quarantine (https://www.dw.com/en/coronavirus-rwanda-imposes-africas-first-lockdown/a-52878787). Kenya introduced a night curfew allowing people to go out for limited hours during the day and completely stay at home during the night. Uganda also practiced a total shutdown and deployed the national armed forces to implement the curfew. The outcome of these strict restrictions in these countries was not impressive. Many acts of intimidations were reported. In Kenya, for example, these strict restrictions had bearings on gender-based violence where women and girls became victims of attack for sexual assaults (Odhiambo, 2020). In Uganda, where Uganda's taskforce for COVID-19 was led by the army, there was public outcry for the excessive use of force to ensure the lockdown is strictly adhered to. The public outcry against military brutality during the lockdown led to public apology of the chief of defense forces and enforcement of legal actions to some military personnel (Namwase, 2020).

The above-mentioned challenges were not reported in Tanzania. This is probably because Tanzania avoided overly restrictions on movements of people. Instead, Tanzania adopted a polite way of implementing standard COVID-19 regulations incorporating religion as a major vehicle. In Tanzania, gatherings were not strictly banned, movement of people was regulated but not strictly restricted, local transportation was carried out but with precautions, and places of worship were not shut down except where religious leaders closed them on their own discretion.

This friendly way of imposing regulations was less painful to the people and, as a result, produced impressive outcomes. Specific guidelines such as self-isolation, physical distancing, hand wash, and use of sanitizers in public places and at home, were readily followed without mandatory supervision. This semi-autonomous imposition of rules motivated people to take additional steps of precautions by devising means for COVID-19 prevention using resources available in their own localities. Tanzania COVID-19 model is an example of how to use social power in times of crisis. Power imposed from above through coercion can generate aggression and emotional outbursts, which are counterproductive. The efficient way is to create awareness through media of socialization such as the family, religion, medical institution, etc. and then let people discipline themselves while central authorities monitoring the effects.

**The role of religion in combating COVID-19 pandemic**

The fundamental importance of religion in combating COVID-19 pandemic appeared in the early WHO guidelines on COVID-19 pandemic with the title: *Practical Considerations and Recommendations for Religious Leaders and Faith-Based Communities in the context of COVID-19. Interim guide* (WHO, 2020a).This document outlines different steps religion and religious leaders can take to effectively deal with COVID-19 pandemic. These include proper education and communication of accurate information about COVID-19; organization of safe faith-based gathering, clean worshipping sites and fight against COVID-19 related stigma; intensifying interfaith collaborations and peaceful coexistence during COVID-19 pandemic; and conducting safe burial services and helping the grieving families or communities to cope with the loss, sadness and distress.

Religion holds a significant place in the lives of any society. It directly or indirectly affects the lives and social activities of the people (Barmania & Reiss, 2020), and therefore, cannot be overlooked on issues which threatens the survival of the society. Tanzania is a multicultural and multireligious society. Religions which have a stronghold in Tanzania are mainly three: Christianity, Islam and African Tradition religions. These religions have inherent elements of differentiation which distinguish them from one another and, therefore, it is naturally not easy to bring them together under one roof. However, during the outbreak of COVID-19 pandemic, Tanzania tried its height by forging them to work together under the theme of COVID-19 prevention.

Religion has an intrinsic duo-character with regard to contagious diseases such as COVID-19 pandemic. It can be an essential vehicle for the spread of the disease but also an important instrument for prevention of the same.

Among the essential assets that religion offers is trust. Religion is a trusted source of information. In fact, in some communities, religion can be the only primary source of information. In times of crisis, people tend to seek in religion and to religious leaders, than even to political authorities or medical institutions, guidance on what to do or how to behave (Iroulo & Boateng, 2020). Thus, if religion is well utilized it can be a useful instrument for the delivery of the right information about the pandemic as information form religion is easily accepted than from other sources.

There are many instances in Africa where religion was used to increase awareness of infectious diseases, reduce stigmatization, and promote safe health behaviors. For example, Muslim and Christian religious leaders were engaged in the fight against Ebola epidemic in West Africa as Ebola infections were largely due to exposure during funerals and burials (Obregón, 2009). A similar practice was done in Tanzania during COVID-19 pandemic where religious leaders were part of a national program for community engagement against the transmission of the virus.

Religious leaders and religious institutions in Tanzania have been in the forefront to implement the COVID-19 standard guidelines issued by the government of Tanzania through the ministry of health. Key areas of prevention emphasized by religion include limiting number of people in prayer sessions by conducting multiple services with limited number of worshippers, reducing the length of homilies, observing sitting arrangements, postponing unnecessary religious group gatherings, encouraging use of soap, water, sanitizers and covering faces with masks, and where possible, organizing services through television or radio (URT, 2020a).

Religion is also a key institution in the provision of social support. A pandemic like COVID-19 can have ramified devastating effects both at the individual and community levels. Factors such as disruption of life, loss of livelihood, self-isolation, working from home, and sudden change of modes of social interaction can generate many problems including worry, loneliness, stress, frustration, and mental health problems (Lucchetti et al., 2020). The consequences of these problems can go beyond an individual to affect the family, neighborhood and community. A holistic approach is usually needed to manage cases of this nature involving psychologists, social workers, and counselors. Religion and religious leaders are well positioned to offer such services. Guidelines on COVID-19 management from the ministry of health in Tanzania lists religious leaders as crucial palliative care providers (URT, 2020b).

Perhaps the most unique contribution of religion to prevention and fight against COVID-19 pandemic is Spiritual and Pastoral care. Religion is the only agency which can offer such services. Individuals affected by the virus and those who are recuperating, together with their families, need support and encouragement. Religious leaders do conduct spiritual and pastoral services to deliver the message of hope.

If there is anything that has united Tanzania during COVID-19 attack is the common act of prayer. Prayers were organized from the national level to all other subsequent lower levels. Political leaders and religious leaders were praying together while observing COVID-19 precautions. The national-level prayer session was conducted on 22 April 2020, where the message of taking precautions against COVID-19 was delivered and emphasized.

Modes and contents of prayer were completely autonomous. Every religion was given space to conduct its prayers according to its own style. Most congregations of prayer were coupled with homilies and songs which emphasized on one or more steps for precautions against COVID-19. Some Christian churches and mosques led special prayers which lasted for months to implore God for protection against COVID-19 pandemic (Mpota, 2020). Traditional religions also conducted rituals to ward off the deadly COVI-19.

Religious organizations have as one of their important mission the commitment to assist people especially the poor, hungry, needy and the sick (Pillay, 2020).Crisis like COVID-19 can drain resources of governments. At such times governments struggle to prioritize and re-allocate resources to save lives and stabilize the situation. The case was the same with Tanzania which could not provide all items of prevention to all citizens at one single time. Consequently, religious organizations took initiatives to assist the government delivering materials required for prevention for public use. The advantage of these organizations is that they can outsource on their own and therefore, they are not a burden to the government. But they have limited coverage. Many could only support at the local level because of limited capacities.

Religious services include Palliative care and bereavement. COVID-19 is a highly contagious disease. Diagnosed patients are quickly isolated and those who are critically ill are put in ventilators. Patients as well as their family members get frightened in such situations (Bakar et al., 2020). Hospitals adopt very strict restrictions for visitation to prevent further transmissions of the disease. In the absence of a real cure, and in a country like Tanzania where the vaccination is still debated, measures to minimize additional transmissions is to intensify restrictions. In fact hospitals in Tanzania have established designated places for COVID-19 patients.

Such restrictions cause immense emotional challenges to family members who would prefer to be at the bedside of their sick relatives and feel connected to them in their time of distress (Chen, 2021). Relatives of patients may not be allowed to enter these restricted areas or may wait for long before they receive updates about the care or treatment of their sick relatives.

This situation is aggravated when COVID-19 pandemic patients die and family members are prevented from conducting normal funeral rites. In Tanzania practices such as viewing the body of the deceased, crying, gathering, and communal funeral are considered as respectful acts of grieving and mourning for the dead. In some communities this may take days and weeks. Shortening such a process of grieving can bring stress to family members who harbor the feelings of underappreciation of the funeral of their loved ones. Inopportunity to grief properly and inability to conduct normal funeral can bring psychological repercussions to the family (Chen, 2021).

Religion help people cope with these uncertainties. Chaplains in hospitals or other religious leaders might not enter patients' room for fear of transmissions but can pray for patients in hospital vicinity or at home with other family members. This brings relief (Bakar et al., 2020). Religious leaders are crucial in times of grieving by ensuring that the departed receive respectful, safe and appropriate burial services according to stipulated guidelines, and by bringing messages of hope to families and communities struggling with loss, anxiety, sadness and despair. In times of stress and anxiety religion acts as an important coping mechanism by offering hope and meaning to people affected by such problems (Barmania & Reiss, 2020). The evidence from a study carried out in Brazil to investigate the association between spirituality and religiosity and the mental health consequences of social isolation during COVID-19 pandemic, indicate that practices of spirituality and religiosity during COVID-19 pandemic was related to positive health outcomes. Participants exhibited increased levels of hopefulness and, at the same time, showing decreased feelings of fear, worry and sadness (Lucchetti et al., 2020).

In Tanzania various religions have been conducting specific rituals for the deceased. The body of the deceased has to be thoroughly prepared and brought to the place of worship for prayers. In some religious services, worshippers either view or touch the face of the deceased as a sign of love, respect and farewell. Condolence expressions continue even after the burial involving large gatherings and frequent occasions of praying together with the bereaved families. During COVID-19 pandemic religion has continued to commit itself to this role but in a new order – that is, with restrictions to traditional practices of mourning.

Apart from its significant role of combating the spread of COVID-19 pandemic, religion can also exacerbate the transmission of the disease such as Corona Virus. In that sense, religion is considered a threat and a risk factor during pandemics. Religion and religious activities involve direct contact with masses of people. In fact, religious leaders entice their followers to attend assemblies of worship and believers can even be made to feel guilty if they don't join the congregation for communal worship (Pillay, 2020).

Religious activities such as prayer meetings, choir, rituals, ceremonies and funerals involve extensive group gatherings. Many acts of worship and devotion solicit the congregation to perform acts of handshakes, kissing, touching and embracing which can aggravate the transmission of the COVID-19 virus to oneself as well as to others.

Religions have symbols and objects which are used for devotion and worship. Worshippers touch and kiss devotional objects before, during and even after the worship. It is common in many religions, for example, to lay hands on peoples' heads as a sign of blessing, receiving Holy Communion in the hands or on the tongue, dipping fingers in a common bowl of Holy water, foot washing, and spreading carpets or mats in a common place of prayer. Religions also have special rites for the deceased. The body of the deceased has to be thoroughly washed and shrouded. In some religious services, worshippers touch the face of the deceased as a sign of love, respect and farewell. In case safety regulations are not properly undertaken, religious gatherings and objects of worship can turn to be causes of transmission for the virus.

There have been instances where religious pilgrimage sites were associated with the spread of the Corona virus. In Iran, for example, many cases of COVID-19 erupted in the Muslim holy sites of Qom and Mashhad in 2020 (Barmania & Reiss, 2020) leading to the sudden closure of these religious centers in order to contain the outbreak (Zamirirad, 2020).Similar cases were observed in South Korea, where the origin of many cases of COVID-19 is associated with the Shincheonji Church of Jesus (Barmania & Reiss, 2020).

## Challenges of religion in preventing the spread of COVID-19 in Tanzania

As mentioned earlier, getting religious leaders to work together in one roof is not an easy undertaking. In spite of the government's effort to bring them together, yet there were some religious leaders who acted on their own way. Some prophesized that through their interventions COVID-19 will not touch the land of Tanzania; others promised outright deliverance of COVID-19 patients. Furthermore, some religious leaders went ahead and closed their places of worship even though the government had not ordered shut down of such places.

Many religions in Tanzania also run social service institutions such as hospitals, schools, universities, and non-profit charitable organization like children's home, homes for institutionalized elderly and disabled. Some of these groups require full-time care and do not have abilities to follow guidelines for precautions by themselves. However, with the disruption of activities due to COVID-19, resources were dwindled and remunerations could not be timely paid and above all care providers could hardly be prevented from regular interaction with people outside the homes carrying the risk of infecting the inmates.

The president of the country and his government came under fierce attack amid apprehensions from neighboring countries and international bodies accusing him for embracing religion as a cover for his political agenda while ignoring regional conventional protocols for combating the disease. Religion was thus viewed as a cheap device of the government used to downplay standard measures of COVID-19 prevention such as masks, physical distancing and vaccines.

It would, however, be misleading to think that by embracing religion, Tanzania gave away adherence to precautions. It should be borne in mind that by taking religion on board the COVID-19 Tanzania prevention program, the government did not ignore standard guidelines for prevention. With the exception of forceful lockdown, Tanzania preserved all other standard measures of prevention and used them in tandem with religion. Religion was an umbrella technique to implement these guidelines in the form of public-private partnership commonly used for the successful implementation of many programs (Roulo & Boateng, 2020).

## Conclusion

The nexus between religion and government of Tanzania for combating COVID-19 has become an eye-opener to the success proposition of government-religion partnership in public health particularly in times of crisis. What is needed even after corona is to see efforts of solidifying this solidarity; steering up collaboration not only in situations of emergency but in general social and economic development of the country. However, utmost care should always be taken to avoid bitter experiences of the fusion of political and religious powers, which historically had negative impacts to many countries in Africa (WBG, 2020).

Tanzania has been exemplary in evaluating its strengths, social structures and localizing standard measures of COVID-19 pandemic according to local conditions and resources available including religion. Religion has played a significant role in appealing to their followers to take safety precautions and also to meet other social and spiritual challenges related to COVID-19 pandemic.

It must also be said that even with all the legitimacy and trust which religion is said to enjoy among its followers, religion did not succeed to make its followers adhere to some COVID-19 pandemic preventive measures. Principles like social distancing and wearing of masks were not relatively easy to apply in comparison to hand wash and use of sanitizers. Moreover, religious legitimacy and authority are not equidistant. They are limited and cannot be applied to all social settings. For example, religion can monitor movement or social distancing during worship but it will not be able to monitor the same people when they are in a shopping mall.

## References

Amon J. (2020). COVID-19 and Detention: Respecting Human Rights. *Health and Human Rights Journal 22(1): 366–370.*

Bakar M., Capano E., Patterson M., McIntyre B., & Walsh C. (2020). The Role of Palliative Care in Caring for the Families of Patients with COVID-19. *American Journal of Hospice & Palliative Medicine 37(10) 866–868.*

Barmania S., & Reiss M. (2020). Health Promotion Perspectives on the COVID-19 Pandemic: The Importance of Religion. *Global Health Promotion 28(1): 15–22.*

Chen C., Wittenberg E., Sullivan S., Lorenz R., & Chang Y. (2021). The Experiences of Family Members of Ventilated COVID-19 Patients in the Intensive Care Unit: A Qualitative Study. *American Journal of Hospice & Palliative Medicine 38(7): 869–876.*

Iroulo, L. C., & Boateng, O. (2020). *African States Must Localise Coronavirus Response.* (GIGA Focus Afrika, 3). Hamburg: GIGA German Institute of Global and Area Studies - Leibniz-Institut für Globale und Regionale Studien, Institut für Afrika-Studien. https://nbn-resolving.org/urn:nbn:de:0168-ssoar-67242-7

Kumar D., Malviya R., & Kumar Sharma P. (2020). Corona Virus: A Review of COVID-19. *EJMO 4(1): 8–25.*

Lucchetti G., et al. (2020). Spirituality, Religiosity and the Mental Health Consequences of Social Isolation during Covid-19 Pandemic. *International Journal of Social Psychiatry 1–8.*

Mpota S. (2020). *The Role of Religion and Traditional Medicines in Fighting COVID-19 in Tanzania.* Blog Shifting Spaces Series—LEAD Research Project. *sl*

Namwase S. (2020). Uganda's Army and Violence: How COVID-19 is Offering Hints of Change. *Conversation Africa, Inc.* (https://theconversation.com/ugandas-army-and-violence-how-covid-19-is-offering-hints-of-change-138331).

Obregón K., Morry W., Bates J., & Galway M. (2009). Achieving Polio Eradication: A Review of Health Communication Evidence and Lessons Learned in India and Pakistan. *Bulletin of the World Health Organization 87: 624–630.*

Odhiambo A. (2020). Tackling Kenya's Domestic Violence Amid COVID-19 Crisis; Lockdown Measures Increase Risks for Women and Girls. Human Rights Watch, Kenya. (https://www.hrw.org/news/2020/04/08/tackling-kenyas-domestic-violence-amid-covid-19-crisis#)

Pillay J. (2020). COVID-19 Shows the Need to Make Church More Flexible. *Transformation 37(4): 266–275.* https://doi.org/10.1177/0265378820963156

URT (United Republic of Tanzania). (2020a). *Mwongozo wa Kinga na Kuzuia Maambukizi katika Jamii Dhidi ya Ugonjwa wa Corona (COVID-19).* Dar es Salaam: Wizara ya Afya, Maendeleo ya Jamii, Jinsia, Wazee na Watoto.

URT (United Republic of Tanzania). (2020b). *Tanzania NCD Prevention and Control Program; Guidance on Provision of NCD and Mental Health Services in the Context of COVID-19 Outbreak in Tanzania (3rd ed.).* Dar es Salaam: Ministry of Health, Community Development, Gender, Elderly and Children.

URT (United Republic of Tanzania). (2020c). *Mwongozo wa Kumfuatilia Mtu aliye karibu na Mgonjwa (Contact) wa COVID-19.* Dar es Salaam: Wizara ya Afya, Maendeleo ya Jamii, Jinsia, Wazee na Watoto.

URT (United Republic of Tanzania). (2020d). *Mwongozo wa Kutoa Huduma kwa Wagonjwa wa COVID-19* kwenye Vituo vya Kutolea Huduma za Afya Nchini. Dar es Salaam: Wizara ya Afya, Maendeleo ya Jamii, Jinsia, Wazee na Watoto.

URT (United Republic of Tanzania). (2020e). *Mwongozo wa Udhibiti wa Maambukizi ya Ugonjw wa Corona (COVID-19) katika Shule, Vyuo na Taasisi za Elimu Nchini.* Dar es Salaam: Wizara ya Elimu.

TCSDF (Tanzania Civil Society Directors' Forum). (2020). *Tanzania Civil Society's Results Based Action Plan on COVID-19 Interventions.* Tanzania: Tanzania Civil Society Directors' Forum.

WBG (World Bank Group). (2020). *Tanzania Economic Update; Addressing the Impact of COVID-19.* Africa Region Macroeconomics, Trade and Investment Global Practice, Issue 14.

WHO. (2020a). *Practical Considerations and Recommendations for Religious Leaders and Faith-Based Ccommunities in the Context of COVID-19. Interim Guide. WHO/2019-nCoV/Religious_Leaders/2020.1*

WHO. (2020b). *Advice on the Use of Masks in the Context of COVID-19. Interim Guide. WHO/2019-nCoV/Religious_Leaders/2020.1*

Zamirirad A. (2020). *Three Implications of the Corona Crisis in Iran* (https://www.swp-berlin.org/en/publication/three-implications-of-the-corona-crisis-in-iran/

# 9 COVID-19 containment measures and 'prophecies' in Kenya

*Julius Gathogo*

## Introduction

Between 13 March 2020 to 25 April 2020, Kenya had tested a total of 17,492 people out of which 343 had tested positive to coronavirus (COVID-19). The country had also posted 98 recoveries and 14 deaths. Although, this is outside the scope of this chapter, Kenya had posted 177,282 infections out of the 1,887,636 cumulative tests by 17 June 2021. The country had also posted 122,018 total recoveries, out of which 88,479 were from the Home Based Care and Isolation Program while 33,539 were from the various Kenyan Health Facilities. By 17 June 2021, the cumulative fatalities stood at 3,434 (Wako, 2021). In the first two weeks of June 2021 however, the positivity rate in Western Kenya region shot up dramatically and now constituted 60% of the national caseload. The Western Kenya region also posted a positivity rate of 25%, which was against the average national positivity rate of 9%. With the entry of the so-called Indian variant (Delta), the rise in infections, in the Western Kenya region, was bound to move upfront. Following the sudden upsurge of COVID-19 cases in June 2021, the government put a partial lockdown to 13 counties from the region. That is, Kisumu, Siaya, Homa Bay, Migori, Trans Nzoia, Kakamega, Kericho, Bomet, Bungoma, Nyamira, Kisii, Busia, and Vihiga (Oketch, 2021). As noted in Angela Oketch (2021, p. 7),

> The surge in infections is higher than in Nairobi and Mombasa, which have been the epicentres of Covid-19 since the first case was announced in Kenya in March last year. Last week, the Lake region recorded 1,320 new cases, with Kisumu taking the lead with 368 cases, followed closely by Siaya (197) and Busia (196). Homa Bay registered 167 new cases, Kericho (102), Kisii (100), Migori (44), Bomet (55), Kakamega (47), Vihiga (27) and Nyamira (17). Kisumu has emerged as Kenya's new Covid-19 hotspot, overtaking Nairobi, which, due to its huge population, had naturally assumed this position since last year.

Such dramatic shifts were also witnessed by 9 October 2020, six months after the initial March-April 2020 entry of COVID-19 in Kenya, as the figures

DOI: 10.4324/9781003241096-9

shot up considerable. That is, Kenya had 40,620 COVID-19 infections out of the 580,039 cumulative tests (Maombo, 2020). The number of fatalities had risen to 755, while the number of recoveries stood at 30,876. And although the first wave of the COVID-19 pandemic had been experienced from March to August 2020, as the locked down country began to open up in September 2020, the second wave had started picking up in early October 2020 as the infections that had flattened began to move upfront. On 9 October 2020, for instance, 442 virus infections were recorded from a sample of 5,327 who were tested (Maombo, 2020). In its highest pick, infection rate would go to about 700 infections, as in the case of 10 July 2020 when 688 infections out of the 4,522 tested cases. By the end of September 2020, daily infections, countrywide, had however gone down to as below 200 infections per day. In my view thus, the second wave appears to have begun in October 2020, as high rate of infections shifted from the traditional bases of Nairobi, Mombasa, Kiambu, Busia, Machakos, and Kajiado to other Kenyan counties which were previously recording lower infections. To this end, Sharon Maombo (2020) has noted thus:

> For the first time, Nakuru takes the lead of coronavirus positives in a day recording 94 cases. Other counties with new cases include: Nairobi with 80 cases, Mombasa 47, Embu 20, Kisumu 20, Meru 15, Garissa 12, Kajiado 11, Kericho 10, Kwale 2 and Bungoma 1.

As positivity rate dropped from 9.1% to about 5% by the end of September 2020 (Tanui, 2020), a general feeling that the first wave in Kenya was over could be felt. The second wave, in my view, was less fatal, even though the opening of schools and other elements of Kenyan economy, still posed a challenge, as the six months' campaign to stop its spread had been done spiritedly. The third wave that can be said to have begun in March 2021, in my view, was more fatal, as the fatality rates shot up.

As noted earlier, the first case of COVID-19 was however confirmed in Kenya on 13 March 2020 (Star 2020). Statistically, the pandemic which was first reported in Wuhan, China, on 31 December 2019, and quickly spread across the world, had infected at least 2,744,614 people by 24 April 2020. While Kenya had registered 14 deaths by 24 April 2020, the global context had registered 191,791 deaths; and while Kenya had registered 95 recoveries, the global context had registered 755,443. In the specific African context, the Worldmeter's count showed that there were 28,351 and 1,301 deaths (Menya, 2020).

In the nature of things, the current crisis, where 2020 experienced Coronavirus epidemic from China, almost replicates the 1918 Influenza pandemic that killed over 100 million people (Andayi et al., 2020). The main difference, however, is that COVID-19 was caused by a different virus, and there was very little likelihood that it could kill such a large number of people, as in the case of the 1918 influenza pandemic. The First World War (hereafter, WWI) was about to end, when the mysterious disease appeared. In order to maintain the morale of soldiers on the battlefield, Britain, Germany and France decided to hide the information. Only the neutral Spain reported about the virus. The constant reports from Spain coupled with the illness of King Alfonso XIII (1886–1941) of Spain finally lifted the lid on the severity of the influenza. This also created the wrong perception that the disease could have originated from Spain; hence the name "Spanish flu." It is worthwhile, at this stage, to appreciate that Alfonso XIII, also known as El Africano or the African, was King of Spain from 1886 until the proclamation of the Second Republic in 1931. Alfonso was monarch from birth as his father, Alfonso XII, had died the previous year (Andayi et al., 2020; Barry et al. 2008).

Thus, while 1918–1919 brought Spanish Flu, the 2019–2020 ushered in Coronavirus, hence it equally threatened the people's lives in a novel way. Put differently, the abundance life (John 10:10) that led to the act of incarnation has found itself under test from different historical times. Was there any prophetic signal and/or any ancestral communication? During the 1918–1919 influenza pandemic, otherwise called Spanish Flu, our African ancestors survived despite lacking the genius of science and technology that obtains to date.

## COVID-19 in Kenya (March–April 2020)

By the end of March 2020, there was no vaccine to prevent coronavirus disease (COVID-19). Instead Citizens were advised to protect themselves and help prevent spreading the virus to others by: Washing their hands regularly for 20 seconds, with soap and running water or alcohol-based hand rub; Covering their noses and mouths with disposable tissues or flexed elbow when coughing or sneezing; Avoiding close contacts (1 meter or 3 feet) with people who are unwell; and were also advised to stay at home and self-isolation from others in the household if one felt unwell. Equally, they were advised not to touch their own eyes, noses, or mouths if their hands were not clean.

Of importance to note is that the first confirmed case of coronavirus in Kenya took place on13 March 2020 (Star 2020). In this case, a 27-year-old Kenyan woman (by name Ivy Brenda Cherotich) who travelled from the United States via London, was confirmed after three consecutive tests (Corona, 2020c). Subsequently, the Kenyan government identified and isolated a number of people who had come into contact with her. Other cases went as follows:

• On 15 March, Cabinet Secretary for Health, Mutahi Kagwe, announced that two people who had sat next to the initial patient on the aircraft in transit from the United States had also tested positive for the virus (Corona, 2020 b; Corona, 2020d). Schools were closed and public gatherings were prohibited. Also, as a result, the country's borders were closed to all except Kenyan citizens and legal residents.

- On 16 March, the government through its spokesman Colonel Cyrus Oguna said on an update that there were another three people who were suspected to be carriers of the virus and that their results were to be released soon (Corona, 2020d).
- On 17 March, it was announced by the Health Secretary that a fourth case had been diagnosed. On 18 March, three more cases confirmed were by the Health Secretary, bringing the total confirmed cases in Kenya to seven (Corona 2020a).
- On 22 March, eight more cases were confirmed by the Health Secretary, bringing the total cases confirmed to 15. The government confirmed it was tracing 363 people who are believed to have had contact with the eight new cases.
- On 23 March, another case was confirmed bringing the total confirmed cases to 16.
- On 24 March, nine more cases reported for a total of 25 nationally.
- On 25 March, the first recovery was confirmed, and three more cases were recorded, bringing the total confirmed cases to 28 (Corona, 2020e).
- On 26 March, three more cases were recorded and bringing the total confirmed cases to 31. In addition to Nairobi, the government confirmed that corona virus cases in Kenya are spread among four other counties, namely Kajiado, Mombasa, Kilifi, and Kwale. On the same date, the first death of a person infected with the corona virus was reported in Kenya. The patient was a 66-year-old Kenyan man who had contracted the virus while traveling from South Africa via Eswatini.
- On March 28, the ministry of health confirmed Seven more cases, bringing a total tally of confirmed COVID-19 cases in Kenya to 38. On the same day, the government announced that two patients who had earlier tested positive had tested negative and were awaiting a second test to confirm they had fully recovered.
- On 29 March, four more cases were recorded bringing the total confirmed cases to 42. During a briefing on a Sunday afternoon, the then Health Cabinet Secretary/Minister, Mutahi Kagwe, said of the four, one was a Kenyan, one American, one Cameroonian and one a Burkinabé. Hon. Kagwe said three of the cases were based in Nairobi and one in Mombasa. The CS said of the 42 cases, 24 are male while 18 are females. Nairobi leads with 31 cases followed by Kilifi (six), Mombasa (Three) and Kwale and Kajiado on each. On 30 March 2020, the number of confirmed cases went up to 50.
- On 30 March, eight positive cases were confirmed, making a total of 50; while on 31 March, nine more cases were confirmed, making a total of 59 cases. On 1 April 2020, 22 cases were confirmed, making a total of 81 cases countrywide. The figure went beyond 100 on 2 April 2020 when an additional 29 cases were confirmed. This brought the total number

to 110 nationally. This led President Uhuru Kenyatta to announce a cessation of movement in and out of The Nairobi Metropolitan Area for a containment period of 21 days, on 6 April 2020. Apart from Nairobi, President Kenyatta ordered the cessation of movement to other highly affected areas such Kilifi, Mombasa, and Kwale in the coastal region of Kenya. On 7th and 8 April, a total of 14 cases each were confirmed, making a total of 179 Kenyans; and by 15 April, the country had registered 225 confirmed cases, with a total of ten deaths, and 53 recoveries. Between 24 and 25 April, 23 cases were confirmed as positive making a total of 343 cases in Kenya, and 98 recoveries.

• Additionally, President Kenyatta announced more measures of combating COVID-19 on 25 April 2020 that included: An extension of the nationwide 7pm to 5am curfew by another round of 21 days; and a further extension of the cessation of movement order affecting Nairobi, Mombasa, Kilifi, and Kwale counties by 21 days. He also announced minimal operations at hotels and other eateries in select counties. Most significantly, he announced a rollout of the National Hygiene Programme on 29 April 2020. This initiative was geared towards creating a healthier environment and jobs. The first phase was envisaged to employ 26,148 workers over 30 days, and more than 100,000 youths progressively (Menya, 2020).

## Response to COVID-19 pandemic

Admirably, the Kenyan context appears to have learnt from the 1918 Spanish Influenza which was contained belatedly thereby taking a global mortality rate of 2.5%. It was responsible for the death of 0.0052% of the world population at one person out of 18,750 (Burnet and Clark, 1942). Thus, in response to the rise of COVID-19 cases, the Government closed all schools and directed that both private and public sector workers to work from home, wherever possible, from 15 March 2020. Additionally, travel restrictions were imposed (Kenyatta, 2020). This was meant to prevent non-Kenyans from entering the country. The Kenyan nationals were also required to self-quarantine for a minimum of 14 days. By then, Kenya had only three COVID-19 confirmed cases, which shows that the steps were taken early enough.

Following the confirmation of an additional eight cases that brought a total figure to 16 nationally on 22 March 2020, the Kenyan Government suspended all international flights with effect from 25 March 2020. Cargo flights were, however, not suspended. Anyone entering Kenya was henceforth compulsorily made to quarantine for 14 days before being allowed to leave the city of Nairobi or any other entry point, though at one's own cost. Other measures taken on 22 March included: All bars were to remain closed from 22 March, restaurants allowed only for takeaway services, all public vehicles were to adhere to passenger-distancing guidelines, all public gatherings in churches, mosques, funerals, political rallies, and wedding gatherings of more than 15 people were banned forthwith (Kenyatta, 2020).

## Economic response

As noted above, the confirmation of three additional cases of COVID-19, on 25 March 2020, sent national panic, as reports of massive deaths in the western world had already reached the country with equal fears. Hence, President Kenyatta announced a nation-wide curfew, from 7pm to 5am, starting from 27 March 2020 (Kenyatta, 2020). Certainly, all these measures had huge negative impact for a country that was struggling to clear debts with international lenders. It was also huge inconvenience to individuals living in fledgling economy. Nevertheless, saving life became a priority rather than saving an economy as President Kenyatta went on to unveil measures to buffer Kenyans against financial hardships arising from the above measures. Such measures included reduction of Pay As You Earn (PAYE) from a maximum of 30% to 25%, 100% tax relief to Kenyans earning USD 228, reduction of resident income tax to 25%, reduction of turnover tax rate from 3% to 1% for all micro, small and medium enterprises, temporary suspension of loan defaulters whose loan account was in arrears effective 1 April 2020, USD 95 million were set aside for vulnerable groups, and the reduction of Value Added Tax from 16% to 14% with effect from 1 April 2020 (Kenyatta, 2020).

The Kenyan government also increased the allocation of funds for health care, plus other fiscal adjustments to the national economy such as: channelling USD 9.5 million from the Universal Health Coverage kitty to the employment of new health workers to combat COVID-19, slash salaries for both the President and the Deputy President by 80%, pay cut for all Cabinet Ministers by 30%, and the Principal Secretaries by 20%. Other government employees, civil servants, lecturers, teachers and others were requested to voluntarily contribute to COVID-19 kitty via a pay cut. Other measures included, requesting State and public officers aged 50 and above, and who have other pre-existing medical concerns to take leave from work or work from home. Those working in the security department were however excluded. Further, the Central Bank lowered the interest rates from 8.25% to 7.25%. The Central Bank or the National Reserve Bank reduced the Cash Reserve Ratio from 5.25% to 4.25% and increased liquidity of Ksh 35 billion to commercial banks (Kenyatta, 2020). The idea here was to help the latter to be in a position to provide loan services to the ordinary citizens.

## Some setbacks

Following the declaration of the national curfew on 25 March 2020, from 7pm to 5am, police brutality akin to the dark days of British colonialism (1920–1963) was witnessed in various parts of Kenya, and especially

Mombasa and Nairobi. In these unfortunate situations, video footages that were disseminated through the social media showed the police giving senseless beatings to people who were unable to get back to their houses by 7pm. In one instance, a truck driver who was caught up with time had his arm broken out of these beatings, after he was accused of daring to fight the police. The police officers who broke his arm were later sacked by the government after both the social and mainstream media exposed the shameful act. The 27 March 2020 clearly contradicted the goal of the curfew especially when the police used teargasses on innocent and oblivious citizens in Mombasa and Nairobi, a phenomenon that caused a huge outcry in Nairobi. As Ferry Services delayed in Mombasa's Likoni area, the innocent people, rather than the Ferry Management, bore the brunt. Equally, the long queues in Nairobi caused delays in getting into the public transport vehicles, yet the police were shown beating huge crowds that were innocently waiting for their turn to get into the public service vehicles.

The 27 March 2020 episode also saw police unnecessarily detaining people who were unable to "obey curfew hours." Worst of all, ordinary people were pushed in crowded areas, contrary to curfew's goals of keeping social distance from one another. Luckily, such brutalities meted across the country were condemned across the political divide, and President Uhuru Kenyatta eventually sacked some of the rogue police officers who treated ordinary men and women with blatant contempt. In the nature of things, Mireri Junior (2020) noted, thus:

> Leaders across the political divide have condemned the brutality meted out on Kenyans by police officers who were enforcing a government's curfew to curb the spread of coronavirus. Led by Senate Majority Leader Kipchumba Murkomen, the leaders said the action of the police as was witnessed on Friday evening defeated the very purpose of the curfew. Police and commuters clashed at the Likoni ferry in Mombasa Friday afternoon, a scenario occasioned by overcrowding as residents rushed to beat the curfew deadline. The situation was not different in Kisumu and Eldoret towns as police teargassed Kenyans for flouting the curfew rules. Photos and clips of police beating up Kenyans who allegedly failed to adhere to the curfew emerged online with netizens condemning the police for using excessive force in handling Kenyans. The Elegeyo Marakwet senator said the police action, endangered the lives of many Kenyans, saying lumping people together could have led to more infections if one of them had contracted coronavirus.

## Economic impact

Apart from the police brutality, noted above, Kenyans suffered in the economic front. Micro and macro businesses suffered alike. There were reports that a family feasted on its own pet, after losing out their economic livelihoods. Apart from hawkers and ordinary vendors who lost out as a result of the lockdown, travel restrictions reduced Kenya's hotel, tourism, and flower industries to nothing (Menya, 2020). Some Kenyans were however able to switch from their urban jobs to rural labour, so as to feed their families. The economic impact thus cannot be explained fully at this stage. Concrete figures will however be explained with time. In the author's Emmanuel Anglican Church, Changamwe, Venerable Geoffrey Guyo Dida employed a creative method of sustaining the Church through online services. A Church pay-bill account was also instituted, as weekly reminders to submit membership fees, love offerings, tithes and other things was set up by the end of March 2020. A message of "Stay Safe" would always conclude the reminder.

## Impact on stewardship of creation

Stewardship of Creation refers to the theological belief that human beings are managers of what God has put in place in the world, for "The earth is the LORD's, and everything in it, the world, and all who live in it" (Psalm 24:1). As such, responsible religious communities, as Kenyans claims to be, will always address environmental challenges in the era of corona virus, the ecological challenges posed by the dumping of plastic masks across Kenya's territorial space, the care of abandoned street children as lockdown denied them 'leftover' food, the rivers that are now left as dumping sites for residues of COVID-19, and animals and birds who relied on human beings and were now affected by the lockdown that had affected various parts of Kenya's territorial space among other concerns (Mugo & Gathogo 2018). Certainly, a lot changed after October 2020 as the national lockdown was being revised, and the economy started to open up.

According to Pkemoi Ng'enoh (2020), tens of stray Cats living around Nairobi City Hall were left with nothing to eat after several hotels closed down in line with the government directive that the restaurants close until further notice to curb the pandemic. Previously, Cats were feeding from leftovers dumped by the joints before they would disappear to their hideouts around Nairobi City Hall and other places around Central Business District. The same case scenario was also witnessed in other Kenyan cities. James Mulwa (quoted in Ng'enoh (2020:7), a security guard in Nairobi explained, thus:

> The Cats are starving. Before, they would roam around searching for food, but that is not the case today since coronavirus came knocking on our doors. Sometimes, we feed them with bread; not long ago, I found a dead Cat around Nyayo house. I think it died out of starvation. For the first time, a dog was spotted along Moi Avenue. It is starvation.

Such stories are in continuum with an early April 2020 announcement by the Kenya Society for the Protection and Care of Animals (PCA) that some animals under their care risk starving during the lockdown (Ng'enoh, 2020). The organization cited lack of food donors and minimum movement across the cities as the real challenge. The society which had 170 Dogs, 105 Cats, four Horses, and nine Donkeys by April 2020 (Ng'enoh, 2020) was already overwhelmed and could do little for the roaming domestic animals, some of whom were dying one by one. A similar scenario, where pets and other domestic animals were abandoned, was visible in India, Philippines and other parts of the world, as lockdown continued to affect the theology of stewardship negatively. With reference to India, Niharika Sharma (2020) has noted that,

> When they found him in an East Delhi locality, towards the end of February, the tall, dark, and handsome Labrador was hungry, weak, scared, and depressed. Apparently abandoned by his owners in the wake of the coronavirus pandemic, the well-bred dog had taken shelter inside a building under construction...Noticing his plight, someone called Ummeed Social Welfare Society, an Uttar Pradesh-based NGO that took him in. While the streets of India emptying out over fears of the novel coronavirus and the lockdown announced in its wake, many localities are witnessing the emergence of a new set of residents: stray pedigree pets.... What's fuelling the fear among the pet owners are news reports of a couple of dogs and a cat being tested positive for the virus in Hong Kong.

As the "creation groans as in the pains of childbirth" (Romans 8:22), in the post COVID-19 Kenya, one wonders how long it would take, and how best it can be handled. Although there were reports from oral sources that pets can contract COVID-19, the World Health Organization (WHO) clarified, in their website that there is no evidence that they can transmit it. Certainly, the care of animals is a religious duty (Genesis 1:28) that cannot be abdicated. In any case, the Psalmist (147:9) is explicit that God "gives to the beast its food; and to the young ravens that cry." The care for the cosmos is undoubtedly the broader message imbedded in COVID-19 pandemic.

## Coronavirus and 'prophecies'

After Kenya's Minister Health, Hon Mutahi Kagwe announced the first confirmed case of coronavirus on 13 March 2020, prophets and their prophetic extravaganza began. This went hand-in-hand with biblical insights, mainly from the Afro-Pentecostal wing of the church, some of which were tried to prove that COVID-19 was a biblical fulfilment; others saw it as prophecies come true, while yet others saw it as a punishment for unrepentant Kenyans. The latter failed to appreciate that it was a global challenge where China, Italy, Spanish, and the United States were some of the most affected. Some of the biblical and/or religious messages that have been circulated through the social media, between March and April 2020, include:

> As the world wide quarantine proceeds of Covid-19, even from the Church, the Holy Mountain where we meet our God of mercy, it is now the moment to quarantine from every kind of sin for God to embrace us back. Let us make Church a place of worship, love one another and fear God. Let us make the world a garden of joy. Let us take a moment with our hearts and ask ourselves individually, what is God feeling about us? Jeremiah 7:3, 8–15.

In rephrasing and 'exegeting' Jeremiah 7:3 which says, "Reform your ways and your actions, and I will let you live in this place," the fulfilment of a prophecy" assumes that COVID-19 was just a punishment from God. In other words, the medical dimension was relegated to the periphery, as the spiritual dimension took a centre stage. The write-up, which was sent to the author via WhatsApp forum, gives a 'clear' impression that if Kenya repented her sins, a chance to live now would be guaranteed. This however turned problematic in that Kenya claims to be an 80% Christian. With very committed Christians in Kenya's territorial space equally bearing the brunt as their businesses were closed down as they obeyed the government imposed curfew and the lockdown that went hand-in-hand, one wondered why they too were under punishment from God. Or was it part of persecutions, martyrdom, and/or trials and temptations that every believer undergoes? Why were the Churches, bars, public gatherings, and schools classed together by the government and were collectively closed down in mid-March 2020? Such happenings did not resonate well with prophet Jeremiah's call for a reformation of ways, as the Holy shrines were not spared as well.

The above 'prophetic' insight that was circulated in Kenya's social media in March and April 2020 is in tandem with another one which was also sent to the author via WhatsApp forum which said thus:

> There is an upcoming disaster worse than COVID-19. Once you are in, you are doomed forever. COVID-19 will soon end, but if you don't put your ways right, and the rapture takes you unawares or you leave this earth without Christ, then the game is over.

While most of these 'prophetic' messages urged revival of the Christians, the pandemic was nevertheless reduced to a mere spiritual (religious) matter without taking cognizance all pillars of culture, that includes economics, politics, kinship, ethics, and aesthetics (Mugambi, 1989). While religion is a critical pillar of culture, working on one pillar alone is inadequate. Further, although the call to wash our hearts, keep a distance from evil, cover oneself with a sneeze of sin, don't shake hands with abomination, don't hug a false teaching (heresy), and sanitize one's life, were some of the 'prophetic' insights that were circulated around the country, the danger remained in that it failed to factor in other pillars of culture thereby rendering it theologically impotent.

Another critical dimension is the numerous 'prophecies' by various well-known afro-Pentecostal leaderships in Kenya. As Damaris Parsitau (2020) says, the

> Self-proclaimed Prophet Owuor has trafficked in fear-mongering threats, and has even claimed that he had prophesied the pandemic. He also said it would kill people in Asia because the continent rejected his prophecy. In Kenya, a section of the public has cajoled him to unleash his "mighty prophetic powers" to fend off the virus. They have also called on him to pray it away.

Parsitau (2020) wonders why there are no spiritual powers to perform miracles and heal coronavirus patients when it is so desperately needed. She goes on to cite some afro-Pentecostal clerics who, in her view, appeared too ignorant of COVID-19; hence they were in a confused state when the government closed the churches. She cites the case of

> Apostles James Maina Ng'ang'a's video on coronavirus – where he is unable to pronounce the word coronavirus – showed not just his sheer ignorance, but also how ill-equipped he and his ilk are when it comes to offering solutions to such complex 21st-century problems.

The ignorance among the afro-Pentecostal leaders was further displayed by Rev. Nathan Kirimi, a Meru-Tigania-based Pastor (Eastern Kenya), of Jesus Winner Ministry, who angered many Kenyans when he dismissed COVID-19 as a global hoax (Muchui, 2020a). He went on to say that God had instructed him not to close his church or terminate services as coronavirus is inexistent and a non-issue. By 18 March 2020 when Pastor Kirimi was dismissing it as a hoax, coronavirus had already claimed 9,800 lives globally. In giving the government directive on banning social gatherings, the Minister for Health, Hon Mutahi Kagwe invoked the Public Health Act (PHA) which gives him broad legal authority to impose various forms of restrictions whenever a public health crisis occurs (Muchui, 2020a).

Nevertheless, Rev. Nathan Kirimi was strongly censured by the main leadership of Jesus Winner Ministry Church who disowned him for misleading the congregants on the coronavirus pandemic (Muchui, 2020b). Kirimi had previously lashed out at Bishops who had suspended worship services by 15 March 2020, as his prophecy had shown that COVID-19 was a hoax. Bishop Edward Mwai, the head of Jesus Winner Ministry, however dismissed Rev. Kirimi's position as personal opinion, unlawful, and against the Government's policy of containing the deadly virus. In a statement through the

Church's Media Channels that came after a huge protest by Kenyans in the social media, Bishop Mwai said that the

> management, Board and the Secretary of Jesus Winner Ministry wish to inform Kenyans that the statements made by Rev Nathan Kirimi of Meru are his personal opinions and do not reflect the official position of the church. The board has already instituted remedies and summoned the pastor to ensure that such an occurrence won't be repeated now or in the future.
>
> (Muchui, 2020b)

As David Muchui (2020a) has comparatively noted,

> The claims by Mr Kirimi come as South Korea's thousands of COVID-19 cases were linked to a religious sect known as Shincheonji Church of Jesus [February 2020]. A new wave of infections in South Korea was also linked to Grace River Church, which had defied calls to suspend services. Media reports indicate that the church finally closed its doors on Sunday after 46 worshippers, including the pastor and his wife, tested positive for coronavirus. South Korea has recorded more than 8,400 cases [by 18 March 2020] with half of them linked to the Shincheonji Church of Jesus.

While Rev Kirimi could be blamed for communicating his "theological" and "prophetic" position openly, he nonetheless spoke for a huge constituency of afro-Pentecostal leaders who did not have the press around them. As noted earlier, various 'prophetic' positions were aired out, some describing COVID-19 as a "non-believer" affair, and others described it as a punishment to "homosexual nations" among other remarks from the leadership that claimed prophetic revelations. Such bizarre positions pointed to an ignorant leadership, especially among the evangelical wing of the Church.

Parsitau (2020) perceptively cautions that "there is a fear that COVID-19 will expose the clergy's dark underbelly and call to question Africa's faith-healing and miracle industry" (Parsitau, 2020). She intuitively cautions that,

> the clergy has been averse to scientific discoveries because science makes their miraculous shenanigans questionable. Prayers for healing have not calmed a shocked and scared populace. Many a clergy has frowned on science, medicine and theological education, instead spiritualising even non-spiritual matters as serious as the coronavirus pandemic. Science shakes the foundation of their spiritual teachings. After all, and in the case of this pandemic, science has proved to be more practical and reliable than faith.

Parsitau's radical position on the practicality of science, as opposed to faith, is certainly driven by this unprecedented act where schools, churches and other social institutions were closed together, globally, following the emergency of the COVID-19. Didn't science appear to be ruling the world as opposed to faith? Or has Goliath won the first battle but lose out to the metaphorical David (faith) in the long run? Has Parsitau failed to be a good judge who listens and observes both the plaintiff and the defendant equally and more keenly? As a good scholar in philosophy and religious studies, Parsitau is partly informed by the global happenings where for instance, the world-renowned Pastor Joel Osteen of Lakewood Church, Houston in the United States had to equally close his church. Osteen Church attracts 50,000 peoples upwards. Additionally, other mega Churches, as in the case of Pastor T. D. Jakes' Potters House also suspended their Church services (Muchui, 2020b) that equally attract thousands of enthusiastic adherents.

## Conclusion

The chapter started by addressing the nature of COVID-19 pandemic in Kenya since the first case was reported on 13 March 2020. In this case, a 27-year-old Kenyan woman by name Ivy Brenda Cherotich, who travelled from the United States via London, was confirmed after three consecutive tests. Although the scope of the chapter was religio-social reaction of COVID-19 pandemic in the months of March and April 2020, it was able to clarify that Kenya had posted 177,282 infections out of the 1,887,636 cumulative tests, 122,018 total recoveries, and the cumulative fatalities stood at 3,434 by 17 June 2021(Wako 2021). The chapter also sought to understand the place of the Kenyan Church in light of all this and explained the dangerous trajectories that were witnessed among some religious leaders who over spiritualised a medical issue.

In its findings, the chapter has ably compared COVID-19 with the Spanish Flu of 1918 which had critical and similar characteristics with COVID-19. The chapter has also underlined the huge fatalities of the 1918, where about 100 million people died. With Kenya responding to COVID-19 without hesitation, the pandemic, may after all not do much damage as envisaged. With good religio-social management, the setbacks noted in this chapter would be eliminated. Likewise, there is need for a sober prophetic voice from religious institutions in delicate matters, as in the case of pandemics. This may drive the religious leaderships to consult experts and professionals in their relevant fields in technical issues such as COVID-19 before making public pronouncements or sending messages.

## References

Andayi, F., Chaves, S. S., and Widdowson, M. 2020. "Impact of the 1918 Influenza Pandemic in Coastal Kenya," *Tropical Medicine and Infectious Diseases*, *Trop. Med. Infect. Dis.* 4, 91. doi:10.3390/tropicalmed4020091 (accessed 21 March 2020).
Barry, J. M., Viboud, C., and Simonsen, L. 2008. Cross-Protection between Successive Waves of the 1918–1919 Influenza Pandemic: Epidemiological Evidence from US Army Camps and from Britain. *J. Infect. Dis.* 198, 1427–1434.

China. 2020. https://www.who.int/docs/default-source/coronaviruse/who-china-joint-mission-on-COVID-19-final-report.pdf (accessed 30 March 2020).

Corona. 2020a. "Kenya confirms first coronavirus case—VIDEO." *Daily Nation*. Retrieved 30 March 2020.

Corona. 2020b. *"Kenya coronavirus cases rises to 3". Capital News. 15 March 2020.* Retrieved 30 March 2020.

Corona. 2020c. "Kenya reports 3 suspected virus cases". *Nation News.* 16 March 2020. Retrieved 30 March 2020.

Corona. 2020d. "Kenya coronavirus cases rise to four." *Daily Nation.* Retrieved 30 March 2020.

Corona. 2020e. "Health ministry confirms 3 more coronavirus cases," *capitalfm. co.ke.* 18 March 2020 (Retrieved 30 March 2020).

Junior, M. 2020. "Coronavirus: Stop bludgeoning Kenyans during curfew, leaders tell police," *Standard Digital*, 28 March 2020, https://www.standardmedia.co.ke/article/2001365989/stop-beating-kenyans-during-curfew-leaders-tell-police (accessed 26 April 2020).

Kenyatta, U. 2020. *Presidential Address on the State Interventions to cushion Kenyans against Economic Effects of COVID-19 Pandemic on 25 March 2020*. Nairobi: State House.

Maombo, S. 2020. "Seven deaths as Kenya's virus cases near 39,000," *Daily Nation*. https://www.the-star.co.ke/news/2020-10-02-seven-deaths-as-kenyas-virus-cases-near-39000/ (accessed 9 October 2020).

Menya, W. 2020. "COVID-19: Uhuru extends curfew by 21 days as cases rise to 343," *Daily Nation*. https://www.nation.co.ke/news/COVID-19-Kenya-cases-rise-to-343/1056-5534198-hookrm/index.html (accessed 26 April 2020).

Muchui, D. 2020a. "Exposed: The Meru pastor courting coronavirus," *Daily Nation*, 19 March 2020, https://www.nation.co.ke/counties/meru/The-pastor-courting-Coronavirus/1183302-5496676-g8qrdc/index.html (accessed 24 April 2020).

Muchui, D. 2020b. "Church disowns rogue Meru pastor courting coronavirus," *Daily Nation*, 19 March 2020, https://www.nation.co.ke/counties/meru/The-pastor-courting-Coronavirus/1183302-5496676-g8qrdc/index.html (accessed 25 April 2020).

Mugambi, J.N.K. 1989a. *African Heritage and Contemporary Christianity*. Nairobi: Longman.

Mugo, M., and Gathogo, J. 2018. "The Use of Indigenous Resources in Environmental Conservation in Ngugi wa Thiong'o's *Murogi wa Kagogo:* A religio-Cultural Perspective," *JJEOSHS*, 1(1), 1–18.

Ng'enoh, P. 2020. "Kanjo Cats starving on deserted streets," *The Nairobian*, No. 1528, 24 April-30 April, 2020.

Oketch, A. 2021. "State declares 13 lake region counties Covid-19 hotspots," *Daily Nation*, 17 June 2021, https://nation.africa/kenya/counties/state-declares-13-lake-region-counties-covid-19-hotspots-3441134 (accessed 18 June 2021).

Parsitau, D. 2020. "Religion in the age of coronavirus," *The Elephant – Speaking the Truth*, https://www.theelephant.info/features/2020/03/23/religion-in-the-age-of-coronavirus/ (accessed 25 April 2020).

Sharma, N. 2020. "Locked out Indians are abandoning their pets on the streets—helpless, scared, and hungry," *QuartzIndia*, 2 April 2020, https://qz.com/india/1826006/coronavirus-scares-indians-into-abandoning-pet-dogs-cats/ (accessed 25 April 2020).

Star 2020. https://www.the-star.co.ke/authors/clairemunde. "First Kenyan dies of COVID-19- CS Kagwe". *The Star.* (Retrieved 31 March 2020).

Tanui, C. 2020. "Kenya: Covid-19 positivity rate drops to 5.4%," *Capital FM*, https://allafrica.com/stories/202010090121.html (accessed 9 October 2020).

Wako, A. 2021. "COVID-19: Kenya records 660 new cases, 10.7 percent positivity rate," *Daily Nation*, 17 June 2021, https://nation.africa/kenya/news/covid-19-kenya-records-660-new-cases-10-7-pc-positivity-rate--3440992 (accessed 18 June 2021).

# 10 Christian religious understandings and responses to COVID-19 in Eswatini

*Sonene Nyawo*

## Introduction

The population of Eswatini (formerly Swaziland) estimated at 1.2 million is struggling to cope with the escalating numbers of confirmed cases of COVID-19 pandemic. This unprecedented health phenomenon has affected all sectors of human and business life. It has also received a lot of attention and interpretations regarding its origins, intentions and eventually, how it is going to recede. In most cases, these have either been economic, biological and or mystical/spiritual. As measures of trying to 'flatten the curve' as many would call it, local and international authorities have come up with strategies and regulations that guide human activities across the globe. The main mandate of such has been to reduce human to human transmission of the virus. This has seen many nations embarking on lockdowns, which have restricted the operation of multiple sectors of business that were deemed as not being essential. Restrictions in people's movement both locally and internationally, and assembling in mass gatherings, amongst a range of other preventative measures, were also introduced. The U.N. Secretary-General, Antonio Guterres, in April 2020 when he was appealing to religious leaders of all faiths to unite in fighting against COVID-19 stated that "[t]he coronavirus pandemic, with its lockdowns and social distancing, has led to a "surreal world" of silent streets, shuttered stores, empty places of worship and of worry" (Guterres 2020). This shows that the pandemic had far reaching effects to different communities, nations and states. Eswatini's first case of COVID-19 was confirmed on 14 March 2020, and infections and deaths have continued to rise drastically.

In terms on religion, legislatively, Eswatini has no official religion, but everyday practices point to Christianity's overriding popularity. Whilst the country's constitution prohibits religious discrimination and provides for freedom of thought, conscience, and religion, including the right to worship, alone or in community with others, and to change religion or belief, most Emaswati identify as Christian (International Religious Freedom Report: Swaziland 2019 International Religious Freedom Report: Eswatini. 2019. Washington: Bureau of Democracy, Human Rights, and Labor, U.S.

DOI: 10.4324/9781003241096-10

Department of State [Google Scholar]). Forms of Swazi Traditional Religion like divination, herbal healing and environmental and ancestral spirit veneration also make up this religious landscape and elide with Swazi culture, a reified set of practices and values shored up by the monarchy in national ceremonies, clothing, tourism, heritage programming and everyday ideations of custom (Golomski & Nyawo 2017). Christian churches affiliate to three ecumenical bodies: the Eswatini Conference of Churches (ECC formerly SCC), the Council of Swaziland Churches[1] (CSC) and the League of African Churches in Eswatini (LACE formerly LACS).

Churches previously established by European and US missionaries founded the SCC in 1929. The overriding aim of SCC had been to foster cooperation among the various mission churches engaged in Christian evangelism and includes several Protestant churches like Church of the Nazarene, Assemblies of God and the Evangelical Church. The SCC experienced a schism in 1976 when liberal members withdrew to form the CSC, which includes the Catholic, Methodist and Anglican churches. While SCC has primary aims in building new churches and conversion, CSC strives to address social concerns in society such as poverty, underdevelopment and injustice. Unlike SCC and CSC, King Sobhuza II formed LACS in the early-1940s in liaison with clergy belonging to African Independent Churches and in response to attempts by the British colonial government and some European missionaries to ban these churches in the then Swaziland. Given Sobhuza's legitimation and mentorship role in the formation of this body, the constitution of LACS recognises the King as its life-long patron, and LACS has been credited with rendering unequivocal support for Swati cultural nationalism (Golomski & Nyawo 2017). Like CSC and ECC, LACE aims to promote fellowship and unity among churches. Aside from a few limited instances (International Religious Freedom Report: Eswatini 2019 International Religious Freedom Report: Eswatini. 2019. Washington: Bureau of Democracy, Human Rights, and Labor, U.S. Department of State [Google Scholar]), there is an overall climate of religious tolerance in Eswatini and between different Christian churches.

People in this predominantly Christian and traditional nation interpret and understand their circumstances in accordance with their religious thought patterns; thus, many fascinating behaviours are performed in the name of religion (Hood et al. 2001). During difficult moments in life, they seek and collaborate with God, in solving both minor and major stressors (del Castillo & Alino 2020); hence Koenig's (2012) submission that numerous empirical studies identify religion as an integral part of human existence. With regard to COVID-19 pandemic, like elsewhere in the world, its dire effects have destabilised Emaswati; it has strained the social fabric, threatened the health care operations, and has put the faith of many Christians to test (del Castillo et al. 2020). However, religious beliefs which are powerful and coherent forces, as described by Barmania & Reiss (2020), become a coping resource (Hart & Koenig 2020). The chapter therefore seeks to establish that whilst Christians in Eswatini hold various religious understandings of the pandemic, which can be a coping resource, the reality is that the pandemic continues to represent a significant stressor for the nation; fear of death and suffering is acutely elevated, Emaswati are ill, hungry and bereaved. The solution lies with church leaders as 'gatekeepers', that they should change their mindset towards COVID-19 and face reality that it is wrecking lives. Thus, they would need to balance religion with practical steps to reduce infections.

## How Christians understand COVID-19[2]

In as much as the drivers of the world economies alongside health practitioners have had a lot to say in response to COVID-19, the Christian community that experience Christ within their traditional thought patterns have also contributed to our understanding of the current situation in Eswatini. Christians have seen it as a punishment for sin; a spiritual warfare; and a fulfilment of biblical prophecies about the end times. The enquiry that then arises is that can Christian responses to the pandemic bind the nation together and contribute to successfully coping with the pandemic, or might they lead to low perception of risk and create a fatalistic attitude in the face of the virus?

### *COVID-19 is God's punishment for sin*

In the Church's response to the COVID-19 pandemic, the most recurring theme has been that the nation has sinned against God, and Emaswati have to fast and pray for God's forgiveness. There have been national prayers convened by the Ministry of Home Affairs, at the King's directive, to carry out this mandate. His Majesty King Mswati III through the Prime Minister of Eswatini Ambrose Mandvulo Dlamini declared a national day of fasting on March 28, 2020, which was followed by the National Day of Prayer the next day. The theme of the prayer was 'God heal our land', whilst the theme verse was 2 Chronicles 2:13–14 which called the nation to repent from wickedness. The prayer was attended by 20 people; pastors and leaders of the three Christian ecumenical bodies; some cabinet ministers; and royalty. The rest of the nation was invited to follow proceedings of service through live broadcast in various media platforms, whilst "they convert their homes into altars, ask for God's forgiveness and seek God's intervention so that no one would die from the virus" (*Eswatini News* March 28, 2020). As every Liswati was urged to observe the fast, "those on medication were advised to take the 'Daniel's fast', which would allow them to eat vegetables", said the Minister of Home Affairs (*Eswatini News* March 28, 2020).

As they were motivating the theme of the national prayer, sermons and prayers by selected church pastors from the three ecumenical bodies made it clear that the nation had sinned against God, hence COVID-19, but now it was repenting and pleading for God's forgiveness. They likened the COVID-19 situation in Eswatini to that of the nation of Israel in the wilderness. The Israelites sinned against God, and He sent snakes to punish them for speaking against him and Moses (Numbers 21:4–9). The people came to Moses to repent and asked him to pray to God to remove the serpents. The bronze serpent on a pole which God told Moses to erect so that the Israelites who saw it would be protected from dying from the bites of the "fiery serpents" was therefore God's response to their repentance. The sermons during the prayer also gave hope to the nation that life and economy shall be restored after the outbreak. One cleric was reported to have claimed that

> no liSwati would die from COVID-19 if the nation would repent and put their trust in God…and the world would ask how we managed to survive the virus and we will tell them that it is because Jesus is our shield as a nation.
>
> (*Times of Eswatini*, 30 May 2020)

Still pursuing the same theme in another forum, one pastor claimed to have received a prophecy from God that brings hope to Emaswati that "they would come out of the coronavirus pandemic without scratches" (*Times of Eswatini* April 14 2020). During this period some Christians would also embark in corporate prayers at the mountains, where they would plead for God's mercy over the nation of Eswatini.

### COVID-19 is a spiritual warfare

There is another perspective advanced by many Christians that the emergence of the pandemic is a spiritual warfare between God and Satan, and that it calls for spiritual strategies to combat its effects and save human life. A publication by a church leader in local print media had this comment about the health crises;

> to understand the Corona pandemic, we have to take into account that there are two Kingdoms presently at war in the earth; the Kingdom of God (Light) and the Kingdom of Satan (Darkness). This war has been playing itself for many centuries and what people have been seeing at times as natural phenomenon has actually been the manifestation of the war between these two Kingdoms. As we draw closer to the end times, the war between these Kingdoms will become even more and more visible. Unfortunately, every war has casualties and this one is no exception.
>
> (Dlamini 2020)

He further suggested that the current phenomenon therefore must be understood from a biblical perspective as the battle between the two Kingdoms which becomes fiercer. At the root of this battle is worship, and Satan's ultimate plan is to get the entire world to worship him (Revelations 13:11).

There are other Christians who share similar sentiments about COVID-19 that it is a spiritual warfare. More arguments in print media emphasise claims that the universe has two kingdoms, the Kingdom of Light which is of God, and that of the darkness belonging to the Satan. At the top of the Kingdom of darkness, there is the devil and he has structured his kingdom (Ephesians 6:12) to mimic that of the Kingdom of God. The devil operates through that structure and unfortunately through people. God also operates through His structure of the believers. There are things in the Old Testament that are a shade of the New Testament while theologians suggest that the New Testament is the Old Testament revealed; hence Christians can learn a lot from the events of the Old Testament to explain events happening in the present times. God used plagues in the Old Testament to pass judgment on the gods of Egypt during or before the Exodus and that God can also use plagues like COVID-19 as judgement on Satan and his demons.

One church was cited in local print media to have said;

> other interesting factors that might also help in understanding the Coronavirus is that we know that when the devil planned to murder Jesus, he thought he was winning the battle but that led to his defeat (1 Corinthians 2:8). God allowed him to believe he is on top only to realize later that he was orchestrating his own demise.
>
> (Dlamini 2020)

According to this argument when the devil had Jesus killed, he must have had a short-lived celebration until he realized the full picture that the title deeds of the earth no longer belonged to him. In the same manner, when the devil used Joseph's brothers to sell him into captivity, he thought he was frustrating God's plan about Joseph yet in actual fact, he was facilitating it. That is why Romans 8:28 says 'and we know that God causes everything to work together for the good of those who love God and are called according to his purpose for them.' "So, if we suppose the Coronavirus is the plan of the devil, then we know that God is one step ahead of him. If the Corona was released by evil people, then they would have been employed by the devil. If the devil is not part of it, then it is purely an act of God", adds the church leader (Dlamini 2020).

### COVID-19 is fulfilment of end time prophecies

Whilst to some Emaswati COVID-19 is a punishment from God, and also a spiritual warfare, to others it is a sign of the second coming of Jesus Christ. Christians have mostly been referring to the scriptures that list the signs of the end times in which the prophecies state that there will be wars, nation against nation, natural disasters and pestilences (Matthew 24 7–8; Luke 21

11). With this being shown from the evidence of the scriptures, they perceive the outbreak of the coronavirus as one of the specific signs of Jesus' coming and of the end of the age which he made reference to at the Olivet Discourse. One pastor who strongly subscribes to this perspective cites Jesus' words that these are the beginning of sorrows (beginning of labour pains);

> If we use the metaphor of a pregnant woman, I believe that the Coronavirus marks the time when the water breaks, a visible sign that a person is now in labor. I use the explanation for the simple reason because, during pregnancy when the water breaks, it marks the very final stages of the pregnancy and generally anxiety begins and the event is notable and gets people to pay attention.
>
> (Simelane 2020)

The pastor further claims that all along there has been agreement that the end times were approaching but there was no specific event people could point at, which marks the very end of the times. He adds that there had been epidemics in the past such as the SARS or the EBOLA, but they did not receive this worldwide attention as COVID-19 has done; hence "I believe COVID-19 is that event, especially since it happens throughout the world, almost all the nations of the world are affected, and are in some form of lockdown (Simelane 2020).

Backing up these sentiments on prophecies there is the perspective that God is using COVID-19 to revive people in readiness for Christ's coming, a revival that was also prophesied. God uses it to judge the gods that are being worshipped at this time. Whether the virus was created or not, it makes no difference. People were so used to worshipping sports, money, lust and perversion. Those evil habits have now been judged. People are not attending sports, businesses are crashing, gatherings and parties have been stopped. The Kingdom of Darkness has therefore been trounced as these gods belong to Satan, and through the confusion of the Coronavirus God passed judgment on the gods. Also, God has used this pandemic to create a space for the revival, such that people who didn't care about God before are now singing a different tune, as Christ's return is approaching.

## Church's response to COVID-19 government regulations

From the analysis of the current situation, concerns rise on how the Christian community respond to the COVID-19 regulations and restrictions by government to help flatten the curve. There are Christians who preach against the spirit of fear and anxiety and that people should trust in God and believe his word than that of men. This is in contrary to the message from government and health authorities on precautionary measures that include being in isolation/ quarantine, practicing social distancing, wearing protective clothing at all times in public places and practicing hygiene through the use of alcohol-based hand sanitisers. It can be seen that the spread of the message from the church is actually a risk to the transmission of the virus since it leads many to be reluctant in obeying lockdown regulations. Many believe that prayer is key to fight demonic forces, and that they should now cleanse themselves in anticipation for the Second Coming of Jesus. Their perception that the pandemic is a spiritual warfare has therefore caused some people to be reluctant in the physical realm with regard to protecting themselves against the pandemic.

Some prominent church leaders in the country have ridiculed Christians that abide by the government regulations on precautionary measures against COVID-19, stating that they are weak in the faith and are carnal believers. In an open letter in one of the local newspapers titled *"Church in bed with the enemy"* the writer accuses the church that they have failed God by not resisting the regulations that prohibit churches from operating during the lockdown. He queries why churches are not being allowed to operate yet they are essential service providers. He notes that other businesses are being allowed to operate during the lockdown, which included bottle stores at the time of publication of the article (Sigwane 2020). The letter openly states that the work of God is being sabotaged and it forcefully states that Christians should be allowed to assemble without fear or favour.

Another article on the local newspaper shows one of the prominent pastors in the country blasting the government and legislators for their persistence that churches should only have 20 members attending in intervals. He blamed the government for the COVID-19 regulations that have still not put the churches on the list of essential service providers. He candidly labelled government's stance about the churches as *'national suicide'* since people are being deprived of what they needed most during the times of COVID-19. According to him, this is a move that is betraying the duty of spiritual care that the people need. The pastor's argument was that churches are essential in providing emotional and social support, spiritual empowerment and it is where the sick would be healed from COVID-19. These churches could also be used for testing, educating and sensitising people about the virus.

Encouraging to Christians as it may sound, evidence from outside Eswatini gives us a different picture to this image. For instance, in Germany, after lockdown was eased, there were 40 new COVID-19 cases that were linked to a church service that was held in Frankfurt on the 10th of May 2020, even though a social distance of 1.5 m was adhered to and there was a provision of hand sanitisers to the congregants (BBC 2020). In California, nine new cases of COVID-19 were linked to two mothers' day church services that were hosted in that state (Wigglesworth 2020). In neighbouring South Africa, just as the pandemic started around March 2020, a Church in Bloemfontein held a conference with some international guests that apparently were infected. There were about 300 people in attendance after which the Free State recorded 18 positive infections, with the bulk being from the church (Shange 2020). These are some of the many examples that provoke thoughts on whether the calls for churches to operate could really bind the nation of Eswatini together to fight this spiritual warfare or it could create elements of ignorance, detrimental to many lives.

Legislators in particular have reacted strongly against relaxing the number of people to attend church, wandering whether pastors of these churches are really concerned about the well-being of their congregations or they had other ulterior motives using the gospel. Evidence to this assertion is grounded on the fact that some of these churches have continued to hold services with 20 members in each service whereas hundreds are seen loitering around the church premises waiting for their turns to get inside. In so doing, the risk of the transmission is heightened, as sources claim that most of these members do not practice social distancing (Mkhonta 2020). However, the government authorities have not been silent but extended the arm of the law towards some of the church leaders that choose to break the lockdown regulations. Four pastors in the country have so far been arrested for defying these regulations. Some church leaders though, have responded positively to the government's directives and they remain at their respective homes and pray with their families. There are also those that access church sermons through online platforms on social media.

The introduction of the live stream services has been referred to by some in the religious community as an opportunity for Christians to practice self-discipline and love in practical ways through adhering to self-isolation. This to the church demonstrates self-value and honour to others. Since God gave to Christians a spirit of power, love, sound judgement and personal discipline, "following the lockdown regulations as a Christian is not an expression of unbelief but rather a definition and expression of wisdom and neighbourly love", claims one cleric (*Times of Eswatini* May 18, 2020).

## COVID-19 as experienced within traditional understanding

Eswatini has a rich history on the interaction between traditional religious thought and Christian thought, since 1844 when Western missionaries first arrived in the country by royal invitation. This encounter marked an interface between two worldviews. B. J. Van der Walt (1994: 337) defines a worldview as "a mental construct that empowers action and endows rhythm and meaning to life processes. It is the foundation of customs, social norms, and law." As "an integrated, interpretative set of confessional perspectives on reality, [it] underlies, shapes, motivates and gives direction and meaning to human activity," adds Kosomo (2009: 35). African theologians have generally argued that the traditional worldview is irreplaceable, despite having interacted with other worldviews. Turner (1977) uses the term primal to explain religious systems that are traditional, saying that they are

> the most basic or fundamental religious forms in the overall religious history of (hu)mankind and that they have preceded and contributed

to the other great religious systems ... thus, they are both primary and prior; they represent a common religious heritage of humanity.

(p. 28)

Oduyoye gives credit to the African primal worldview which she says comprises religious beliefs and practices that it has provided and continues to provide Africa with a philosophical fountainhead for the individual's life and for the ordering of society" (1979: 112). The thesis that this chapter therefore advances is that the response of the church in Eswatini to COVID-19 is largely shaped by the coexistence of two religious orientations that conform to one another; that is the traditional religious thought and the Christian thought. African theologians like Mbiti (1995); Bediako (1979); Turaki (1977); and Dickson (1984), amongst others explain the relationship between the two traditions as continuity. According to Walls (2002) it is continuity in the sense that the material of the Christian tradition is applied to already existing maps of universe shaped by the traditional worldview. Thus, the Christian impact on the pre-existing categories is not completely changed but reordered. However, Turaki is quick to give this caution concerning the parallels, that "to speak of continuity is not to imply a full convergence of ideas, for there is also a discontinuity between the two traditions; thus, this dialectic relationship must be recognized, and wrong conclusions must not be drawn".

Recurring in the responses of Christians to COVID-19, as presented earlier were that the epidemic is a punishment from God because of evil or sins that Emaswati are committing; it is a spiritual battle between two kingdoms, one headed by God and the other by Satan; and that it is a fulfilment of the end time prophecies. The following discussion seeks to explain why Emaswati have this perspective of COVID-19.

### As a punishment for sin

Kosomo (2009) comes out with different classifications of evil, and one of them is moral evil. Accordingly, moral evil which he also calls sin is an act or an action performed by a free human person. Sin to Kosomo is an act of the will because it is a decision and indeed a free decision. Crenshaw (1983) adds another category of evil, namely, religious evil. According to him, religious evil signifies an inner disposition that perverts authentic response to the holy God. This perversion may assume the form of idolatry, where worship is directed away from God to a pale reflection of the ultimate. This type of evil operates on the vertical plane; it concerns human relationship with God and thus extends to the innermost recesses of imagination (Crenshaw 1983: 3). Notably, religious evil (sin) is more hidden than moral evil (sin), given that it operates on the vertical plane. It is therefore more pernicious since its presence can easily be concealed from human eyes (Kosomo 2009).

The notions of sin or evil are existent in African religious consciousness. Magesa (1997) asserts that what in Christianity, is conceptualised and explained as "sin" or "evil", is better expressed in African religion by the concept of "wrong-doing", "badness", or "destruction of life." According to African traditional thought patterns, sin is always associated with humans; it cannot exist in the human experience except as perceived in people. Emphasising this point Kosomo (2009) states that it is people who are evil or sinful, whether or not they are aided by invisible forces.

However, according to Sawyer (1964) in traditional thought patterns sin is seen within the context of community life (as opposed to individualism), and any breach which punctures this communal relationship amounts to sin. This makes the corporate solidarity of the family, the clan or the nation a fundamental factor of life. Relating this observation to the thesis of this chapter, we noted earlier that amongst the responses of the church in an Eswatini to COVID-19 was the call to national prayer and fasting, at the King's directive. The theme of the service (God heal our land), and the trending Bible verses suggested that Emaswati as a nation, collectively, have sinned before God. The pandemic comes as a punishment from God over the nation, hence the call to repentance as a community. Underlying this response from the church is the fact that Emaswati Christians experience the faith within the context of their traditional understandings. As noted by Nyawo (2017) when two religious orientations interact, the new orientation is only able to enlarge the traditional one; thus, a Swati Christian remains undeniably Swati in his or her perception of space (p. 372).

### As a spiritual battle between two kingdoms

In Christianity there is a dualistic understanding which sees evil to be originating from or associated with spiritual beings other than God. Here, evil is personified, and the argument is that there is an evil divinity which God created good, but later turned against him and began to do evil. This evil divinity is assisted by evil spirits known as demons and all evil now comes from that lot. Thus, a kind of duel exists, between good and evil forces in the world (Kosomo 2009), and calamities like death, epidemics, locusts and other major catastrophes are caused by these evil forces. However, the power of Jesus released through prayer confronts the hollow powers of demons and spirits, and those of sickness, poverty and death (Hock 1995). It is for this reason that some Emaswati Christians view COVID-19 with spiritual lenses that it is a manifestation of the struggle between God and Satan. With regard to the traditional religious frameworks, the belief in mystical powers is dominant, and that they influence the course of human life. Mbiti calls these frameworks a worldview with a spirit world that is very densely populated with spirit beings (1969: 75). Designated as positive and negative, good and evil, the powers are said to bring blessings and curses. For safety and protection against the wrath of the evil powers people need a spiritual guidance and practical efforts for control, protection and security. The understanding and response of some Christians to COVID-19 therefore show that these categories of evil are interpreted within the frameworks of their traditional religious worldview; hence Hock's claim that at the bottom of traditional African concepts of demonic powers are specifically African concepts of evil (1995: 62).

### *As a fulfilment of end time prophecies*

As noted earlier, another recurring theme in the Church's response to COVID-19 has been that there is nothing sinister about the virus, but rather, it is a sign of the Second Coming of Jesus Christ. For Christians the centre of their hope is Christ and His glorious appearing or Second Coming. They are waiting in anticipation of this future hope because, amongst other benefits, it will ultimately bring to an end the life of hardships on earth. Also, it will reunite community of Christians who died in Christ with those who will be living when Jesus returns. Thus, the reunion with loved ones and promised crowns by Jesus for demonstrating an upright life on earth, provide Christian an element of hope. Understanding COVID-19 as a fulfilment of prophecies about the end of times is popular amongst Christians and it is taken positively. This understanding resonates with the traditional tenets about life after death, which still confirms that some Emaswati Christians experience COVID-19 within the context of their traditional understanding. Life after death is a core belief in the traditional frameworks. It is believed that when a person dies, he transcends into another realm which is not as physical as earth, and he or she is conferred with supernatural powers; hence death is not the end but the beginning or in some cases continuation of life. This explains why death in most African traditions is not viewed as a tragedy; rather it is celebrated with several rites of passage (Hick 1976).

### Conclusion

"The silent streets, shuttered stores, empty places of worship and of worry" birthed by COVID-19, as expressed by U.N. Secretary-General Antonio Guterres in the opening quotation of this chapter, have provoked different reactions in societies. This chapter has shown that Emaswati perceive the phenomenon as a God's punishment, a spiritual warfare and a fulfilment of prophecies. This kind of thinking is informed by their primal religious orientation which views the nation as a community, the universe as populated by both malevolent and benevolent spirits and life after death as a futuristic hope. However, whilst the people's understandings and responses to COVID-19 have the potential to bind the nation together and enable them to cope with the pandemic, it may also lead to fatalistic risks as infections and death rate continue to escalate.

As noted above Emaswati Christians experience COVID-19 within their traditional frameworks, which are irreplaceable despite having interacted with other worldviews. Thus, it is imperative to balance their religious thought patterns as a coping mechanism, with practical approaches to the pandemic. The discussion has shown negative attitudes of some church leaders towards the COVID-19 compliance programme initiated by Eswatini Government. Barmania & Reiss (2020) use the word 'gatekeepers' to describe the role played by religious leaders at their communities. This is to say they play a vital role in setting an appropriate tone for the church's response to life stressors and uncertainties. Church leaders are well-respected and trusted by the people in their own communities. When they talk to their church members, they listen because they (church members) believe in them, and their communities become anchors of social solidarity. So, if they demonstrate that they are taking seriously the facts of the situation and they adhere to all COVID-19 precautions, their followers will emulate them. If they model those acts of love that keep people safe, which include wearing a mask when in a public place, social distancing, and staying at home when feeling ill, church members will follow suit. Thus, their response to COVID-19 will be 'flying with both wings'; one wing being religion as a coping resource, whilst the other represents the practical steps to deal with the pandemic.

## Notes

1 The Council of Swaziland Churches ecumenical body has not yet changed its official name to reflect Eswatini.
2 The discussion captured in this section comes from content analysis gathered from secondary sources.

## References

Barmania, S., & Reiss, M.J. (2020). Health promotion perspectives on the COVID-19 pandemic: The importance of religion. *Global Health Promotion.* doi:10.1177/1757975920972992
BBC. (2020). *Coronavirus: Over 40 Covid-19 cases traced to church service in Germany.* Retrieved from https://www.bbc.com/news/world-europe-52786242, 07 June 2020.
Bediako, K. (1979). "Continuity and discontinuity between the old testament and African life and thought." In African Theology en Route: Papers from the Pan-African Conference of Third World Theologians, December 17–23, 1977, Accra, Ghana, Kofi Appiah-Kubi and Sergio Torres (eds.), 59–65. Maryknoll, NY: Orbis Books, 1979.
Golomski, C. & Nyawo, S. (2017). Christians' cut: Popular religion and the global health campaign for medical male circumcision in Swaziland. *Culture, Health & Sexuality.* doi:10.1080/13691058.2016.1267409.
COVID-19 Eswatini Dashboard pioneered by UNESWA for daily updates on the development of Coronavirus in Eswatini, Africa and the world. Retrieved

from https://datastudio.google.com/reporting/b847a713-0793-40ce-8196-e37d1cc9d720/page/2a0LB, 6 June 2020.

Crenshaw, J. (1983). *Theodicy in the Old Testament*. Philadelphia, PA: Fortress Press.

del Castillo, F.A., & Alino, M. (2020). Religious coping of selected Filipino Catholic youth. *Religions, 11*, 462.

del Castillo, F.A., del Castillo, C.D., & Clyde Corpuz, J. (2020). Dungaw: Re-imagined Religious Expression in Response to the COVID-19 Pandemic. April 2021. https://link.springer.com/article/10.1007/s10943-021-01266-x, 28 May 2021.

Dickson, K.A. (1984). *Theology in Africa*. Maryknoll: Orbis Books.

Dlamini, I. (2020). The coronavirus, a biblical perspective. *Eswatini News*. March 28, 2020.

Guterres, G. (2020). https://globalnews.ca/news/6807879/coronavirus-religious-leaders-united-nations/, 13 April 2020.

Hart, C.W., & Koenig, H.G. (2020). Religion and health during the COVID-19 pandemic. *Journal of Religion & Health, 59*, 1141–1143. doi:10.1007/s10943-020-01042-3.

Hick, J. (1983). *Death and Eternal Life*. London: MacMillan.

Hock, K. (1995). "Jesus Power–Super-Power" On the Interface between Christian. Fundamentalism and New Religious Movements in Africa. *Mission Studies*, 12(1), 56–70.

Holy Bible. New International Bible Version.

Hood, R., Hill, P., & Spilka, B. (2009). *Psychology of Religion* (4th ed.). New York: Guilford Press.

International Religious Freedom Report: Swaziland. 2019. Washington: Bureau of Democracy, Human.

Koenig, H. (2012). *Religion, Spirituality, and Health: The Research and Clinical Implications. ISRN Psychiatry, 2012* (278730), 1–34. doi:10.5402/2012/278730.

Kosomo, D. (2009). An investigation of sin and evil in African cosmology. *International Journal of Sociology and Anthropology, 1*(8), 145–155.

Magesa, L. (1997). *African Religion: The Moral Traditions of Abundant Life*. Nairobi: Pauline Press.

Mbiti, J.S. (1969). *African Religions and Philosophy*. London: Macmillan.

Mkhonta, S. (2020). *Elijah Fire's Church Defiant*. Eswatini Observer, Tuesday, April 14, 2020, p. 2.

Nyawo, S. (2017). "Praying for Rain? African Perspectives on Religion and Climate Change." In *The Ecumenical Review*, Chitando, E. & Conradie, E. (eds.). 69.3 A World Council of Churches Publication. Oxford: John Wiley & Sons Ltd.

Oduyoye, Mercy Amba. (1979). "The Value of African Religious Beliefs and Practices for Christian Theology." In *African Theology en Route: Papers from the Pan-African Conference of Third World Theologians*, December 17–23, 1977, Accra, Ghana, Kofi Appiah-Kubi and Sergio Torres (eds.), 109–116. Maryknoll, NY: Orbis Books.

Sawyer. (1968). Sin and forgives in Africa. *Frontier, 7*, 60–63.

Shange, N. (2020). *Covid-19: Bloemfontein Church that Hosted Infected Guests Says They Were Screened on Arrival in SA*. Retrieved from https://www.timeslive.co.za/news/south-africa/2020-03-24-covid-19-bloemfontein-church-that-hosted-infected-guests-says-they-were-screened-on-arrival-in-sa/, 07 June 2020.

Sigwane, B.B.J. (2020). Church in Bed with the Enemy? *Times of Eswatini*, Wednesday, April 22, 2020. p. 27.

Simelane, B. (2020). PM Lobbies MPs for Support *Times of Eswatini* April 14, 2020.

*Times of Eswatini*, May 18, 2020.

Turaki, Yusufu. (1999). *Christianity and African Gods: A Method in Theology.* Potchefstroom, South Africa: Potchefstroomse Universiteit vir CHO.

Turner, Harold W. (1977). "Primal Religions and Their Study." In *Australian Essays in World Religions,* Victor Hayes (ed.), 27–37. Bedford Park: Australian Association for World Religion.

United Nations Secretary-General Antonio Guterres Speech. Retrieved from https://globalnews.ca/news/6807879/coronavirus-religious-leaders-united-nations/. 13 April 2020.

Van der Walt, B.J. (1995). *The Liberating Message: A Christian Worldview for Africa.* Potchefstroom: IRS, 1994, Series F3, no. 44: 337.

Walls, A.F. (2002). *The Cross-Cultural Process in Christian History.* Edinburgh: T&T Clark.

Wigglesworth, A. (2020). *More COVID-19 Cases Linked to California Church Services.* Retrieved from https://www.latimes.com/california/story/2020-05-24/more-coronavirus-cases-linked-to-california-church-services, 07 June 2020.

## 11 Standing together in faith through the time of COVID-19

### The responses of Church umbrella bodies in Zambia

*Nelly Mwale and Joseph Chita*

### Introduction

The global outbreak of COVID-19 which was first reported in Wuhan, China and in Zambia on 18 March 2020 affected all spheres of life including religious communities. While the interaction of religion and the pandemic attracted media attention, religion and public health interface continued to receive limited scholarly attention. This was despite the fact that religion manifested its presence in public health not only as a provider of health-care, but as part of the emergency response team. The immediate scholarly engagement with COVID-19 in the country was grounded in education as Sintema (2020), Mulenga and Marbán (2020) focused on the effect of the pandemic on the performance of Grade 12 learners with reference to STEM subjects and COVID-19 as a gateway for digital learning in Mathematics education, respectively.

This chapter focuses on the place of religion in the COVID-19 pandemic as exemplified by the Church umbrella bodies in the country. It specifically addresses how Church umbrella bodies responded to COVID-19 in relation to emerging solutions, challenges and suggestions in the early phases of the pandemic in Zambia. This was deemed significant in a context with a multi religious landscape which implied that people's orientation to public health messages was, by and large shaped by religious beliefs and the response of the religious leaders.

Given that COVID-19 was a new pandemic, the chapter sought to not only indirectly contribute to the discourses of religion and public health in Zambian scholarship that has been preoccupied with other pandemics, but also take stock of religion's complex role during pandemics and consequent contribution during a crisis. Acknowledging that different religious actors were involved in the fight against COVID-19, the interconnectedness of religion and public health in Zambia during the COVID-19 pandemic is purposively situated in the institutional setting of the Christian umbrella bodies, commonly referred to as Church Mother bodies. This is because although the Zambian religious landscape is multireligious (with representation of other religions like Islam, Hinduism, Zambian Indigenous Religions, Bahai

DOI: 10.4324/9781003241096-11

and Sikhism which account for smaller percentages in terms of following), Christianity remained the dominant religion. Zambian Christianity is often spoken of as represented by the Church umbrella bodies. These are the Zambia Episcopal Conference (ZEC), now the Zambia Conference of Catholic Bishops (ZCCB), the Council of Churches in Zambia (CCZ), the Evangelical Fellowship of Zambia (EFZ), Independent Churches Organisation of Zambia (ICOZ) and the Bishops Council of Zambia (BCZ).

Officially instituted in 1963, the ZEC [ZCCB] is the administrative body of all Roman Catholic dioceses (Hinfelaar, 2004) and member of the Association of Member Episcopal Conferences in Eastern Africa (AMECEA) and Symposium of Episcopal Conferences of Africa and Madagascar (SECAM). The CCZ was established in 1945 as the umbrella body of mainline Protestant churches. The EFZ was officially formed in 1964 to oversee evangelical churches. In 2001 a fourth umbrella body, ICOZ, was formed to bring together charismatic churches, ministries, fellowships, and centres. The latest Pentecostal Church umbrella body is the BCZ.

The involvement of religious actors in public health was not new in Zambia. Apart from religious institutions forming the bulk of the health delivery systems as part of national health service delivery, the Church umbrella bodies have often collaborated on different fronts in health related ventures. For example, in the wake of HIV and AIDS, the umbrella bodies partnered with other religions to form the Zambia Interfaith Non-Governmental Organisation (ZINGO). The Church umbrella bodies were also key actors during national epidemics like cholera. For example, during the recent cholera outbreak of 2017 that was declared by the Ministry of Health (MoH) on 6 October 2017, with 547 cases of which 15 deaths were recorded with a case fatality rate of 1.8% (WHO, 2017), the Church umbrella bodies were part of the response team. With the underprivileged living in poorly serviced communities mostly affected by cholera, the majority of this population was served by both religious bodies and government.

With a background of engagement in pandemics and epidemics, it became imperative to understand the responses of the Church umbrella bodies during the COVID-19 outbreak. The chapter unfolds by situating the responses of the Church umbrella bodies in existing scholarship, highlighting the context of COVID-19, approach to religion and public health and research design before exploring the responses of the Church umbrella bodies to the pandemic.

## Religion and pandemics in existing literature

The chapter situates the responses of the Church umbrella bodies to COVID-19 in discourses of religion and pandemics, especially that which is centred on religious or faith leaders. This scholarship has partly engaged with the role of religious leaders in curbing pandemics. For example, with reference to Cholera, Braley (2017) drew on the history of the 1854 cholera epidemic in London to highlight how histories of cooperation between religion and public health could help focus thinking about the potential for intersectoral cooperation in response to modern epidemics concluded that responses to contemporary epidemics continued to involve local religious entities and global religious networks.

In the case of Ebola, Jansen (2019) concluded that the unified voice and collective action from faith leaders around infection prevention activities decreased the fear and stigma about Ebola. This was through the religious leader's communication of messages of hope to the population. Jansen observed that the Muslim and Christian faith leaders drew lessons from their own religious texts to support the recommended infection control and prevention measures for Ebola. These included seeking medical care when sick, avoiding contact with bodily fluid, and routine hand washing after contact with the sick or with dead bodies. Faith leaders emphasized the need for safe and dignified burials, acceptance and appreciation of Ebola workers and validated the need for psychosocial support for those impacted by the disease, rather than stigmatising them.

Similarly, with reference to the Ebola outbreak in 2014–2015 that profoundly disrupted three west African countries (Guinea, Liberia, and Sierra Leone), Marshall and Smith (2015) also recognised that religious beliefs and practices shaped (positively and negatively) ways of caring for the sick, patterns of stigma, and gender roles and affirmed that throughout the crisis, religious institutions provided services including health, education, and social support.

With regard to COVID-19, emerging scholarship has also been centred on religion's role in the spread of the pandemic and religion's response to the pandemic. For example, Jala *et al.* (2020), while focusing on social distancing, examined how religion, culture, and burial ceremonies undermined the efforts to curb COVID-19 in South Africa. They observed that during funeral rites, social distancing was not necessarily followed while cultural practices (such as those relating to washing of hands in one basin after the funeral) presented an opportunity for guests to contract the virus. Using the context of Nigeria, Tanzania and Ethiopia, Lichtenstein *et al.* (2020) also observed that while many religious leaders had complied with government regulations and policies, others had spread religious ideology and doctrine supporting the notion that faith or belief would protect one from the virus. Similar conclusions were drawn in South Korea (Wildman *et al.*, 2020).

The focus on COVID-19 and religion in emerging scholarship has also been on the positive responses of religion through mediatisation in addressing the pandemic. For example, Aluko (2020) from the Nigerian context analysed the various responses of the Christian denominations to the emergence of the COVID-19, and subsequent lock down of the whole country. Aluko observed that some churches devised a means of worshipping through the services provided over the Internet (such as streaming their services online), through the use of Facebook, WhatsApp, YouTube, Instagram, Twitter, Mixlr, Zoom and Vimeo among others. Wildman *et al.* (2020) also concluded that most religious groups were innovating in response to opposing demands of collective worship and social distancing by conducting online services, stretching the world's data bandwidth at certain times of the week to stream live videos of suitably modified rituals, sermons, and prayers, including disseminating practical health information and offering urgent financial help in the wake of rapidly degrading economic conditions.

Similar observations were made in the Philippines context, where Catholic congregations took steps to provide the public with online-based Church masses, community prayers, spiritual recollections and retreats and eucharistic adoration and processions, including people dealing with issues about mortality, coping and recovery were provided via online formative counselling and pastoral guidance (del Castillo *et al.*, 2020).

While acknowledging the complex role of religion during pandemics, the foregoing studies affirm how pandemics can be positively or negatively shaped by religion and religious actors in different contexts. However, the responses of religious leaders to the pandemic in the Zambian context were yet to receive scholarly attention, thus this chapter seeks to contribute to emerging scholarship on religion and COVID-19 with specific reference to the Church umbrella bodies in Zambia.

## Brief context of COVID-19 in Zambia

First reported on 31 December 2019, in a wet market in Wuhan, China, it became a global threat as cases of the virus were confirmed in numerous countries and territories worldwide. The WHO consequently declared the disease as a pandemic on 11 March 2020.

In Zambia, the first reported cases were a couple that travelled to France for a short holiday. The two cases were announced a day after the Government of the Republic of Zambia (GRZ) announced the shutting down of all educational facilities as a preventative measure against the pandemic. Since 18th March 2020, cases of the COVID-19 were on the increase. The hot spot was initially Lusaka, the country's capital, before the pandemic soon spread to other parts of the country such as Nakonde in Northern Zambia, the Copperbelt, North-Western, Muchinga and Southern provinces.

According to the MoH, as of 27 May 2020, the country had recorded 1,057 confirmed cases, 779 recoveries, seven fatalities and 271 active cases (MoH Ministerial update, 27 May 2020). To prevent the spread of the disease, measures such as social distancing and lockdowns in certain towns were implemented as supported by the Public Health Act Cap 295 of the Laws of Zambia through two statutory instruments (SI) 21 of 2020 which designates COVID-19 as a notifiable disease and SI 22 of 2020 which provides additional regulations to facilitate management and control of COVID -19 (MoH, 17 March 2020). The outbreak of the pandemic had diverse impacts on the well-being of people. For example, besides the socio-economic impacts, the pandemic took a toll on people as they underwent different forms of suffering such as sickness, dying and death, grief and mourning among other aspects.

## Analytical lens: approach to religion and public health

As shown in the selected existing literature on religion and pandemics, the response of religion to public health, particularly pandemics, is not new in scholarship. For example, besides the role of religion in the Cholera and Ebola outbreaks, religion was also identified as one of the multifaceted approaches through which the HIV and AIDS pandemic could be addressed as shown by different scholars (such as Iyakaremye (2015)).

In linking religion and other spheres like health, different approaches to religion are used, the most popular being aligned to notions of religious assets. For example, the African Religious Health Assets Programme (AR-HAP) identified religious assets for addressing health matters expressed in six assumptions, some of which include the wide presence of Faith-Based entities on the ground in many contexts where health crises are most urgent and having a public impact on health (ARHAP, 2005:2). Thus, the intangible and tangible religious health assets include infrastructure; funding agencies and healers; prayer; health seeking behaviour and relationship for care; choirs, rituals and leadership skills and faith, time, and power as identified by scholars like Olivier (2011) and Chitando (2007) among others.

These perspectives are closely related to notions of religious capital as expounded by Verter (2003) who offered a model of religious capital. Verter's (2003) 'spiritual capital', included religious knowledge, competencies, and preferences as 'positional goods' within a competitive symbolic economy. Religious capital relates to the skills and experiences specific to one's religion including religious knowledge, familiarity with ritual and doctrine and friendliness with fellow worshippers (Iannaccone, 1990). This perspective takes the view that capital also exists in symbolic forms (Verter, 2003). Similarly, ter Haar's notion of religious resource can be closely related to these concepts of religious assets and religious capital. Religious resources consist of ideas, practices, organisation, and experiences (ter Haar, 2005).

Given the interconnectedness of concepts of religious assets, capital, and resource, the chapter links religion and public health through the concept of religious resource. In doing so, this chapter takes the view that religion through its resources that are located in the ideas, practices, organisation, and experiences could be deemed significant to understanding the responses of the Church umbrella bodies to COVID-19 pandemic especially as expressed by the religious leaders. It acknowledges the constructive and destructive tendencies inherent in religion as a social construct with the potential to be used positively or negatively during any pandemic. Indirectly, the religious resources are linked to theological perspectives that have emerged as tools for religion's response to pandemics especially the theology of life (Dibeela, 2007), compassion (Dube, 2007), and healing (Hadebe, 2007).

## Research design and methods

The chapter draws on insights from an interpretative case study because there was little known in a particular research area (Barker *et al.*, 2002), and that the interest was to explore in depth the responses of the Church umbrella bodies to the COVID-19 pandemic. The primary method of data collection was content analysis, which included institutional reports, postings, and newspaper articles in the public sphere. Given that non-probability sampling is more appropriate in interpretative case studies (Kothari, 2004:56), the Church umbrella bodies were purposively selected as the case study was situated in an institutional context.

Similarly, the avenues for data were purposely selected. Limiting the notion of media to its technological uses in which the media was a conduit for the transmission of messages from religious leaders in the face of COVID-19, the content analysis was situated in different forms of media, such as television, newspapers, and photographs in the public space. Since social media was an area of research, just as religious websites were dynamic archives of religious worlds (Hackett *et al.*, 2014), it was used as a supplementary source of data. The data were collected between April and May 2020.

The collected data were inductively analysed using the general framework for interpretive qualitative research suggested by Elliott *et al.*, (1994). In this case, the data were thematically analysed through a search for common themes that transcended the data alongside an interpretation of the themes. This involved the generation and application of codes to the data, and the identification, analysis, and report of patterns (themes) (Braun and Clarke, 2006:77–101).

## Response of Church umbrella bodies to COVID-19 in Zambia

The Church as a part of societal structures not only recognised that it was impacted by COVID-19, but also positioned itself as a tool in navigating through the pandemic by way of providing some solutions during the crisis.

### *Solutions offered by the Church umbrella bodies during the pandemic*

The Church umbrella bodies contributed towards providing solutions through their response to the pandemic. This was largely by offering solidarity through: Suspending public worship; offering public health education and service provision; pastoral care and advocacy so as to address different forms of suffering resulting from the pandemic.

### *Offering solidarity in the fight against the pandemic*

The Church umbrella bodies recognised the dangers associated with the pandemic in the country.

> As Church of our Lord Jesus Christ, we understand the effects of this outbreak on the people of Zambia and the world at large. We liken this scenario to that found in the Gospel according to Matthew 8:23 where the storms hit the boat on which the disciples were, while Jesus Christ

was asleep on the same boat. The storms were very strong and almost overpowered the boat. But the disciples knew who was with them in the boat and they cried out to him and he woke up and rebuked the storms. We wish to encourage everyone that we will be secure because there is hope in the Lord; we will take our rest in safety (Job 11:18).

(Church Mother Bodies Statement, 28th March 2020)

As such, the Church umbrella bodies called for unity of purpose among Zambians in an effort to address COVID-19. This was through a joint press briefing at the Catholic Secretariat at Kapingila House in Lusaka where they also pledged to work with the government in the fight against the pandemic.

Zambia Conference of Catholic Bishops (ZCCB) and other Church Mother bodies have called for unity of purpose among Zambians in an effort to address COVID-19. The ZCCB, Evangelical Fellowship of Zambia and Independent Church of Zambia at a joint press briefing held at the Catholic Secretariat at Kapingila House in Lusaka on the 28th of March, 2020, pledged to work with government in the fight against Coronavirus.

(Mukuka, AMECEA News, 3rd April 2020)

By pledging to offer solidarity and support to the government during the COVID-19 pandemic, this did not mean that the Church umbrella bodies were always in support of government as they had often critiqued the government on numerous national issues as was the case on the recent closure of the private TV station (Ncube, News diggers, 7 March 2020).

The Church umbrella bodies also called for stringent measures to control the spread of the pandemic such as calling for a lock down.

We are privy to the fact that this move will negatively affect our economy but given the current scenario, we do not have a choice but to close all our borders in order to preserve human life. In addition to closing borders, we also advocate for a shutdown of all public gatherings and stringent measures to limit physical contact in markets, bus stations and restricting numbers in public transport vehicles.

(Chisanga, Mast Newspaper, 29th March 2020)

As observed by the General Secretary of CCZ, the Zambian churches collaborated in response to COVID-19 through issuance of 'pastoral statements to the nation calling for the church to follow and abide by government guidelines regarding the fight against COVID-19' (Fr. Emmanuel Yona Chikoya, May 2020). The Church umbrella bodies' response through offering solidarity during the pandemic is line with conclusions by Deguma *et al.* (2020), that different Catholic congregations were in solidarity with the poor by drawing on the Catholic Church's Social Teachings which resonated with the Liberation Theology' of Gustavo Gutiérrez in the Philippines in their responses in mitigating the experience of the crisis among Filipino poor amid COVID-19 pandemic. As observed by O'Brien and Shannon (1992:421), solidarity entailed persevering determination to commit oneself to the common good; that is to say, to the good of all and of each individual, because we are all really responsible for all.

## Suspending public physical worship

Apart from pastoral statements, the Church umbrella bodies practically undertook preventive measures as informed by MoH and WHO guidelines on the pandemic. These included holding an online national prayer on 29 March 2020 as opposed to physical prayers. The Church umbrella bodies held a National Day of Prayer and fasting under the theme "standing together in faith through the times of the coronavirus".

> During this National Day of Prayer and fasting, people were advised to fast and pray in the comfort of their homes as no gathering would be held in any church for the prayers. The National Day of Prayer was aired on the national TV while other churches conducted their church meetings online as a preventative measure to address the virus.
>
> (ZNBC TV News, 29th March 2020, 19:00 GMT)

Thus, faith became a uniting force amid the pandemic through which religious communities readily engaged in acts of solidarity that built community resilience. The national online prayers were accompanied by suspending church gatherings.

> We wish to inform the nation that as Church Mother bodies we have instructed all our membership across the country to be proactive and channel all energies in preventing the spreading of the disease. Given the rising numbers of confirmed cases of COVID-19 in Zambia, we have resolved to suspend Church gathering for at least 14 days. For some Church Mother bodies, this will take effect on Sunday 29th March 2020 while for others the commencement date as already communicated will be Monday 30th March 2020.
>
> (Church Mother Bodies Statement, 28th March 2020)

Even after the Presidential directive that places of worship could reopen after a month of lock down (Presidential address, ZNBC TV 24 April 2020), the Church took a stance to maintain the closure of their churches. The churches directed their members to await further communication from the Church leadership. For example, the ZCCB leadership emphasised that no 'mass or service' would take place:

> the suspension of all public church gatherings and communicable liturgical celebrations will remain in effect... In the meantime, the Church

remains desirous of protecting the lives and health of its members and pastoral agents. Allow me to exhort you to religiously and judiciously follow the rules of hygiene especially those of washing your hands with soap regularly, and thoroughly; avoiding physical greeting and contact; observing social distancing; avoiding to touch your eyes, nose and mouth; avoiding to spit in public; covering your mouth and nose with a bent elbow or tissue when coughing or sneezing and wearing face masks whenever you are in public…Once more give heed to the extortion of St. Paul; we must never get tired of doing good because if we don't give up the struggle, we shall reap our harvests at the proper time (Galatians 6:9).

(ZCCB Memo, 25th April 2020)

Other Church umbrella bodies also reacted in the similar manner. The rituals of death, mourning and burial were also limited to few people so as to manage the pandemic. This response signified the authority of the religious actors and concern for safety of the people during the pandemic. This was significant given that in other contexts, the spread of the pandemic was linked to church gatherings (Wigglesworth, *Los Angeles Times*, 24 May 2020). The Church umbrella bodies' suspension of public worship was consistent with how other faith leaders had responded to the pandemic as concluded by Aluko (2020), Wildman *et al.* (2020) and del Castillo *et al.* (2020) among others. This was also similar to how the Church had responded to the cholera outbreak by suspending some religious rites as affirmed by Becket (2018) and Mwale and Chita (2020) that Catholics were advised to stay away from funeral houses as only a priest could go there for prayers.

*Public health education and service provision*

Besides reorienting Church operations, the Church umbrella bodies further responded by providing public health education on the pandemic. The Church umbrella bodies also instructed their members to adhere to preventative messages.

Adhere and follow all instructions and guidelines being shared by the government and other authentic stakeholders and pray for God's intervention. It was time that science and gospel worked together to save the world from calamity. Encourage people to go for medical attention while you pray for them. Avoid telling your members to depend on prayer alone. Let them get both prayer and medical attention from health facilities. The Church must avoid being an obstacle in the fight against the spread of the coronavirus disease.

(Church Mother Bodies Statement, 28th March 2020)

Additionally, the mother bodies provided medical facilities and financial and material resources towards the fight against the pandemic. CCZ offered their structures (David Livingstone College of Education) to be used as quarantine facilities by the government; and like other Church mother bodies led the way by stopping large gatherings, changed the way of worship and how religious rites were conducted; offered food and other necessities to the very vulnerable families (aacc-ceta.org, 2020). Similarly, the ZCCB were involved in setting up a COVID-19 Response Fund (CRF). CRF was meant to fund prevention programmes in Zambia and to offer support to 59 health facilities working to curb COVID-19 in the ten Provinces of Zambia (Agenzia Fides, 2020). This was accompanied by pastoral care within the context of the pandemic by emphasising that physical distancing did not mean spiritual isolation and pledging to help provide pastoral care to communities especially the vulnerable, the dying and bereaved, the elderly and psychologically distressed. This demonstrated that the Church bodies were not only playing their prophetic role through issuing press statements and pastoral letters but also through service delivery and programmes.

The Church umbrella bodies' responses resonated with the manner in which the Church umbrella bodies had responded to the cholera and HIV and AIDS crisis and therefore affirmed faith leader's role in relying preventative messages and providing service during the pandemics (Featherstone, 2015; Marshall, 2016). Additionally, the responses of the Church umbrella bodies were related to Mendoza (2020)'s observation from the Philippine context in which the pandemic was seen as a trying time which called the Church to move by doing concrete acts of charity by sharing resources with those who need it the most. Similarly, Deguma *et al.* (2020) affirmed that through putting its social teaching into practice, the Church was not only for the poor but more substantially, a Church of the poor and by preferring the poor, the Church strengthened the whole community by assisting those who were the most vulnerable.

*Advocacy and call for accountability*

The Church umbrella bodies further advocated for the wellbeing of the poor by urging the government to give priority to those who lived in poverty as well as the marginalised and refugees living in the country.

> We urge the government to come up with mechanisms such as economic stimulus packages and mitigating measures as well as incentives to help the industry and citizens in coping with the adverse effects of the Coronavirus.
> (Chisanga and Chisenga, Mast Newspaper, 29th March 2020)

The stance by the Church umbrella bodies to advocate for the plight of the poor resonates with the observations (with reference to) of the Catholic Church made by Phiri (1999) that ZEC challenged the government to look into the plight of the poor,

> the Church cannot be silent in the face of this suffering of our people. The word of God challenges us: 'If you refuse to hear the cry of the poor, your own cry for help will not be heard' (Proverbs 21:13).
> (1999:346)

The advocacy for the poor was also accompanied by calls for accountability on COVID-19 resources. In this regard, they urged the government to ensure that there was proper stewardship and accountability of all donations and allocated funds for the COVID-19 control programme. This was similar to the Philippines context in which the pandemic was viewed as another oppressor of the poor as it slowed down the economic sector and the poor bore the brunt of the crisis (Mendoza, 2020), thus the Church had to safeguard the interest of the masses by calling for accountability and transparency.

## The challenges and Nature of Church umbrella bodies' response to COVID-19

The response of the Church umbrella bodies to COVID-19 revealed both the challenges that emerged during the pandemic and religion's potential to be used as a resource during a crisis. The challenges revolved around the themes of debates on the existence of COVID-19 and Pastoral care among the faithful, increased vulnerability of vulnerable groups, distress and limited health infrastructure.

### *Debates on the existence of COVID-19 and pastoral care*

To start with, the Church bodies' response to the pandemic was characterised by the challenge surrounding the debates on the existence of the pandemic the country. Soon after the breakout of the pandemic and the introduction of the prevention and management measures, there were some expressions of doubts as to whether the pandemic was real or not, including non-compliance of the preventative measures. For example, the UN Office for the Coordination of Humanitarian Affairs (2020) observed that poor compliance by the public to recommended prevention measures such as use of masks, hand hygiene and limited laboratory testing, remain key challenges to the COVID-19 response. This made the voices of the religious leaders significant as they urged the population to heed the advice from the medical practitioners (Church Mother Bodies Statement, 28 March 2020) and took a lead in following the guidelines on social distancing and stay home campaign by resorting to virtual worship among other measures.

The debates on the existence of COVID-19 in the country were also accompanied by misconceptions on how COVID could be prevented and managed. The Church umbrella bodies encouraged people to seek both medical and divine interventions during the pandemic. This could not be detached from the lessons and experiences they had gained over time in the country. This stance on approaching the pandemic with medical and divine intervention could also be easily linked to narratives of the HIV and AIDS pandemic in which people had abandoned Antiretroviral therapy in favour of prayers. Therefore, this guidance was posed to make a positive contribution at the onset of the COVID-19 pandemic. This is because social resistance to medical interventions had implications on the spread of infectious diseases, hence the Church umbrella bodies preached a message of linking science and religion by emphasising that it was time that science and gospel worked together to save the world from calamity.

Additionally, the response to the pandemic was associated with challenges relating to pastoral care in the moment of suffering. For example, the COVID-19 prevention measures entailed controlled rituals associated with sickness and death. This was a challenge given the nature of community as understood in the Zambian setting where for instance, one person's grief becomes a concern to every member of the community. Therefore, the limits posed on mourning and burial rituals remained the challenge the religious leaders and their communities had to deal with in the context of the pandemic. In this regard, the religious communities encouraged the community to reorient the way in which mourning was done by advising people to stay away from funeral houses as only a priest and religious officials could go there for prayers. This signified how religion was a resource, asset or capital towards navigating through the pandemic. This is because as opposed to using religion to frustrate the efforts to prevent and manage the pandemic, the Church umbrella bodies adhered to public health messages and took steps to provide leadership during the crisis. This was underpinned by the Church umbrella bodies' reinterpretation of their Christian dogma on worship to prevent and manage COVID-19 by suspending public worship and stressing that physical distancing did not entail spiritual isolation. These actions could not be detached from the teaching on human life as expressed by the Church Mother bodies. 'Our faith in the God of life compels us to protect life by doing all that we can to avoid transmitting this virus (Church Mother Bodies Statement, 28 March 2020). As observed by Muzaffar (2005), the transformative potential of religion lies in the shared spiritual and moral heritage of humankind.

### Increased vulnerability of vulnerable groups and distress

The response to the pandemic was further characterised by the challenge of increased vulnerability of the vulnerable groups of people. For example, the lock down and stay home halted not only church gatherings but also businesses thereby worsening the socio-economic situation of the vulnerable. This explains the Church's stance to advocate for the well-being of the population. Closely related to the theology of life (Dibeela, 2007), the drive for the response also shows that the Church umbrella bodies continued to be compelled by their teachings on life. In so doing, they tapped into their role of reinterpreting religious ideas according to the social context which ter Haar (2005) argues is their prime responsibility. The Catholic social teaching that emphasised that while every person had a right to share in the benefits of the common good, everyone also had a right and duty to contribute one's share to the welfare of others, to the whole community, and even to the global community of humankind, especially the least well-off and most vulnerable (Cahill, 2007). The foregoing can easily be seen as a teaching shared among the Church umbrella bodies but also that which was related to the manner in which they responded to the pandemic. Thus, the responses were anchored on teachings on the option of the poor and vulnerable groups of society as COVID-19 had also revealed the long-standing inequalities entrenched in society. In a context characterised by high levels of poverty, the outbreak of the pandemic entailed that the poor would be negatively impacted, hence the religious leaders' concern for the poor.

The response of the Church umbrella bodies was also characterised by challenges of distress. The Church umbrella bodies used their scripture to provide hope to the people during the pandemic. By this, the Church bodies continued to be a source of meaning during the moment of grief and suffering. While this was part of the pastoral ministry of healing, this could be deemed significant during a time when people were filled with uncertainties. For example, through Bible passages like Matthew 8:23; Galatians 6:9, the Church provided assurance to their faithful in ways that pointed to their attempts to stand together in faith in the fight against the pandemic. The Church umbrella bodies' tapping into scripture during the crisis was therefore in line with conclusions drawn by scholars such as Jansen (2019) and Marshall and Smith (2015) during the Ebola outbreak. As observed by Marshall (2020), millions of people worldwide look more to religious authorities than health officials for guidance on how to behave and what to believe during a crisis.

### Health infrastructure

Limited health infrastructure was another challenge in dealing with the pandemic. This was a challenge given that the health context of the country was already shaped by the burden of HIV and AIDS (the prevalence of HIV among adults aged 15–59 was 12% (MoH, 2019). The country's healthcare was the responsibility of state and non-state actors including Faith-Based Organisations (FBO). Challenges such as limited funds for health care, high burden of diseases and staff shortages, the rates of poverty, inequality and poor distribution of resources especially in rural areas continued to impact the healthcare system as these were intrinsically tied to economic policies and infrastructure development (Sopitshi and Van Niekerk, n.d:7). Thus, the pandemic could only strain the already overburdened health system in the country. In this regard, the Church umbrella bodies used their structures and networks to navigate through the pandemic. This implied that the public health education efforts in the context of the pandemic were conveyed given the wide presence of the Church in various parts of the country, both urban and rural, pointing to the strength shared by faith communities in public health centred on their widespread presence (ARHAP, 2005). The

Church umbrella bodies also used their network to provide practical interventions during the pandemic. Closely related to their religious behaviour centred on theologies of compassion, these responses also demonstrated the trust and authority associated with the religious leaders. In this way, religion was positively used to contribute towards the fight against the pandemic in ways that revealed how the Church umbrella bodies stood together in faith to fight the COVID-19 pandemic.

## Suggestions on religion's place in a pandemic

The responses of the Church umbrella bodies ultimately pointed to a collaborative relationship between the church and state during the pandemic with isolated moments of disagreement on the course of action. The voice of the Church umbrella bodies remained significant during the crisis as affirmed by Marshall (2020) that people tend to look more to religious authorities for guidance on how to behave and what to believe during a crisis. This brings to the fore lessons which include the need to safeguard and promote human life, as both the church and state exist to serve humanity; and need to recognise and appreciate the vital roles of religious actors during pandemics so as to draw on religious ideas and behaviour since cultural and religious practices are very often crucial in curbing the spread of pandemics; and incorporating faith leaders in emergency response teams during pandemics.

Given the largely positive utilisation of religion as a resource during the pandemic, the chapter points to suggestions centred on the religious teachings, practices, organisation and experiences. In relation to religious teachings and practices, the chapter suggests the continued use of scripture to draw lessons on how pandemics ought to be managed and reorienting rituals in ways which promote life. This is deemed significant as existing studies have affirmed that when exposed to a threat such as a pandemic, people resort to various strategies of survival, faith being one of them, which allows them to keep hope and feel a sense of security (Kowalczyk et al. 2020).

Since religious leaders were a trusted source of information in the country, with a presence in every part of the country, the chapter suggests continued capacity building of religious leaders and utilising their structures to foster the communication of vital information and facts on the pandemic across the country. Religious leaders were long standing partners in public health as the church has been effective in reaching the most destitute in the country (Mwale, 2013). Given the vast experiences of the Church in public health, the chapter suggests the recognition of religious leaders as critical players in a crisis as they are the bridge between science and spirituality in the context of the pandemic. As affirmed by Hart and Koenig (2020), religious faith will likely make an important difference in how many make it through this challenging time in the history of nations and the world.

## Conclusion

The chapter explored the place of religion during a pandemic using the responses of the Church umbrella bodies to the COVID-19 pandemic in Zambia. Given that the Church umbrella bodies utilised their teachings, networks (structures), religious behaviours and experiences to respond to COVID-19, the chapter concludes that the response of Church umbrella bodies showed that constructive use of religion could be instrumental during pandemics. This implied that efforts of preventing and managing pandemics needed to embrace religious actors for effective and far-reaching responses to public health. The chapter also concludes that religious actors remained key stakeholders in public health since the response of the Church umbrella bodies demonstrated how religion could be mobilised as a tool to navigate through a pandemic and thus contribute to the promotion of life.

## References

African Religious Health Assets Programme (ARHAP). 2005. Background and a Conceptual Framework for Contributors, in *An Invitation: International Case Study Colloquium,* by ARHAP, Pretoria, South Africa, 13–16 July: 1–3.

Aluko, Oluwasegun Peter. 2020. COVID-19 Pandemic in Nigeria: The Response of the Christian Church. *African Journal of Biology and Medical Research* 3(2):111–125.

Barker, Chris, Nancy Pistrang, and Robert Elliott. 2002. *Research Methods in Clinical Psychology: An Introduction for Students and Practitioners.* England: John Wiley and Sons.

Barnett, Tony, and Alan Whiteside. 2002. *AIDS in the Twenty-First Century: Disease and Globalization.* New York: Palgrave Macmillan.

Becket, Adam. 2018. 'Cholera Epidemic in Zambia Shuts Churches.' *Church Times.* 19th January.

Braley, Matthew Bersagel. 2017. Recovering Religion: Practising Intersectoral Co-operation in a Time of Cholera. *Development in Practice* 27(5): 745–749.

Braun, Virginia, and Victoria Clarke. 2006. Using Thematic Analysis in Psychology. *Journal of Qualitative Research in Psychology* 3: 77–101.

Cahill, Lisa Sowle. 2007. Global Health and Catholic Social Commitment. *Health Progress* 88(3):55–59.

Chitando, Ezra. 2007. *Living with Hope: African Churches and HIV/AIDS 1.* Geneva: WCC.

Church Mother Bodies. 2020. *Statement by the Church Mother Bodies on the Coronavirus Disease – COVID-19 Pandemic.* 28th March.

Deguma, Jabin J., Melona C. Deguma, Jemima N. Tandag, and Harlene Marie B. Acebes. 2020. Where Is the Church in the Time of COVID-19 Pandemic: Preferring the Poor via G. Gutierrez' 'Liberation' and the Catholic Church's Social Teaching in the Philippine Setting. *Journal of Social and Political Sciences* 3(2): 363–374.

del Castillo, Fides A., Hazel T. Biana, and Jeremiah Joven B. Joaquin. 2020. ChurchInAction: The Role of Religious Interventions in Times of COVID-19. *Journal of Public Health* 42(3): 633–634.

Dibeela, P. Moiseraela. 2007. Module 6: A Theology of Life in The HIV & AIDS Context, in *Theology in the HIV & AIDS Era* Series, edited by M. W. Dube. Geneva: WCC.

Dube, Musa W. 2007. Module 7: A Theology of Compassion in the HIV & AIDS Era, in *Theology in the HIV & AIDS Era Series,* edited by M. W. Dube. Geneva: WCC.

Featherstone, Andy. 2015. Keeping the Faith: The Role of Faith Leaders in the Ebola Response. London: *CAFOD.*

Hackett, Rosalind, Anne Melice, Steven Van Wolputte, and Katrien Pype. 2014. Interview: Rosalind Hackett Reflects on Religious Media in Africa. *Social Compass* 61(1): 67–72.

Hadebe, M. Nontando. 2007. Module 8: A Theology of Healing in the HIV & AIDS Era, in *Theology in the HIV & AIDS Era Series,* edited by M. W. Dube. Geneva: WCC.

Hart, Curtis. W., and Koenig, Harold. G. 2020. Religion and Health During the COVID-19 Pandemic. *Journal of Religion and Health* 59: 1141–1143.

Hinfelaar, Hugo. 2004. *History of the Catholic Church in Zambia:1895-1995.* Lusaka: Bookworld Publications.

http://www.fides.org/en/news/67770    AFRICA_ZAMBIA_A_Church_fund_to_ fight_Covid_19_the_solidarity_of_the_Bishops_of_Malawi_Zambia_and_Zimbabwe

https://www.oikoumene.org/en/press-centre/news/knowing-covid-19-was-on-its-way-africas-churches-prepared

https://www.who.int/csr/don/11-december-2017-cholera-zambia/en/

Iannaccone, Laurence R. 1990. Religious Practice: A Human Capital Approach. *Journal for* the *Scientific Study of Religion* 29: 297–314.

Iyakaremye, Innocent. 2015. Neglecting Religious Health Assets in Responding to HIV and AIDS. An Assessment of the Response of the Free Methodist Church of Southern Africa to HIV and AIDS. *Missionalia* 43(1): 23–44.

Jaja, Ishmael Festus, Madubuike Umunna Anyanwu, and Chinwe-Juliana Iwu Jaja. 2020. Social Distancing: How Religion, Culture and Burial Ceremony Undermine the Effort to Curb COVID-19 in South Africa. *Emerging Microbes & Infections* 9(1): 1077–1079.

Jansen, Perry. 2019. The Role of Faith-Based Organizations and Faith Leaders in the 2014–2016 Ebola Epidemic in Liberia. *Christian Journal for Global Health* 6(1): 70–78.

Kothari, Chakravanti Rajagopalachari. 2004. *Research Methodology: Methods and Techniques.* New Delhi: New Age International.

Kowalczyk, Oliwia, Roszkowski, Krzysztof, Montane, Xavier, Pawliszak, Wojciech, Tylkowski, Bartosz and Bajek, Anna. 2020. Religion and Faith Perception in a Pandemic of COVID-19. *Journal of Religion and Health* 59(6): 2671–2677.

Lichtenstein, Amanda, Rosemary Ajayi, and Nwachukwu Egbunike. 2020. Across Africa, COVID-19 Heightens Tension Between Faith and Science. *Pandemic Response and Religion in the USA: Doctrine* 1.

Marshall, Katherine, and Sally Smith. 2015. Religion and Ebola: Learning from Experience. *The Lancet* 386(10005): e24–e25.

Mendoza, Ruben C. 2020. What If: COVID-19 in the Philippines in the Light of the Catholic Social Tradition. *Journal of Dharma* 45(2): 201–222.

Ministry of Health. 2020a. Ministerial Update: *Press Briefing on COVID-19 and Additional Preventive and Control Measures,* 17 March, Lusaka.

Mukuka, Mwenya. 2020. Church Mother Bodies Come Together in Support of Government Amid COVID-19. *AMECEA News*, 3 April.

Muzaffar, C Chandra. 2005. Religious Conflict in Asia: Probing the Causes, Seeking Solutions, in *Bridge or Barrier: Religion, Violence and Visions for Peace*, edited by G. Haar ter and J.J. Busuttil. Leiden: Brill: 57--79.

Mwale, Nelly. 2013. Religion and Development in Zambia: The Role of the Roman Catholic Church in the Political Development of Zambia 1890–1964. *Interdisciplinary Journal for the Study of the Arts and Humanities in Southern Africa* (Alternation) 1: 110–133.

Mwale, Nelly and Chita, Joseph. 2020. The Catholic Church and Epidemics: Safeguarding People's Wellbeing in the Advent of the 2017/18 Cholera Outbreak in Zambia. *Alternation Special Edition* 30: 295–310.

Mulenga, Eddie M., and José M. Marbán. 2020. Is COVID-19 the Gateway for Digital Learning in Mathematics Education? *Contemporary Educational Technology* 12, 2: ep269. https://doi.org/10.30935/cedtech/7949

Ncube, Sipilisiwe. 2020. Mother Church bodies SHAME Government over Prime TV Closure. News Diggers, 7 March.

O'Brien, David. J., and Shannon, Thomas. A. 1992. *Catholic Social Thought: The Documentary Heritage*. Maryknoll: Orbis Books.

Olivier, Jill. 2011. Religion and Policy on HIV and AIDS: A Rapidly Shifting Landscape, in *Religion and HIV and AIDS: Charting the Terrain*, edited by B. Haddad. Scottsville: University of KwaZulu-Natal Press: 81–104.

Olivier, Jill, and Gillian Margaret Paterson. 2011. Religion and Medicine in the Context of HIV and AIDS: A Landscaping Review, in *Religion and HIV and AIDS: Charting the Terrain*, edited by B. Haddad. Scottsville: University of KwaZulu-Natal Press: 25–51.

Phiri, Isaac. 1999. Why African Churches Preach Politics: The Case of Zambia. *Journal of Church & State* 41: 323–347.

Sintema, Edgar John. 2020. Effect of COVID-19 on the performance of Grade 12 students: Implications for STEM Education. *Eurasia Journal of Mathematics, Science and Technology Education* 16, 7: em1851. https://doi.org/10.29333/ejmste/7893

Ter Haar, Gerrie. 2005. *Religion: Source of Conflict or Resource for Peace?*. Bridge or Barrier: Religion, Violence and Visions for Peace. Leiden: Brill, 303–320.

UN Office for the Coordination of Humanitarian Affairs. 2020. Zambia Situation Report. 29 July.

Verter, Bradford. 2003. Spiritual Capital: Theorising Religion with Bourdieu against Bourdieu.' *Sociological Theory* 21(2), 150–174.

Wigglesworth, Alex. 2020. *More Coronavirus Cases Linked to California Church Services*. Los Angeles Times, 24 May.

Wildman, Wesley J., Joseph Bulbulia, Richard Sosis, and Uffe Schjoedt. 2020. Religion and the COVID-19 Pandemic. *Religion, Brain & Behaviour* 10(2): 115–117.

Zambia Conference of Catholic Bishops. (2016). *Strategic Plan 2017–2026*. ZCCB: Lusaka.

Zambia Conference of Catholic Bishops. (2020). Memo: Extension of the suspension of Church gatherings and Liturgical Celebrations in View of the Continued Fight against COVID-19. 25 April.

# 12 Churches and COVID-19 in Botswana

*Tshenolo J. Madigele and James N. Amanze*

## Introduction and background

COVID-19 pandemic is a contagious disease that is also known as corona virus. It is caused by the SARS-CoV2 virus. The virus was first identified in Wuhan, China in 2019. From there the virus spread across the world. The first cases of COVID-19 to be reported in Botswana on 30 March 2020 were three. As of 1 June 2020, there have been 35 confirmed cases and one death (Worldometers, 2020). On 31 March, President Dr Mokgweetsi Eric Masisi of Botswana declared a 28-day State of Public Emergency in order to curb the spread of the COVID-19 pandemic. The legislators later approved an extension of State of Public Emergency to last up to six months (Mmegi Online, 30/03/2020). Extreme social distancing or the lockdown started on 2 April 2020 in Botswana.

During the lockdown period, people in Botswana were expected to stay home except for essential services such as going for medical care, pharmacies, buying groceries, petrol and collection of social grants during certain hours only. Thus religious, educational and social activities were suspended. People that violated lockdown rules could be imprisoned for a period lasting not more than two months or would be asked to pay a fine (Gazette, 2020a). The move towards extreme social distancing and its restrictions were influenced by the effects of the virus in all aspects of human existence. The virus is attacking humans, economy, social and spiritual aspects. It is more than a health crisis. It has been declared a pandemic by the World Health Organization as it is affecting societies at their core (WHO, 2020).

COVID-19 affects all segments of the population, it does not exclude anybody. However, people who are mostly affected are those in vulnerable positions such as the poor, elderly, unemployed youth, people with disabilities, some businesspeople, women and children. *Mmegi Newspaper* reports that Botswana has a population of 2.26 million. Of these, women are 1.17 million while men are 1.09. These statistics show that there are more women in Botswana than men. Moreover, women dominate the informal sector at 88.1%. The informal sector is identified as the activities of the poor. These people include those who work in hotels, restaurants and self-employed. Most

DOI: 10.4324/9781003241096-12

are working in unregulated sectors. Extreme social distancing took away many women's financial ability. During lockdown, many household helpers returned to their homes and many mothers were further faced with a duty of caregiving and increased chores as everybody was home on fulltime basis (Mmegi, 2020b).

Moreover, the newspaper reports that domestic and gender-based violence cases escalated during lockdown. Those included intimate partner femicide and attempted murders. It was difficult for women under lockdown restrictions to seek for help. Hence, many stayed home with their perpetrators who were mainly primary earners in the family. Social workers were not able to deal with psycho-social impacts of COVID-19 since their focus was mainly on the role of food provision (Mmegi, 2020a).

Meanwhile, UNICEF on the 15th of April 2020 reported concerning alarming numbers of children who had been raped since the beginning of COVID-19 lockdown in Botswana. Twenty-two rape cases of children aged between 2 and 13 were reported within 14 days of extreme social distancing. It is further reported that rape and defilement offences during lockdown were committed by family members of the victims (UNICEF, 2020). Still on child rape and defilement, on April 14, Yarona FM News reported that Deputy Police Commissioner Dinah Marathe shared that they recorded 23 defilement cases and 22 rape cases of children under 13 years of age. The Commissioner did not rule out the possibility of more incidents of this nature as it mainly involves family members hence secrecy at the expense of children (Yarona FM News, 2020). The above reports show that confinement is a nightmare for children in Botswana hence the need for protection during and post COVID-19 era.

The era of extreme social distancing has not only denied children's sexual and reproductive rights, and it has also denied them the right to nutrition. Schools in Botswana do not only serve as education institutions, and they are also places that provide food and nutrition for the survival of many children. The economic hit has direct effect on families with larger membership. Therefore, there is a need of intervention (Sunday Standard, 27th April 2020).

The San community had also been devastated by the COVID-19 pandemic. The community is communal in nature and sharing of food and other good is a cultural value and norm. In other words, communalism is a necessity. COVID-19 had further exacerbated economic loss as those that had been retrenched now rely on monthly government food ration that is not enough for larger households. Health information and advice issued by the government is mainly in Setswana. This fails to take into account other local languages and the cultural specifications and the conditions under which the San community live (Naturaljustice.org, May 21st, 2020).

At the time of writing this chapter, Botswana had recorded one death case due to the pandemic. This victim was an elderly woman who was 79 years old. Meanwhile, information moving around on different media platforms in Botswana reveals that elderly people are among the most vulnerable groups in the COVID-19 pandemic especially if they are physically unfit and suffering from respiratory illnesses, heart disease or high blood pressure. More news reveal that the death rate of COVID-19 increases for those aged 70 or higher (Garg et al. 2020; Promislow et al. 2020). There is currently no information on effects of COVID-19 on the elderly people in Botswana. However, literature shows that extreme social distancing cut-off extended family and traditional community support systems that older persons depend on for survival (Promislow et al. 2020). Most of the elderly live in rural areas where health care systems, sources of income and access to information are poor (Promislow et al. 2020; Volpato et al. 2020). Changes to operational infrastructures including transport systems to support the curbing of the pandemic put older persons at increased health risks. It has been revealed that elderly people experience ageism, discrimination, neglect abuse and violence at family, community and society levels (Ingstad et al. 1992; Mudiare, 2013). However, their challenges received no attention during lockdown.

Studies further reveal that, because of their frailty, elderly people depend on their families and other caregivers for care and in the process, they are abused (Ingstad et al. 1992; Mudiare, 2013). Also, in the absence of institutional care, adult children who are too busy to take care of their parents hire caregivers who also maltreat them. Unfortunately, the elderly are unable to challenge their abusers and have no way of reporting their abuse, and so many suffer in silence (Mudiare, 2013). COVID-19 had obviously aggravated the situation of the elderly but there is currently nothing on the awareness on the situation of the elderly, neither is there tailor-made information on COVID-19 to older persons in rural areas using community structures and local languages so that older persons are fully informed about the disease, prevention, protection and treatment measures.

The youth of ages 15–24 are among people who are vulnerable to COVID-19 pandemic. Youth unemployment had always been a concern in Botswana as it leads to social ills such as drug and alcohol abuse, poverty and crime (Mogomotsi & Madigele, 2017). Statistics Botswana 2018 reveals that national youth unemployment rate in Botswana was 25.1% in the year 2016. The numbers escalated to 37.52% in 2019 (Statistics Botswana, 2019). Due to COVID-19, the unemployed youth are likely to be among those whose jobs have come to an end in formal and informal employment as a result of the pandemic. After just less than a month of restrictive measures, most of the youth are struggling to survive, meet their basic needs and adhere to orders and guidelines set up by the government of Botswana. Some were brutally assaulted by members of Botswana's armed forces (the police and soldiers), while on the streets. However, the president of Botswana, Dr Mokgweetsi Eric Masisi warned the country's law enforcers not to abuse people during the lockdown, as the nation fights COVID-19 pandemic (The Botswana Gazette, April 2020b).

*Mmegi Newspaper*, article titled, "Possible Economic Impact of COVID-19 on Botswana" reports that currently, unemployment stands at 29%. In this report, 57% are employed in the formal sector while 43% are in the informal sector (Mmegi, 2020a). The pandemic has hit hard the informal sector, small business owners and the unemployed. The issue is likely to cause social unrest if not attended to (Mmegi, 2020a).

It is worth noting that the government of Botswana had established a COVID-19 relief fund with a 2 billion Pula to finance wage subsidy amounting to 50% of salaries of affected businesses. The government subsidy ranges from 1,000 to 2,500 pula for a period of three months (Mmegi, 2020). This means that those left out are from informal sectors, Non-profit organizations and companies which are not registered with Botswana Unified Revenue Services (BURS). Botswana Council of Churches (BCC) Secretary General Rev Gabriel Tsuaneng says the church is amongst the hardest hit institutions by the Coronavirus (COVID-19) pandemic in the country. There is currently no solution on the economic status of pastors and church employees during this period (Gazette, 2020a). Therefore, the Church remains a victim of COVID-19 pandemic and extreme social distancing. The cancelling of religious gatherings might have negative impact on the mental health of people. Religious gatherings contribute to the healthy sense of community, tradition and national identity (Gazette, 2020b). During these times, many people are being fired and that is a risk factor for the development of mental health issues. Religious leaders are equally facing mental health issues as

> The Church relies on offerings and tithes, and since there are no church services, things are now very difficult. Pastors' welfare has significantly changed as a result of the outbreak of the pandemic and also since the extreme social distancing protocols were put into effect.
>
> (Gazette, 2020a)

Moreover, if there are no offerings and tithes, congregations will not be able to provide basic needs to the poor.

This chapter provides an overview of how the religious fraternity in Botswana has responded to COVID-19 by identifying the strengths and challenges of these responses as well as outlining lessons learnt for the future in terms of the interface of epidemics, religion and politics.

## Method

A qualitative research method was adopted to understand the impact of COVID-19 on Christian communities falling under three church organizations namely Evangelical Fellowship of Botswana (EFB), Botswana Council of Churches (BCC) and Organization of African Instituted Churches (OAIC). These organizations fall under the Botswana Network of Christian Communities (BONECO). Adopting a phenomenological design, a structured telephonic interview was used targeting 30 pastors from different congregations who fall under the umbrella BONECO. At least ten pastors from congregations that fall under each umbrella organization were interviewed. The interview comprised six questions:

1   Explain the impact of COVID-19 on you and your congregation and discuss adjustment you made in your congregation?
2   Do you have any diaconal programs prior or and during the pandemic? Discuss the adjustment you had to make because of COVID-19.
3   How have extreme social distancing affected your ministry?
4   Kindly share with us congregational written guidelines to address the above if you have them.
5   How are you reaching out to your congregants under COVID-19 restrictions?
6   Which methods of communication are you using to uplift people's spirits under realities of COVID-19?

A questionnaire was sent to 45 pastors who were requested to send their responses within a period of two weeks. Thirty questionnaires were sent back on time hence the number of participants is enough to gather valid information (Crouch & McKenzie, 2006). The data collected were coded and thematized according to literature review findings and the interview questions. This chapter was also guided by the practical considerations and recommendations for religious leaders and faith-based communities in the context of COVID-19 from the World Health Organization's (WHO). On the 7th of April 2020, WHO came up with an interim guidance on how religious leaders, faith-based organizations, and faith communities can play a major role in saving lives and reducing illness related to COVID-19.

## Findings and discussion

### *COVID-19 fear, anxiety and panic*

Given the impact of COVID-19 on health, financial, social, religious, political and travel aspects, there is a likelihood of increasing anxiety, fear and panic. The rise of other infections such as flu might exacerbate more concern and panic. Moreover, ungoverned media coverage on COVID-19 that talk about this pandemic as unique and deadly has added more stress and panic. On the other hand, uncertainty, social isolation may contribute to stress and breakdown (Shigemura et al., 2020).

When deliberating on how the Church in Botswana managed to deal with the psychological, emotional and social impacts of the pandemic, most of the respondents maintained that they used technology such as videos, audio tapes, phones, social media to reach out to their congregants and the wider society. The Evangelical Lutheran Church in Botswana (ELCB) Ramotswa Congregation created a WhatsApp group for its members called

"A Sermon" as a platform of sharing messages of hope during these difficult times (Interview with Deac. Bachomi, 2020).

The advantage of technology is that pastors managed to reach out to the wider society. Botswana national Television (BTV) recorded messages available online or handed to them by different churches and organizations such as Botswana Council of Churches (BCC). Even though the church could not measure the impact of media evangelism, people could hear the gospel with their families and people are being reached out without any possibility to gather. Those who do not have the internet and mass media orbit were encouraged to have household and family worship sessions.

A guide by the World Health Organization (WHO) outlines the critical role of religious leaders in disseminating accurate information, reducing fear and stigma and ensuring safe worship spaces and practices in the wake of COVID-19. As indicated, conspiracy theories that unsettled people were rampant and were coming from all angles including religious angles. What might have further caused confusion, anxiety, panic and stress were religious teaching that looked at COVID-19 as the end of the world, punishment from God or a tool of anti-Christ (Calys- Tagoe, 2020).

It is however part of human life to panic when people realize dangers which can threaten our lives. John 16: 33 says, "...fear not, I have overcome the world." Teachings such as these should liberate and strengthen people to develop responsible ways for dealing with the pandemic. People therefore need to hear words of hope and encouragement in order to deal with the fears that are caused by COVID-19. The Church should further reach out to those who are struggling to understand the meaning of life and questioning the existence of God in order to help them discover the meaning of their lives, and gain hope.

It is argued that religion is very important for COVID-19 health promotion. It contributes to better health and wellbeing (Hart & Koenig, 2020; Kowalczyk et al., 2020). In that regard, religion should not be viewed as a problem but as an important part of the worldview and lifestyle of the people. It is associated with the enhancement of health and it is an essential coping mechanism during these stressful times of COVID-19. Religion could further be a wheel that drives behavioural change, disease management in all levels including the revision of policies that are not favourable to the people (Kowalczyk et al., 2020).

In this era forward, therefore, the church should deliver hope where there is no hope instead of aggravating hopelessness. Church bodies such as BCC, EFB, OAIC and the umbrella body BONECO should be encouraged to examine the information from their member churches before circulation. The Church could also work alongside other service providers and the Ministry of Health and Wellness to ensure that people receive accurate information. In their sermons and messages, they should counter and address misinformation and misleading teachings which aggravate pain and stress. Moreover, the Church could translate accurate information to the language that could be understood by their members. The WHO has provided guidance that could be replicated and shared on different faith platforms. Ministry of Health and Wellness in Botswana has websites and different information channels that could be accessed for guidance.

## COVID-19 and abuse of other persons

According to the letter written by the Synod Chairman of the United Congregational Church in Southern Africa (UCCSA), COVID-19 has put stress on the ministry and mission of the denomination. It demands for strong support system, prayer circles, counselling networks and prayer. The Chairman encouraged members of the UCCSA to be each other's keepers during these trying times. He further advised that the doors of the Church should be open as isolation centres, accommodation for the homeless during lockdown. The Church was further advised to extend the psychosocial and spiritual support of the distressed members of our society (Global Ministries, 7th April 2020).

Moreover, Botswana Council of Churches (BCC) in collaboration with the Ministry of Nationality, Immigration and Gender Affairs Department in Botswana has called for all COVID-19 responses to include tactics to stop sexual and gender-based violence. BCC stated that services for survivors are harder to access during the lockdown. The Church and the whole religious sector were not regarded as essential during lockdown; therefore, it was not easy to go out promoting messages of gender justice and provide counselling and support services. The church was not able to address the pain and suffering of others because of different reasons such as lack of finances. One of the respondents cited Matthew 25:39–40 to prove that the church failed dismally to reach out to the needy during the lockdown. The text reads '... when was it that we saw you sick or in prison and visited you?' And the king will answer them, 'Truly I tell you, just as you did it to one of the least of these who are members of my family, you did it to me.'

Different churches in Botswana had similarly extended their facilities and resources to the needy during these trying times. However, there is a general concern of inadequate infrastructure and health facilities, posing higher risks for the spread of the disease. There is also a concern on lack of funds to enable the setting up of facilities for hand washing, manufacturing and distributing face masks as well as other hygienic measures. The Church is therefore challenged to promote collaboration and coexistence with relevant service providers during the COVID-19 pandemic. Through its close contact with local realities, the Church could direct action through advocacy.

Collaboration between religious and medical communities has been described as a smart move in the response to COVID-19. Community centred care that includes all stakeholders such as religious leaders, social workers, psychologists and social scientist should be encouraged in order to promote holistic healing (Winiger, 2020).

The World Health Organization recommends the use of technology to maintain connection and support people who need pastoral care, small-group interactive prayers and other forms of accompaniment (WHO, 2020). The organization highlights the increase of gender-based violence under the restricted environment. The Church is encouraged to actively speak against violence against women, children and marginalized people. It is also encouraged to provide support and encourage the abused persons to seek for assistance.

Another important role of the Church highlighted by WHO is advocacy. The Church is not only expected to provide a supportive environment, and it is also expected to advocate for the rights of the vulnerable people such as the elderly, youth, women, children and the San community. The World Council of Churches issued a Statement on the dual pandemics of COVID-19 and sexual and gender-based violence on the 23rd of April 2020. In the statement, the Church is advised to look beyond the current crisis and address the root causes of sexual and gender-based violence rather than wishing for a return to "normal." The Church is called upon to promote justice and peace that ultimately reduce vulnerabilities for all (WCC, 2020).

## COVID-19 and grieving

There is little knowledge about impacts of COVID- 19 related grieving on all those who had endured loss, but it is common knowledge that COVID-19 leave children orphaned and people without their loved ones everywhere including in Botswana. This adds to the abovementioned multiple stressors which are likely to contribute to mental health problems. "Grief is a normal reaction to loss. It is experienced as feelings and emotions, while it preoccupies the mind in the form of thought and worries" (UNICEF, 2002). This implies that grieving has to do with a process of accepting the reality that the relationship to a significant person is gone. People go through an intense sense of loss when a loved one dies. Louw (2008:560) advises that grieving people should be allowed to cry and talk about their grief as this will speed recovery. Unfortunately the nature of the pandemic and regulations that surround it could not make it possible for pastors to take people through the grieving process. However, if there is little or no social support, people may suffer depression. Their loss could be more heart-breaking if they had witnessed their loved going through pain and if they were not able to bury their loved ones.

People should therefore be empowered on grieving. More support groups who meet using different platforms should be formed to facilitate spiritual and religious coping and move through the grieve process towards healing. Individual counselling is also very essential during this time of need (Schoulte, 2011; Jeffreys, 2011).

## Diaconia and COVID-19

COVID-19 has affected all aspects of our lives; it has disrupted the socio-economic, psycho-emotional and the spiritual aspects of life. In a context of inequalities, promotion of self-interest and profit making such as ours, human lives are likely to suffer. The Church is also a victim of such context but has generally been engaged in humanitarian or diaconal services. During lockdown, some churches made contacts with their members through phone calls, WhatsApp calls and messages and emails. They used these platforms to pray, share uplifting reflections and to reach out to the concerns of their parishioners. Members were encouraged to donate food, shelter, clothing and share resources with those that had been affected by the pandemic. Communality and solidarity were attributes or values that were encouraged among members. In a joint message, the World Council of Churches, World Communion of Reformed Churches, Lutheran World Federation, and Council of World Mission urged governments to bolster support for healthcare and social protection, the Church is called to advocate against ineffective and corrupt governance at national levels that has exacerbated the inability to support those who are most vulnerable to the pandemic (European Christian Environmental Network, 2020). Hence suffering is structural and addressing its root cause brings sustainable development.

However, the government of Botswana has made a national call to contribute funds (or in-kind) to the COVID-19 Relief Fund. Individuals, companies, organizations and churches are making contributions towards the fund in order to cushion the economic status of the affected. The Seventh-Day Adventist Church (SDA) has donated the sum of P200, 000.00 to the COVID-19 Relief Fund and thus encouraged its members "who are financially able to voluntarily support this government initiative over and above what the SDA Church as an entity has contributed," (Guardian, 2020). As indicated, this palliative approach to address the socio- economic impacts of the pandemic is not sustainable. A sustainable approach is the one that restores inequities and justice; that acknowledges the intrinsic interdependence of humanity and all aspects of human existence. Economic success, peace and tranquility can only prevail if people are treated well.

## The challenge to the church

The idea of closing churches was not welcomed by some Christians during national lockdowns. According to lockdown regulations, a maximum number of 50 is expected to gather. This regulation was disregarded by some congregants who were constantly dispersed by the police officers (interview, 20/08/2020). In other instances, protesting campaigns were being organized. An "Open Churches" campaigns were brewing in some churches against the idea of the regulated number of the people gathering for worship. The campaigns were however silenced by the escalating numbers of the deaths that were COVID-19 related. The main argument behind those attempted protests was that as much as public transport and places selling liquor were in full operation, the Church should also be allowed to operate as normal; they wanted a waver in numbers of people who gather at Church to be lifted (interview, 20/08/2020).

The other argument posed was that the government of Botswana did not give the Church an ample opportunity to play their role especially in mobilizing their members to take part in relieving those who were financially affected by COVID-19. Although in some churches, congregants pledged some money towards that noble cause, other churches experienced dwindling financial contributions as their members were affected financially by the pandemic (interview, 22/08/2020).

In as much as preaching the gospel, caring for the poor and attacking injustices has been the role of the Church (Newbegin, 1960:911), the Church has been forced to belong to the private spaces; to belong to a digital mediated space that excludes the poor and vulnerable. These spaces have immensely impacted on the offerings. Not all could do online money transfers hence congregations are not able to provide for the needy during these trying times (interview, 20/08/2020).

Digital mediated platforms further exclude those who cannot access pastoral services because they cannot afford technological and internet devices. Furthermore, not all afford observing COVID-19 protocols such as social distancing and constant washing of hands with soap and clean water. For people who do not have the means to access clean water, soap and who are living in crowded spaces, it is near impossible to observe all COVID-19 protocols. The Church is therefore challenged to come up with new ways of reaching out to the poor in the context of COVID-19.

Notwithstanding, the Church was not even enabled to voice their concern when they saw the negligence of the economic needs of the poor people (interview, 22/08/2020). However, solidarity and liberation of the poor has always been the essence of being Church. The Church is looked upon as a moral compass, 'inspiring, transforming, life-giving work of the Holy Spirit' (Kim, 2009:30). The issue of poverty, injustices and inequalities are structural, and it affects the whole community, not a local church. Therefore, the Church during these times is forced to extend the services to all the people and address those structures that had long normalized pushing other people to the margins of the society. It is forced to be in solidarity with the poor through playing its transformative role (Kim, 2009:30).

## A challenge or an opportunity?

In fact the Church in Greek is referred to as *ekklesia* which means "gathering" (Magezi, 2012:4). It refers to the gathered people rather than a physical building. In that manner therefore, it is the buildings of the Church that are constantly closed as per the precautionary measures of COVID-19, but the

Church is never closed. It is rather unfortunate that the Church had confined itself in its walls when it is not supposed to be limited to a particular space. COVID-19 therefore has created an opportunity for the Church to re-evaluate its mission, mandate and further fully embrace its identity. Prior to COVID-19, the church has been unfaithful to its identity and calling.

Maybe the Church should start off by being contextual and adopt a culture of listening to people in their specific context and time towards societal change and transformation (Baron & Maponya, 2020:3). Being missional entails portraying God's glory in a transformative way. A missional Church therefore should find alternative ways of thinking about the church and an alternative hermeneutic to read the Bible in context (Niemandt, 2012:8; 2019:3). It should further be present to all people in all circumstances.

Digital mediated communication platforms such as video calls, zoom, emails, WhatsApp, Facebook provide opportunities for ministries that are not confined by space and time. Sermons are not necessarily prepared only for Sundays but are also prepared daily for all to follow in their space, be it at home with their families, while driving or at work. People grow spiritually whenever and wherever they are. In this case, ministers are forced to be innovative and adopt practical ministerial skills that are relevant for ministry during the COVID-19 era. Therefore, even though virtual space that excludes the poor and vulnerable, it makes it possible for people to be reached in all corners of the globe. Being missional, relevant and contextual entails using any available tool to be present, active and transformative in all circumstances. It entails coming up with long-term strategies to address poverty and domestic violence; focusing its mission to the needy and exploring new ways of being church as we try to transition to the new normal.

There is an urgent need for material support, financial and logistic resources. There is further need for advocacy for human rights and equity. A crisis like this demands for collaboration between the Church and other stakeholders such as the Ministry of Health and Wellness and civic organizations in providing justice, education services and psycho-social care to all. Liberation theologies should engage with scientists and policy makers to ensure that the Church rediscovers its identity and calling which is transformative and restorative in nature.

## Conclusion and recommendations

COVID-19 pandemic continues to ravage our social, religious and economic structures. Though being victim of the pandemic, not regarded as essential during this crisis, the Church is expected to be a part of finding long-term solutions. The visibility of the Church has become minimal during and after extreme social distancing. Other challenges such as domestic or gender-based violence and poverty were further aggravated by the lockdown. The Church focused more of its energies trying to maintain its visibility upon the suspension of physical and public gatherings. It has since succeeded hence Christians would continue to hear God's word in other ways. This means that the Church had opened itself to the paradigm shift. The only area that is lagging is advocacy for human rights and equity. When the economy is business not people based, more unrest is yet to come. Poverty is structural and should be dealt with amicably. Issues of abuse are also structural. Marginalization is deeply rooted in patriarchy, racism, ageism and corruption. Dealing with the structures that influence inequality may consequently bring sustainable long-term development.

## References

Baron, E., & Maponya, M.S. (2020). The recovery of the prophetic voice of the church: The adoption of a "missional church" imagination. *Verbum et Ecclesia* 41(1), a2077. https://doi.org/10.4102/ve.v41i1.2077.

Calys- Tagoe, J. (2020). *Theological Reflections on the COVID-19*. All African Conference of Churches (AACC-CETA), Kenya.

Crouch, M., & McKenzie, H. (2006). The logic of small samples in interview-based qualitative research. *Social Science Information* 45(4), 18. doi:10.1177/0539018406069584.

European Christian Environmental Network. (2020). Retrieved from https://www.oikoumene.org/en/press-centre/news/european-christian-environmental-network-releases-assembly-statement on the 20/04/2020.

Garg, S.K.L., & Whitaker, M., et al. (2020). Hospitalization rates and characteristics of patients hospitalized with laboratory-confirmed Coronavirus disease 2019—COVID-NET, 14 states, March 1–30, 2020. *Morbidity and Mortality Weekly Report* 69: 458–464. doi: 10.15585/mmwr.mm6915e3.

Gazette. (2020a). *Emergency Powers and COVID 19*. Gaborone: The Botswana Gazette.

Gazette. (2020b). *The Church Clashes with Gov't over COVID-19 Relief Fund*. Gaborone: The Botswana Gazette.

Global Ministries. (2020). Pastoral Ministry in the Wake of COVID-19: A Message from UCCSA Synod of Botswana. Retrieved from, https://www.globalministries.org/pastoral_ministry_in_the_wake_of_covid_19_a_message_from_uccsa_synod_of_botswana on the 28/05/2020

Guardian. (2020). *Seventh-Day Adventist Church (SDA) has Donated the Sum of P200,000.00 to the COVID-19 Relief Fund*. SDA. Gaborone: Guardian Newspaper.

Hart, C.W., & Koenig, H.G. (2020). Religion and health during the COVID-19 Pandemic. *Journal of Religion & Health* 59, 1141–1143. https://doi.org/10.1007/s10943-020-01042-3.

Ingstad, B., Bruun, F., Sandberg, E., & Tlou, S. (1992). Care for the elderly, care by the elderly: The role of elderly women in a changing Tswana society. *Journal of Cross-Cultural Gerontology* 7(4): 379–398.

Jeffreys, S. (2011). *Helping Grieving People When Tears Are Not Enough: A Handbook for Care Providers. Series in Death, Dying, and Bereavement*. New York: Brunner-Routledge.

Kim, K. (2009). *Joining in with the Spirit: Connecting World Church and Local Mission*. Epworth, London.

Kowalczyk, O., Roszkowski, K., Montane, X. *et al.* (2020). Religion and faith perception in a pandemic of COVID-19. *Journal of Religion & Health* 59, 2671–2677. https://doi.org/10.1007/s10943-020-01088-3.

Magezi, V. (2012). From periphery to the centre: Towards repositioning churches for Meaningful contribution to public health care. *HTS Teologiese Studies/Theological Studies* 68(2), a1312. https://doi.org/10.4102/hts.v68i2.131.

Mmegi. (2020a). *COVID 19: Masisi Declares State of Emergency, 28-Day Lockdown.* Gaborone: *Mmegi Newspaper.*

Mmegi. (2020b). *Possible Economic Impact of COVID 19 on Botswana.* Gaborone: *Mmegi Newspaper.*

Mogomotsi, G.E.J., Madigele, P.K., & Chamberlain, J.M. (2017). A cursory discussion of policy alternatives for addressing youth unemployment in Botswana. *Cogent Social Sciences* 3(1), 455–469: 1356619. https://doi.org/10.1080/23311886.2017.1356619.

Mudiare, P.E.U. (2013). Abuse of the aged in Nigeria: Elders also cry. *American International Journal of Contemporary Research* 3(9), 79–87.

Niemandt, C.J.P. (2012). Trends in missional ecclesiology. *HTS Teologiese Studies/Theological Studies* 68(1), a1198. https://doi.org/10.4102/hts.v68i1.1198.

Promislow, D. (2020). A geroscience perspective on COVID-19 mortality [published online April 17, 2020]. *Journals of Gerontology Series A Biological Sciences and Medical Sciences.* doi:10.1093/gerona/glaa094

Schoulte, J.C. (2011). Bereavement among African American and Latino/a American. *Journal of Mental Health Counseling* 33(1), 11. 2.

Shigemura J, Ursano RJ, Morganstein JC, Kurosawa M, Benedek DM (2020). Public responses to the novel 2019 coronavirus (2019-nCoV) in Japan: Mental health consequences and target populations. *Psychiatry and Clinical Neurosciences* 74(4):281–282. doi: 10.1111/pcn.12988.

Statistics Botswana. (2019). Labour Statistics Report 2011, Statistics Botswana, Gaborone, Botswana.

Sunday Standard. (2020). *WHO, UNICEF joins hands with Botswana as child rape continues to rise.* Retrieved May 28, 2020, from http://www.sundaystandard.info/who-unicef-joins-hands-botswana-child-rape-continues-rise.

UNICEF. (2020). *COVID-19: Children at heightened risk of abuse, neglect, exploitation and violence amidst intensifying containment measures.* Accessed at www.unicef.org. 22nd of May 2020.

Volpato, S., Landi, F., & Antonelli-Incalzi, R.A. (2020). Frail health care system for an old population: Lesson from the COVID-19 outbreak in Italy [published online April 21, 2020]. *Journals of Gerontology Series A Biological Sciences and Medical Sciences.* doi: 10.1093/gerona/glaa087.

WCC. (2020). *Statement on the dual pandemics of COVID-19 and sexual and gender-based violence.* Retrieved from https://www.oikoumene.org/en/resources/documents/wcc-programmes/women-and-men/statement-on-the-dual-pandemics-of-covid-19-and-sexual-and-gender-based-violence/view.

WHO. (2020). *Technical guidance #1. Strengthening the health systems response to COVID-19.* Copenhagen: WHO Regional Office for Europe. http://www.euro.who.int/__data/assets/pdf_file/0007/436354/strengtheninghealth-systems-response-COVID-19-technical-guidance-1.pdf, accessed 22 May 2020.

Winiger, F. (2020). "More than an intensive care phenomenon": Religious communities and the WHO guidelines for Ebola and Covid-19. *Spiritual Care* 9(3), 245–255. https://doi.org/10.1515/spircare-2020-0066.

World Health Organization. *Coronavirus disease (COVID-19) outbreak*. Available from: https://www.who.int/emergencies/diseases/novel-coronavirus-2019 [cited May 25, 2020].

Worldometers. (2020). *COVID-19 coronavirus pandemic*. Available from: https://www.worldometers.info/coronavirus/. Accessed 20 May 2020.

Yarona FM News. (2020).

# 13 The coronavirus pandemic and persons with disabilities

## Towards a liberating reading of the Bible for Churches in Southern Africa

*Makomborero Allen Bowa*

### Introduction

The COVID-19 pandemic has caused very serious social suffering across the globe and has exposed just how vulnerable our communities are. Societies are struggling to absorb the unfolding devastating consequences of the pandemic. In the context of Southern Africa, as is the case across the globe, the pandemic has severely disrupted public life and has had a devastating and ruinous impact on the formal and informal economy (UN 2020b:8; Paul et al. 2021:2). The implications of the coronavirus are much more far-reaching in the context of disability as the pandemic is triggering and exacerbating several challenges for persons with disabilities, particularly those who have always been vulnerable to economic discrimination. Developments from many Southern African countries including Zimbabwe, Zambia and South Africa strongly indicate that persons with disabilities continue to be the forgotten vulnerable community in the wake of the COVID-19 pandemic. Their challenges have been compounded by the impact of the pandemic which continues to threaten lives and livelihoods in ways that have not been seen or experienced before (UNPRPD and IDA 2020:2). The pandemic has deepened and heightened the marginalisation of persons with disabilities by increasing the risk of poverty in their lives. Recognising the unprecedented challenges that persons with disabilities are facing in the Southern African context, this article advocates for a more comprehensive and inclusive response from the Church in partnership with other stakeholders if the retrogressive impact of the pandemic is to be minimised.

Historically, the Church has a long history of reading the Bible poorly in response to disability resulting in the marginalisation of such persons in the broader societal context. A climate of exclusion in the context of disability characterises the Church in Southern Africa and the broader African society. The Church has contributed substantially to the stigmatisation and marginalisation of persons with disabilities through its faulty interpretation of biblical texts on disability. Certainly, the Church has contributed to the continuum of negative perspectives towards disability prevailing in

DOI: 10.4324/9781003241096-13

contemporary society, which perspectives nurture and perpetuate the nexus between disability and poverty in the Southern African context. This chapter engages and interrogates the beliefs in the Church that fuel negative perspectives on disability in Zimbabwe, Zambia and South Africa with the view advocating for a liberative approach to biblical texts on disability. The major implication of this way of thinking is that there must be a paradigm shift in the way the Church has addressed the issue of disability as suggested by Ndlovu (2016:36). This should result in the development of a liberative theology of disability, which theology is rooted in the positive perspectives on disability found in the Bible. The chapter further argues that the Church must champion a disability response to the coronavirus pandemic and any other future calamities of a similar magnitude and nature. The Church in Southern Africa has a huge role to play in serving the needs of persons with disabilities during and in the aftermath of the pandemic by taking appropriate action to guard against their marginalisation and stigmatisation through a liberative reading of biblical texts on disability. Therefore, this chapter assesses the potential risks for persons with disabilities during and in the aftermath of pandemic and articulates the measures that the Church in collaboration with other stakeholders can put in place to mitigate processes that may further marginalise persons with disabilities from the mainstream structures of society thereby exposing them to poverty.

## The Church in Southern Africa and disability: critical reflections on the Churches' interpretation of biblical texts on disability

The Church in the Southern African context, as is the case globally, has a long history of excluding persons with disabilities and this practice is rooted in its interpretation of biblical texts on disability. Osukwu (2019:61) indicates that the exclusion of persons with disabilities in the Church is a common practice that continuously negates the purpose of a "Church of All and for All". Respectively, writing in the context of Zimbabwe, Sande (2019:3) observes that when it comes to the integration in the mainstream of the Church, persons with disabilities continue to experience very serious exclusion and stigmatisation. This exclusion is nurtured and perpetuated by negative and discriminatory perspectives on disability, which perspectives are rooted in the Church's interpretation of biblical texts on disability. For Sande (2019:3), biblical interpretation is undoubtedly at the centre of denigrating persons with disabilities in the Church and consequently in the broader Zimbabwean society. Accordingly, Matsebula (2012:414) observes that there is a serious disparity in the recognition of disability as a human right and social development paradigm in South African Churches and this has been a great injustice to persons with disabilities. This disparity emanates precisely from the manner in which the Church interprets texts on disability. As Machingura (2019:212) indicates, the discriminatory attitudes towards persons with disabilities prevalent in the Southern African context manifest primarily from the intersection of cultural traditions and biblical texts on disability. As such, the Church has always provided the ideological funding which fosters the marginalisation of persons with disabilities. Consequently, the Church's interpretation of biblical texts on disability, particularly those found in the Old Testament, has been detrimental to the inclusion of persons with disabilities.

Scholarship on disability has established that the Old Testament contains texts such as Leviticus 21:16–23 depicting discrimination against persons with disabilities as well as texts such as Leviticus 19:14 and Deuteronomy 27:18 that call for non-discrimination (Vengeyi 2016:151,152,161; Nyamidzi and Mujaho 2016:78–90). What is surprising is that the Church in the Southern African context has tended to focus on those texts that depict disability negatively and yet there are several other texts that depict positive perspectives on the experience of disability. In their ancient social setting, both perspectives on disability had a bearing, particularly on the inclusion and exclusion of persons with disabilities in the mainstream structures of social organisation (Bengtsson 2014:290). The positive and non-discriminatory perceptions fostered the inclusion of persons with disabilities. Conversely, the negative and discriminatory perspectives promoted the exclusion of such persons from the mainstream structures of society. The Church in the Southern African context seems to have ignored this fact and has continuously focused on negative texts on disability which foster the exclusion of persons with disability. For example, in the Zambian context, the understanding of disability as the consequence of social-cultural and religious misfortunes directed to the family emanates partly from the Church's interpretation of biblical texts on disability (Banda-Chalwe et al. 2012:922). This idea has resulted in the exclusion of persons with disabilities. Therefore, as rightly pointed out by Machingura (2019:220), it is quite unfortunate that the Bible is intermingled with texts that have been interpreted in oppressive ways and these continue to reinforce the marginalisation, discrimination and exclusion of persons with disabilities from the mainstream structures of society

The fundamental implication of the Church's interpretation of biblical texts on disability has been the development of a theology that fosters the exclusion of persons with disabilities. The Church's approach to these texts has led to shrinking attitudes towards persons with disabilities. As Togarasei (2019:147) indicates, the Church's interpretation has informed its response strategy to the realities of disability through the ministry of charity and healing. Certainly, the perception of persons with disabilities as cases of charity has been prevalent in the Church. Historically, this has been the Church's approach to disability in Southern Africa but while this approach seems plausible, it has been quite problematic in that it reinforces the discrimination of persons with disabilities. It is in this respect that Mugeere et al. (2020:66–67) argues that even though charity may offer much needed help, it also promotes segregating and demeaning attitudes, rather than justice, equality and participation. Accordingly, Eiesland (2009: 240) is convinced that the Church has for too long provided the ideological funding and charitable practices which result in the marginalisation of persons with disabilities. For Wolfenberger (1998:15–16), persons with disabilities are often marginalised when society views them as objects of charity. Certainly, the lived experiences of persons with disabilities in many Southern African countries including Zimbabwe, Zambia and South Africa strongly indicate that persons with disabilities are marginalised and excluded from the mainstream structures of society.

Accordingly, Togarasei (2019:136, 137) stipulates that it is quite unfortunate that the Church has concentrated on the theology of healing since several problems arise from this theology in the context of disability. This theology develops from a faulty understanding which associates disability with sin, which system of thought has been very common in the Church from time immemorial. Throughout history, the Church has interpreted Biblical texts on disability in ways that subtly or explicitly reinforce the idea that disability is caused or is rather a consequence of sin (Satterlee 2010:34; Machingura 2019:214). For instance, Mugeere et al. (2020:75) highlights that in Zambia, some of the pastors portray persons with disability as testimony to God's punishment to the "wicked and spiritually cursed" and this has resulted in the development of a disabling theology which has been problematic for persons with disabilities. For Gosbell (2018:9) and Mugeere et al. (2020:75), the alleged association between sin and disability contributes substantially to the marginalisation and rejection of persons with disabilities in the broader societal context. Therefore, as Sande (2019:4) demonstrates using the example Apostolic Faith Mission in Zimbabwe, the faulty belief that disability is associated with sin is problematic as it fosters and perpetuates the discrimination of persons with disabilities and often encourages their withdrawal from the Church. Accordingly, this belief creates problems for persons with disabilities and results in their stigmatisation and exclusion (Chitando and Phiri 2016:471; Togarasei 2019:138,142). This faulty system of thought causes a lot of pain, embarrassment and disaffection on the part of persons with disability as they are often accused of being sinners or lacking faith in the event that their disabilities are not healed (Kabue 2016:228; Togarasei 2019:138). Consequently, this system of thought often disqualifies persons with disabilities from actively participation in the Church. For instance, Mugeere et al. (2020:75) highlights cases of pastors and other leaders who tend to exploit the plight of persons with disabilities in the name of performing healing in the Zambian context. Consequently, it is because of such developments that persons with disabilities withdraw themselves from actively participating in the institution of the Church.

Mueleman and Billiet (2012:173) argue that religious outlooks continue to structure the values, behaviour and attitude patterns in the broader society. In this respect, the use and interpretation of biblical texts on disability provides insights regarding how disability is constructed in the context of the Church and the broader Southern African context. As has been indicated, the Church has contributed immensely to attitudes towards disability prevalent in Southern African societies through its interpretation of biblical texts on disability. Certainly, by implication the negative and discriminatory perspectives on disability prevalent in these countries have emanated from the Church's teachings and attitudes towards persons with disabilities. It is in this respect that Masango (2019:4–6) argues that the church in the southern African context has not only neglected persons with disabilities but has also discriminated against them, and reinforced their exclusion from the mainstream structures of society. As suggested by Machingura (2019:220), biblical texts just like African traditions, beliefs and cultures must never be taken for granted when it comes to how they shape attitudes, values and beliefs towards disabilities. Thus, the Church plays a significant role in shaping attitudes towards disability, which attitudes filter into the broader society. What this means therefore is that, if the Church's perspectives on disability are predominantly negative and derogatory, as is common in most Churches in Southern Africa, the same attitudes are fostered in the broader communities thereby subjecting persons with disabilities to discrimination and marginalisation.

The fundamental implication of the Church's response to disability has been the exclusion of persons with disabilities from the mainstream structures of the Church and society. The negative perspectives on disability that develop from the Church's interpretation of texts on disability have given rise to the systematic segregation and oppression of persons with disability. In Osukwu's (2019:62) view, this explains why persons with disabilities are rarely considered in the larger scheme of things of the Church. Similarly, persons with disabilities are hardly considered in the mainstream activities of the Church in Zimbabwe. For instance, Sande's (2019:3,4) study demonstrates that there exists no disability focused subject in the pastoral training curriculum of most Churches and that a very few Churches in Zimbabwe have Braille Bibles and other facilities like ramps for persons with disabilities to use. Osukwu (2019:62) also indicates that it is extremely difficult to find any mainline Church in which persons with disabilities are ordained as priests. Respectively, it is extremely difficult to find persons with disabilities occupying positions of leadership in mainline Churches in Zimbabwe, Zambia and South Africa. For instance, Matsebula (2012:414) one of the major challenges is that the institution of the Church in South Africa has not accepted that disability is a human right that requires mainstreaming in all respects. This evidence clearly suggests that the exclusion of persons with disabilities from the structures of the Church emanates from the negative perceptions and ideologies relating to disability prevalent in the Church. The same negative and discriminatory perspectives are perpetuated in societies and foster the marginalisation and exclusion of persons with disabilities from the mainstream social, political and economic structures of social organisation. These negative attitudes transform into the discrimination of persons with disabilities, which discrimination is often exacerbated in crisis situations

## Social exclusion in the context of disability: implications on the poverty-disability nexus

Generally, social exclusion is a process that involves the marginalisation, systematic disadvantaging and discrimination of certain groups of people from mainstream society on the basis of their disability, ethnicity, etc. (Tobias and Mukhopadhyay 2017:25). In the context of disability, social exclusion involves the marginalisation of persons with different categories of disabilities from the mainstream society to the extent that such persons are systematically disadvantaged on the basis of their disability (ibid). Research has established that in any given context, social exclusion through marginalisation leads to poverty and deprivation (ibid). As such, social exclusion in the context of disability has the same effect. Ramachandran (2016:30) indicates that the relationship between social exclusion and poverty is such that poverty is seen as a consequence of social exclusion and social exclusion as a vulnerability factor leading to poverty. Research has also demonstrated that social exclusion confers disadvantage on certain groups and involves the inability to participate in the normal relationships and activities available to the majority of people in society, whether in economic, social, cultural and political arenas (Ramachandran 2016:26). Tobias and Mukhopadhyay (2017:26) also stipulate that social exclusion is a complex phenomenon that is closely linked with the complexity of powerlessness that often results from inadequate social participation. Certainly, social exclusion in the context of disability becomes a form of disempowerment, particularly for persons with disabilities, especially considering the fact it inhibits their integration into the mainstream structures of society. Consequently, it is this lack of participation that disempowers persons with disabilities and renders them helpless as well as incompetent.

This development makes persons with diverse disabilities powerless and susceptible to the very extreme levels of the social and economic condition of poverty in all its multi-faceted dimensions. As such, the poverty among persons with disabilities in contemporary Southern African societies especially in Zimbabwe and Zambia is one element that is ultimately associated with their powerlessness, which powerlessness is the primary result of exclusionary tendencies. When considering the relationship between poverty and disability, focus should be on the negative perspectives on disability since it is commonly acknowledged that such perspectives provide the foundation for the stigmatisation and discrimination of persons with disabilities (Nyamidzi and Mujaho 2016:78). In Southern Africa, the bulk of negative perspectives on disability which fuel the exclusion of such persons in society are rooted in the Church's faulty interpretation of Biblical texts on disability. Consequently, this social exclusion becomes the primary mechanism that connects disability and poverty. It becomes the very mechanism that perpetuates this vicious and disruptive connection. Given that research on poverty has generally established that social exclusion leads to poverty through fostering the marginalisation of certain categories of people in society (Tobias and Mukhopadhyay 2017:26), it therefore follows that the nexus between poverty and disability in contemporary African societies is rooted in the exclusion of persons with disabilities from mainstream structures of the Church and society.

Accordingly, the persistence of negative perspectives and attitudes towards disability in any given context confers great disadvantage on the lives of persons with disability. This is evidenced in the context of the Church in Southern Africa which continues to view disability in negative and discriminatory ways which emanate primarily from its interpretation of biblical texts on disability. Such perspectives have the power to influence the exclusion of persons with disabilities from both the mainstream structures of the Church and society. In other words, negative perspectives on disability confer disadvantage on persons with disabilities in that they establish the limits to the inclusion of such persons within the mainstream structures of Church and broader society. In fact, negative perspectives on disability establish the limits to the Church's social ideology of inclusion in the context of disability, resulting in the alienation of persons with disabilities from its mainstream structures. Therefore, negative perspectives on disability in the Church occasion the exclusion of persons with disabilities, which exclusion leads to marginalisation and discrimination of such persons in the broader society exposing them to serious conditions like poverty. In his study on disability in Southern Africa, particularly in Zimbabwe, Machingura (2019:212) attests that historically, persons with disabilities have experienced discrimination and poverty as a result of societal interpretation of scriptures on disability, which interpretation is often championed by the Church. As such, the institution of the Church has nurtured and perpetuated the nexus between poverty and disability prevailing in most Southern African countries through its interpretation of scriptures on disability.

## The COVID-19 pandemic and the increased risk of vulnerability and poverty among persons with disabilities in Southern Africa

Having established how social exclusion in the context of disability leads to poverty, this chapter advances the argument that the COVID-19 pandemic has increased the risk of vulnerability and poverty among persons with disabilities. Generally, crisis situations such as the COVID-19 pandemic magnify and exacerbate the challenges of all vulnerable groups in society including the constituency of persons with disabilities (UN 2020a:2). Peek and Stough (2010:1262,1268) argue that from a social vulnerability paradigm, persons with disabilities are most at risk during and in the aftermath of a disaster and have concluded that disasters often lead to unfolding adverse effects on the lives of persons with disabilities since such persons already face many developmental challenges. Respectively, the COVID-19 pandemic and its related socio-economic consequences is exacerbating the challenges of persons with disabilities (UNPRPD and IDA 2020:2). The negative perspectives that foster the exclusion of persons with disabilities are still in effect during the coronavirus crisis. For instance, in the context of Zimbabwe, the available evidence strongly indicates that persons with disabilities continue to be largely ignored in the responses to the pandemic. As Rambiyawo (2020) indicates, disability organisations such as the Centre for Disability and Development, Deaf Zimbabwe Trust and the Zimbabwe National League for the Blind have expressed concern over the unprecedented social exclusion of persons with disabilities in the government's Covid-19 response process and have advocated for a response that is not homogeneous, but disability category specific, corresponding directly to identified COVID-19 disability needs.

Generally, the response of many African countries is feeding on preexisting social and economic inequalities associated with disability and threatens to exacerbate them (UN 2020a:4). Certainly, Zimbabwe, Zambia and South Africa are not an exception. Generally, as Peek and Stough (2010:1264) indicate, the stigma and institutional exclusion often experienced by persons with disabilities can further threaten their physical health in the context of a crisis. In this respect, many persons with disabilities in the Southern African context are at a high risk during the Covid-19 era and their risk is twofold. First, persons with disabilities are at a high risk of contracting the coronavirus since gathering information can be more difficult for such persons in the context of a crisis as information changes so quickly, and yet that information is not made readily available in formats accessible, especially to persons with hearing, vision and even cognitive disabilities (UN 2020a:5). This the situation prevailing in the context of Zimbabwe to the extent that organisations representing persons with disabilities have sued the government and the Zimbabwe Broadcasting Corporation (ZBC) demanding accessible formats on all COVID-19 related information.

Respectively, in the context of Zambia and South Africa such organisations have emphasized the need for all other official communications by government ministries involved in the fight against coronavirus to be produced in formats which are accessible to persons with disabilities, through the use of Braille pamphlets, and audio versions, large print versions, and digital readable-text versions of official communications (IDA 2020). The unavailability of COVID-19 related information in formats accessible to persons with disabilities increases their vulnerability to the coronavirus, which vulnerability emanates precisely from their lack of sufficient information relating to the pandemic. Accordingly, most of the methods that have been recommended for preventing the spread of the pandemic prove to be ineffective in the context of disability as persons with certain types of disabilities struggle to adopt to social distancing and washing of hands regularly (WHO 2020:2). Such approaches are not always feasible for persons with certain types of disabilities and yet there are no specific initiatives that take into account such limitations and realities in the context of disability. Therefore, it is in this respect that the IDA (2020) has recommended that African countries, including Zimbabwe, Zambia and South Africa come up with holistic and integrated disability inclusive Covid-19 responses that meet the needs of people with disabilities across the entire COVID-19 prevention, treatment, mitigation, care and support spectrum (Rambiyawo 2020).

Secondly, persons with disabilities are at high risk of falling into extreme poverty during and in the aftermath of the pandemic. Tragically, the pandemic has plunged the world economy into recession and risks reversing decades of progress in the fight against poverty (UN 2020b:8–9). The pandemic threatens to derail the progress that has been made with regards to addressing the challenge of poverty among persons with disabilities in Southern Africa. The relationship between poverty and disability has been evident in a number of studies conducted around the world, especially in developing countries including Zambia and Zimbabwe (Mitra et al. 2011). This chapter contends that in Zimbabwe, Zambia and South Africa persons with disabilities belong to the vulnerable populations that are at a high risk of falling into abject poverty as a result of the pandemic. This argument is not far-fetched because persons with disabilities continue being excluded and their perspective is barely being included in the response to the pandemic. Writing in the context of South Africa, Trani et al. (2020:2) highlight that, persons with disabilities face high risks of poverty and their inclusion in humanitarian interventions and development policies remains elusive. As such, the pandemic threatens to exacerbate the levels of poverty experienced by persons with disabilities in South Africa especially considering that such persons with disabilities in South Africa have been disproportionately represented amongst the poor and many of them live in circumstances of poverty (Graham et al. 2013: 325).

The pandemic has had a devasting impact on the formal and informal economies (UNPRPD and IDA 2020: 2) and Southern African countries have not been spared especially considering the fact that the economies of countries such as Zimbabwe and Zambia have been fragile for a very long time. For instance, Paul et al. (2021:2) indicate that the economic consequences of pandemic have been felt most strongly by persons with disabilities and other vulnerable groups in Zambia and they argue that the pandemic has indeed exacerbated the poverty levels in the country. Respectively, Darren Sharpe (2021:15) et al. indicate that the high level of poverty in Zambia was already one of the major problems prior to the pandemic, especially for unemployed youth and people with disabilities. As such, the pandemic threatens to exacerbate this problem by increasing the risk of vulnerability and poverty among persons with disabilities. Certainly, the

COVID-19 shock has further aggravated the poverty and inequality situation in Zambia, whose economy has been increasingly fragile over the years (Paul et al. 2021:18). In the context of Zimbabwe, persons with disabilities are also among those worst affected by the COVID-19 pandemic and the national lockdown as many of them are unemployed with no stable income (Masenyama 2020).

Therefore, in the Southern African context, the pandemic is taking a heavy toll not only on the health of all people, but also on people's ability to earn a living, to feed themselves and their families. The pandemic has caused very serious human and economic devastation such that persons with disability are enduring great hardships. For instance, the majority of persons with disabilities in Zimbabwe, Zambia and South Africa survive on informal trading and most of them have been unproductive and continue to be unproductive until the lockdown measures are relaxed, a development that is largely devastating to their economic well-being. Consequently, the COVID-19 has become a food security issue in these countries as most persons with disabilities are food insecure since their livelihoods are informal and thus affected by the lock down measures (IDA 2020). This has impacted negatively on the financial situation of persons with disabilities such that if nothing is done to assist them their poverty will inevitably rise to extreme levels. As such, the pandemic is posing very serious challenges in terms of income security for persons with disabilities (UNPRPD and IDA 2020: 2), which financial challenges are likely to worsen even in the aftermath of the pandemic.

According to Peek and Stough (2010:1261), disaster risk is socially distributed in ways that reflect pre-existing inequalities in that some groups are more vulnerable and prone to economic loss in the wake of different hazards. It is quite unfortunate that this is exactly the pattern witnessed in the context of disability during the era of the COVID-19 pandemic. Generally, as has been indicated before, the response to the pandemic is feeding into pre-existing social and economic inequalities associated with disability and threatens to exacerbate them (UN 2020a:4). In the Southern African context, the pandemic has exposed a climate of exclusion and inequality in the context of disability, which often characterises most African societies in normal times. For instance, the government of Zimbabwe announced a ZWL600 million financial package to assist vulnerable households during the lockdown but it is unclear whether persons with disabilities are beneficiaries of this programme (ZimRights 2020:13). Thus, it is apparent from the government of Zimbabwe's response to the pandemic that there is no specific package to cater for persons with disabilities (Masenyama 2020). The absence of a disability specific financial package attests to the exclusion of persons with disabilities in the government's response strategy.

This is a disturbing development especially considering that the pandemic is surely affecting persons with disabilities more significantly than the rest of the population in Southern African context. Consequently, persons with disabilities have undoubtedly become a more vulnerable group within a vulnerable population, especially considering that they are already excluded and are subjected to very serious social suffering which is largely felt in relation to poverty. Generally, persons with disabilities are rarely considered in the larger scheme of things even though such persons constitute a significant part of the population (Osukwu 2019:62). Similarly, this pattern is witnessed in Zimbabwe, Zambia and South Africa where persons with disabilities are being excluded particularly in measures to mitigate the devasting economic impact of the pandemic on the population. It is also unfortunate that the pandemic has exacerbated the challenges faced by persons with disabilities as the barriers to their inclusion have become even more complex and heightened. It has become extremely difficult for persons with disabilities to navigate many community, institutional and attitudinal barriers, which barriers are even challenging for them in the absence of any pandemic or crisis (UN 2020a:9). Such persons are certainly struggling against negative and discriminatory perspectives on disability which are perpetuating their exclusion in the wake of the pandemic. In essence, the pandemic is negatively impacting on the health and economic well-being of persons with disabilities resulting in the increased risk of vulnerability and poverty among such persons, not only in the context of Zimbabwe, Zambia and South Africa but across the African continent as well.

## Positive perspectives on disability and the social ideology of inclusion: lessons from the old testament for Churches in Southern Africa

Historically, the Church's interpretation of biblical texts on disability has tended to focus on the negative and discriminatory perspectives on disability, which perspectives have always led to the exclusion of persons with disabilities. Fundamentally, this has created the impression that positive perspectives on disability are absent in the Bible, and yet the reality is that texts such as Job 29:15, Leviticus 19:14 and Deuteronomy 27:18 exist and clearly articulate positive perspectives on disability that contest the stigmatisation and marginalisation of persons with disabilities. Certainly, in their original context, such texts commanded the Israelites to treat persons with disabilities as one would treat those without (Vengeyi 2016:135). The positive perspectives captured in texts such as Leviticus 19:14 and Deuteronomy 27:18 were designed to respond to prevailing discriminatory social attitudes that led to the stigmatisation and marginalisation of persons with disabilities in the ancient society (Frick 2003:229; Olyan 2008:1; Vengeyi 2016:160). In most cases, such exhortations acted as mechanisms for the inclusion of persons with disabilities. The objective of such measures was that of protecting persons with disability against stigmatisation and discrimination which would ultimately culminate into their exclusion from the main structures of social organisation.

This exclusion was a threat to the concept of social justice in that it fostered the stigmatisation and discrimination of persons with disabilities violating the maintenance of social solidarity in ancient Israel. As such, texts in the category of Leviticus 19:14 offered an alternate perspective on disability. This alternate perspective protected persons with disability against discrimination and indeed fostered their inclusion into the mainstream structures of society. The logic of this line of inquiry leads to the conclusion that the exhortations expressed in the texts were social protection measures that were meant to eliminate or mitigate against the exclusion of persons with disabilities which resulted from the actions that the texts strongly speak against. The behaviours that are discouraged in such texts had the potential of inhibiting the participation of persons with disabilities in the mainstream structures of society. As a result, persons with disabilities were excluded on the basis of such negative perspectives and this increased their risks of falling into poverty.

Having indicated that positive perspectives on disability exist in the Bible, this chapter argues that there has to be a paradigm shift in the way the Church in the Southern African context has addressed and dealt with the issue of disability. As Ndlovu (2016:36) rightly puts it, there is need to rethink all religious attitudes, doctrines and practises emanating from Christianity that militate against full participation of the persons with disabilities in the mainstream activities of society. Given that in the past the Church has nurtured negative perspectives through its faulty interpretation of biblical texts on disability, it now has the mandate to cultivate positive perspectives through the same process. Writing in the context of South Africa, Masango (2019:4–6) argues that there is need for a theology that will help us to reconstruct a full understanding that persons with disabilities are also created in the image and likeness of God, and thus they can and must fully participate in society. Machingura (2019:220) argues that the theological engagement of the Bible must help challenge our theological understandings and misunderstandings that promote the exclusion of persons with disabilities. This calls for the development of a theology of disability in the context of Churches in Southern Africa, which theology must be informed by a liberative reading on Biblical texts on disability, particularly texts that express positive perspectives on disability. This theology of disability should seek to liberate persons with disabilities from all oppressive structures and systems that contribute to their material deprivation and discrimination (Ndlovu 2016:37).

The Church's mission towards persons with disabilities should not necessarily be limited to healing and charity, but their empowerment and integration into our societies (Satterlee 2010:37; Togarasei 2019:136,138). Togarasei (2019:138,147) further argues that the mission of the Church in the context of disability, must not only be limited to what happens in the Church, but to go as far as advocating for the welfare of persons with disabilities in society and ensure that such persons are included and participate fully in all activities of their societies. This is exactly what the Church in the Southern African context and across the African continent needs do during and in the aftermath of the coronavirus pandemic. To achieve this, the Church has to seriously endorse all positive perspectives on disability in the Bible that can be appropriated in the creation of a more just and inclusive society (Ndlovu 2016:36,37). Respectively, Churches in Southern Africa must engage such positive perspectives on disability to counter to prevailing negative and discriminatory social attitudes towards disability that are subjecting persons with disabilities to various forms of stigmatisation and marginalisation exposing them to extreme levels of poverty during and in the aftermath of the coronavirus pandemic.

It is evident that the COVID-19 pandemic is deepening pre-existing inequalities, exposing the extent of exclusion in the context of disability (UN 2002a:2). As such, it is imperative that the Church, as an institution that commands moral authority, must ensure that persons with disabilities are not isolated and ignored in any initiatives. The Church has to champion the inclusion and integration of persons with disabilities during and in the aftermath of the COVID-19 pandemic. Swinton (2012:172) argues that the idea of including persons with disabilities does not go far enough in overcoming the alienation, stigmatisation and exclusion of such persons and he thus advocates that the Church should move from ideas of inclusion to the practices of belonging. The thinking of belonging should therefore be at the centre of the Church's theology of disability to ensure that persons with disabilities are accepted for who they are without having to conform to some kind of faulty relational social and legal norms that are defined society (Swinton 2012:184). This thinking of belonging in the context of disability must therefore inform the Church's response during the period of the pandemic. The integration of persons with disabilities should find its roots in the Church's interpretation of Biblical texts on disability, which interpretation should be inclined towards exploiting the positive perspectives that foster a social ideology of inclusion and belonging in the context of disability. The Church in Southern Africa must provide an alternative social ideology of inclusion which contests the stigmatisation of persons with disabilities. This social ideology of inclusion must be engaged as a mechanism to protect persons with disabilities against stigmatisation and discrimination which consequently leads to their exclusion from the mainstream society. Respectively, this social ideology of inclusion based on the liberative interpretation on Biblical texts on disability can be the primary mechanism that the Church can use to break the connection between disability, vulnerability and poverty in Southern Africa especially considering that historically this connection is nurtured by negative perspectives on disability which emanate primarily from a poor reading of the Bible.

## Conclusion

This chapter has established that COVID-19 pandemic has disrupted many aspects of people's lives, but its impacts are especially acute for persons with disabilities. Historically, the Church in Africa has contributed largely to the continuum of attitudes towards disability which are predominantly negative and discriminatory through its interpretation of biblical texts on disability, Consequently, such negative attitudes have fostered the exclusion of persons with disabilities from the mainstream structures of the Church and broader society. This exclusion has nurtured the correlation between disability, vulnerability and poverty in the Southern African context. The chapter has argued that the COVID-19 pandemic has increased the risk of vulnerability and poverty among persons with disabilities in Zimbabwe, Zambia and South Africa. In these countries, persons with disabilities are subjected to very serious social suffering, during the era of the COVID-19 pandemic and their suffering is heavily felt in relation to the social condition of poverty. The chapter has argued that the positive perspectives on disability in the Bible can be quite resourceful for the Church in Africa in its fight against the systematic and institutionalised marginalisation of persons with disabilities in the wake of the COVID-19 pandemic. The pandemic has created an opportunity for the Church to revise its approach to biblical texts on disability and embrace a more liberative reading of these texts to enforce positive social attitudes towards disability. In essence, this inevitably leads to the inclusion of persons with disability in the mainstream structures of the Church and the broader Southern African societies during and in the aftermath of the pandemic. Essentially, such positive perspectives emanating from the Church will reduce the chances of persons with disabilities being seriously disadvantaged, socially and economically thereby breaking the causal intersection between poverty and disability in many African countries including Zimbabwe, Zambia and South Africa.

## References

Banda-Chalwe, M., Nitz, J.C. & Desleigh de Jonge. 2012. "Globalising Accessibility: Drawing on the Experiences of Developed Countries to Enable the Participation of Disabled People in Zambia", *Disability & Society*, 27:7, 917–934.

Bengtsson, S. 2014. "On the Borderline-representations of Disability in the Old Testament", *Scandavian Journal of Disability Research*, 16:3, 280–292.

Chitando, E. & Phiri, L. 2016. "Religious response to multiple layers of exclusion against people with disabilities, and HIV in Africa", In Kabue S., Amanze J., Landman C. (eds), *Disability in Africa, Resource Book for Theology and Religious Studies*. Kenya: Acton Publishers.

Eiesland, N. 2009. "Sacramental Bodies", *Journal of Religion, Disability & Health*, 13:3–4, 236–246.

Frick, F. 2003. *A Journey Through the Hebrew Scriptures*. USA: Thompson Wadsworth.

Gosbell, L. 2018. *The Poor, the Crippled, the Blind and The Lame": Physical and Sensory Disability in the Gospels of the New Testament*. Germany: Mohr Siebeck.

Graham, L., Moodley J. & Selipsky, L. 2013. "The Disability–Poverty Nexus and the Case for a Capabilities Approach: Evidence from Johannesburg, South Africa", *Disability & Society*, 28:3, 324–337.

International Disability Alliance. 2020. When Accessible Information is Far From a Reality: Zimbabwe during COVID-19. Accessible at https://www.internationald-isabilityalliance.org/covid19-story-zimbabwe

Kabue, S. 2016. Disability: Post-modernity Challenges to the Theology. In Kabue S., Amanze J. & Landman C. (eds), *Disability in Africa: A Resource Book for Theology and Religious Studies*. Nairobi: Action Publishers.

Machingura, F. 2019. "The 'Unholy Trinity' Against Disabled People in Zimbabwe: Religion, Culture and the Bible", In Chataika T. (ed), *The Routledge Handbook of Disability in Southern Africa*. London and New York: Routledge Francis and Taylor.

Masango, M.J. 2019. 'Neglect of People with Disability by the African Church', *HTS Teologiese Studies/Theological Studies* 75:4, a5631, 1–6.

Masenyama, M. 2020. "Govt Forgot Plight of People with Disability During Lockdown', *New Zimbabwe*. Accessible at. https://www.newzimbabwe.com/govt-forgot-plight-of-people-with-disability-during-lockdown/

Matsebula, S.P. 2012. "Persons with disability in South Africa", In Kabue Samuel and Mombo Esther (eds), *Disability, Society and Theology*; Zapf Chancery Publishers Africa.

Mitra, S., Aleksandra, P. and Vick, B. 2011. "Disability and poverty in Developing Countries", *World Development*, 20:10.

Mueleman, B. & Jaak, B. 2012. "Religious Involvement: Its Relations to values and Social attitudes", In Eldad Daridor, Peter Schmidt, Jaak Billet (eds), *Cross Cultural Analysis: Methods and Applications*. London: Routledge.

Mugeere, A.B., Omona, J. State, A.E., & Shakespeare, T. 2020. "Oh God! Why Did You Let Me Have This Disability?": Religion, Spirituality and Disability in Three African Countries", *Journal of Disability & Religion*, 24:1, 64–81.

Ndlovu, H. 2016. "African Beliefs Concerning People with Disabilities: Implications for Theological Education", *Journal of Disability & Religion*, 20:1–2, 29–39.

Nyamidzi, K. & Mujaho, Z. 2016. "Disability and the Beauty of Creation: An Analysis of the Old Testament Perceptions on Disability", In Kabue S., Amanze J., & Landman C. (eds) *Disability in Africa, Resource Book for Theology and Religious Studies*. Kenya: Acton Publishers.

Olyan, S. 2008. *Disability in the Hebrew Bible: Interpreting Mental and Physical Differences*. New York: Cambridge University Press.

Osukwu, C. 2019. "Disability, Performance, and Discrimination", *International Review of Mission*, 108:1, 53–64.

Paul, B.V., Finn, A., Chaudhary, S., Gukovas, R.M. and Sundaram, R. 2021. "COVID-19, Poverty, and Social Safety Net Response in Zambia", *Policy Research Working Paper 9571, World Bank Group: Social Protection and Jobs Global Practice*. Accessible at: https://elibrary.worldbank.org/doi/pdf/10.1596/1813-9450-9571

Peek, L. and Stough, L. 2010. "Children with Disabilities in the Context of Disaster: A Social Vulnerability Perspective", *Child Development*, 81:4, 1260–1270.

Ramachandran, M. 2016. "Poverty, Social Exclusion and the role of a Comprehensive Human Rights Framework", *ILI Law Review*, 24–25.

Rambiyawo, L. 2020. Zim needs disability Covid-19 Response. *The Herald*. Accessible at https://www.herald.co.zw/zim-needs-disability-covid-19-response/

Sande, N. 2019. "Pastoral ministry and Persons with Disabilities: The Case of the Apostolic Faith Mission in Zimbabwe", *African Journal of Disability*, 8, pp. 1–8.

Satterlee, C. 2009. ""The Eye Made Blind by Sin": The Language of Disability in Worship", *Liturgy*, 25(2), 33–41.

Sharpe, D., M, Rajabi, M., Chileshe, C., Joseph, S.M., Sesay, I., Williams, J. and Sait, S. 2021. "Mental Health and Wellbeing Implications of the COVID-19 Quarantine for Disabled and Disadvantaged Children and Young People: Evidence from a Cross-Cultural Study in Zambia and Sierra Leone", *BMC Psychology*, 9:79, 1–15.

Staffan, B. 2014. "On the Borderline-Representations of Disability in the Old Testament", *Scandavian Journal of Disability Research*, 16(3), 280–292.

Swinton, J. 2012. "From Inclusion to Belonging: A Practical Theology of Community, Disability and Humanness", *Journal of Religion, Disability & Health*, 16(2), 172–190.

Tobias, E. and Mukhopadhyay S. 2017. "Disability and Social Exclusion: Experiences of individuals with visual impairments in the Oshikoto and Oshana regions of Namibia", *Psychology and Developing Societies*, 29(1), 22–43.

Togarasei, L. 2019. "Paul's "Thorn in the Flesh" and Christian Mission to People with Disabilities", *International Review of Mission*, 108(1), 136–147.

Trani, J.F., Moodley, J., Anand, P., Graham, L. and May, T.T.M. 2020. "Stigma of Persons with Disabilities in South Africa: Uncovering Pathways from Discrimination to Depression and Low Self-Esteem", *Social Science & Medicine*, 265, 1–12.

United Nations. 2020a. Policy Brief: A Disability-Inclusive Response to COVID-19. Accessible at https://www.un.org/development/desa/disabilities/wp-content/uploads/sites/15/2020/05/sg_policy_brief_on_persons_with_disabilities_final.pdf

United Nations. 2020b. Shared Responsibility, Global Solidarity: Responding to the Socio-Economic Impacts of Covid-19. Accessible at https://www.un.org/sites/un2.un.org/files/sg_report_socio-economic_impact_of_covid19.pdf

United Nations Partnership on the Rights of Persons with Disabilities and International Disability Alliance. 2020. Disability Inclusive Social Protection Response to Covid-19 Crisis. Accessible at http://unprpd.org/sites/default/files/library/2020-04/SP%20inclusive%20leaflet_COVID%2019_2.7_fin.pdf

Vengeyi, O. 2016. "The Interpretation of Biblical Texts on Disability: Then and Now", In Kabue S., Amanze J., & Landman C. (eds), *Disability in Africa, Resource Book for Theology and Religious Studies*. Kenya: Acton Publishers.

Wolfensberger, W. 1998. *A Brief Introduction to Social Role Valorization: A High-Order Concept for Addressing the Plight of Societally Devalued People, and for Structuring Human Services.* Syracuse, NY: Training Institute for Human Service Planning, Leadership and Change Agentry (Syracuse University).

World Health Organisation. 2020. Disability Considerations during the COVID-19 Outbreak. Accessible at https://www.who.int/publications-detail/disability-considerations-during-the-covid-19-outbreak

Zimbabwe Human Rights Association. 2020. "Their Voices Matter" Community Responses to Covid-19 Measures in Zimbabwe. Accessible at https://www.zimrights.org.zw/download/Their%20Voices%20Matter%20Week%203%20Report.pdf

# 14 The influence of health perceptions on Zimbabwe Muslim responses to COVID-19 restrictions over Ramadan, pilgrimages and funeral rites in 2020

*Edmore Dube*

## Introduction

Serious debates have raged on pertaining to whether faith communities do not endanger public health with respect to such rituals as "touching, kissing and washing of bodies" (Winiger 2020: 246). This debate is particularly important because faith communities claim a large majority of the world population; directing their interactive and health perceptions according to religious values (Sulkowski & Ignatowski 2020: 1). Anthropological studies on viral diseases such as Ebola and influenza have long demonstrated the dangers associated with such rituals both with respect to those living with the infections and corpses of victims of such diseases. Early epidemiological studies on the spread of COVID-19 in Shia Muslims shrines observed similar dangers, noting that earlier studies on Ebola and influenza ought to be utilized. By February 2020 it was already known that those who visited "Shia Muslim holy sites of Qom and Mashhad" in Iran were partly associated with the spread of the initial cases of COVID-19 in the Middle East (Barmania & Reiss 2021: 16). In early March 2020 South Koreans traced nearly 5,000 patients (two thirds of all known cases) to 'Patient 31' who had attended a church gathering in which touching and disregard of masks and registers were openly encouraged by the church leadership (Wildman et al. 2020: 115). The case demonstrated that faith communities defying regulation endangered other communities well beyond their borders. The World Health Organization (WHO), however, tends to reject the perception that faith communities are a great risk to public health, preferring to see them as invaluable partners in health promotion instead. Needless to say, that the three rituals are part of the Muslim traditions with respect to touching and kissing shrines, and corpse ablutions. The necessary temporary suspensions of these rituals can safely be done with the faith communities taking the lead in the interest of health promotion.

Scientists and anthropologists have also put overcrowding during rituals including worship, pilgrimage and funerals, among super-spreaders of

DOI: 10.4324/9781003241096-14

viral diseases. By deemphasizing human touch and spontaneity in gatherings for acts of worship and bereavement, COVID-19 has not only affected human bonding with each other, but has inevitable communicated itself as "a sickness of solitude" (Winiger 2020: 252). Despite the barring of worshippers from accessing prayer houses, shrines and severe limitation to funeral attendances, Muslim communities in Zimbabwe rejected the position of Mantineo emphasizing that the overwhelming emotions remained those of "sorrow, grief and loneliness" (Mantineo 2020: 29). Muslims were convinced that though such feelings could not be ruled out there was mitigation provided by the Quran and the *Sunnah* (traditions) of Prophet Muhammad, which made pandemics liveable experiences. The Muslim public health perceptions discussed below demonstrate why Muslims have not been overwhelmed by the banning of religious assemblies during the important times of Ramadan, pilgrimages and funeral services in the year 2020. That was especially after demonstrations that funerals in South Africa and Indonesia had been noted among the early spreaders, with ritual corpse ablutions at the centre (Barmania & Reiss 2021: 18). In this case religious leaders become essential in selecting the relevant traditions that can take people out of the crisis. Religious leaders have the power to proscribe or alter certain traditions in the face of both the marauding pandemic and severe state limitation of citizen freedoms in the public interest (Consorti 2020b: 15), as will become apparent. The discussion on public health perceptions below demonstrates that religious world views may help believers overcome such problems of freedom limitations.

## Muslim perceptions on public health

Muslims in Zimbabwe, as elsewhere, emphasise a worldview dominated by the Quran and the *Sunnah* of the Prophet in their discourses on public health and pandemics. Mandatory reference to these sources in all matters makes all decisions subject to religion. Consequently, Muslims and Muslim organisations deploy Islam for their understanding of health issues (Al-Khayat 2004: 7). Though the Quran is not a book of prescriptive medicine, it is revered for its overall guidance on health and disease control. That it makes reference to healing in Surah 17:82 legitimises not only healing, but all forms of surveillance meant to forestall sickness including vaccinations and lockdowns. Parents are strictly charged with the immunisation of their offspring to forestall the outbreak of preventable epidemics (Al-Khayat 2004: 23). Vaccination is read in light of a *hadith*[1] attributed to Muhammad, which praises the removal of obstacles on the road in order to ease life: "To remove a harmful object from the road is an act of benefaction" (Al-Bukhari, as cited by Al-Khayat 2004: 23). The physical act of removing objects from the environment is generalised to include all environmental pollutants, including viruses for which immunisation becomes necessary. Since dirty environments are the key causes of disease outbreaks, one *hadith* puts Muhammad on record as stressing: "Clean your houses" (Al-Tirmithi, as cited by Al-Khayat 2004: 24). A clean environment is therefore the first stage to a healthy community, because "there shall be no contagion and no evil omen" (Al-Bukhari, as cited by Al-Khayat 2004: 24).

Muslims in Zimbabwe adopted the world *ummah*'s normative position of emphasising active participation (Ayatollahi 1992: 117), to facilitate both "health promotion and health protection" (Al-Khayat 2004: 7). In that regard Surah 17:82, is read together with Surah 17: 70 arguing that health as an honour to humanity is inevitably "a basic human right" (Rahman & Mahmud 2014: 2). Public health and the right to life are further read in light of Surah 5:32: "And if anyone saved a life, it would be as if he saved the life of the whole people." Muslim public health professionals who answer calls to save lives through their services count themselves in the service of God, dispensing religious calls.

Muslims communities noted that 'hand washing procedures' were pristine Muslims' traditions adopted by WHO on account of merit. It has been found out that religions which emphasize cleanliness as next to godliness are better placed to handle regular hand-washing, "a key strategy in the defence against COVID-19" (Barmania & Reiss 2021: 19). In that regard Muslim scholars contend that "in health, cleanliness is considered one of the basic and cheap prevention and control methods in disease occurrence. Cleanliness is also an essential part of Islamic life" (Rahman & Mahmud 2014: 4). To Muslim (2010), is also attributed a *hadith* which equates cleanliness to 'half of faith.' This *hadith* is read together with Surah 2: 222, which states that "Truly, Allah loves those who turn to Him constantly and He loves those who keep themselves pure and clean." These "hygienic teachings of Islam" observed since the days of Prophet Muhammad (Ayatollahi 1992: 117), need religious leadership with sufficient knowledge and skill to communicate them now that they are needed most to roll back the pandemic. Ritual purity and cleanliness are important for the Muslims as specified in Surah 5:6:

> O ye who believe! When ye prepare for prayer, wash your faces, and your hands (and arms) to the elbows; rub your heads (with water); and (wash) your feet to the ankles. If ye are in a state of ceremonial impurity, bathe your whole body.

Bathing is commendable for ridding the body of pathogens capable of causing disease. Such pathogens may not be taken into the mosque where people may spread them through contact. Those parts most capable of carrying and transmitting them are recommended for thorough washing before prostration with the rest (Abdalati 1986: 60). Though the same rules are enforced for lone worship, their physiological impacts become more pertinent during mass prayers. The relevant carrier parts of the body receive thorough attention, with at least three water rinses each. In practical terms, when using modern sewer systems, the believer uses running water so that the same water may not be reused. Reusing untreated water may pass dangerous pathogens to the next user. WHO (2020: 2) advises that modern ablution facilities be sanitised regularly. In the absence of modern water reticulation, the worshipper uses a container to get water for ablutions out of the natural water system. One is not supposed to do the ablutions into the natural water system (stream, river or oasis) (Al-Khayat 2004: 25).

It is important to note that Muslim scholars who compiled the *Hadiths* back in the 9th century were already sensitive to pandemics; and more so that Muslim scholars in Zimbabwe demonstrate clear exposure to such *hadiths*. The *Hadiths* compiled by Al-Bukhari (1996) and Muslim (2010) proposed lockdown and exclusion for the containment of disease outbreaks. The relevant hadith says, "When you hear about a break of plague in any area, do not enter there and when it has broken in a land where you are, then do not run away from it [and spread elsewhere]" (Rahman & Mahmud 2014: 5). This *hadith* was the most widely cited text by Muslims in Zimbabwe. It helped with the comprehension of the statutory lockdowns affecting pillars of Islam in 2020. The understanding was that in case of a plague on the *hajj* (pilgrimage) route, or in the holy city of Mecca, affected pilgrims have always been advised to cancel the pilgrimage (Mandivenga 1983: 28). Prophet Muhammad stated: "Do not let those infected transmit their disease to those who are healthy" (Al-Bukhari and Muslim, as cited by Al-Khayat 2004: 29). Further traditions helped Muslims comprehend the lockdowns which affected the economy and the majority of the wealth-seeking enterprises. Those were read in line with another *hadith* attributed to Muhammad: "Wealth is of no harm to a God-fearing person, but to the God-fearing, health is better than wealth" (Ibn Majah et al., as cited by Al-Khayat 2004: 14). Making wealth subservient to health helped in the spiritual and psychological comprehension of the proscriptions to wealth-seeking enterprises in light of COVID-19.

## Lockdown and the celebration of Ramadan in Zimbabwe

The 2020 edition of Ramadan was celebrated in individual household *ummahs* despite it being the Muslim "annual season of worship, comradeship and relationship" (Shaban 2020: 1). Like their fellow Abrahamites (Christians) who had for the first time celebrated an "Easter of the heart", the Muslims went on to experience the first Ramadan without public ceremony between April 23 and May 23 2020 (Picciaredda 2020: 113). Mosques and collective worship places had been placed out of bounce by the successive government statutory instruments meant to legalise lockdowns for the rolling back of COVID-19. Through these statutory instruments the formal ritualistic activities of normal worship were proscribed severely limiting the fundamental rights to worship. The limitations were accepted on the grounds that they were the last resort and that consequences would be dire if they were not implemented. There was general agreement that there was necessity for the regulations "of such a gravity as to trump the exercise of religious liberty" (Hill 2020: 3). There was no other law capable of achieving the same with a lesser gravity on the rights of citizens in line with international standards (Rivers 2006: 198). Of necessity was that "the SARS-CoV-2 is a virus that is transmitted with tremendous facility, mutates fast, and is proving to be particularly resilient" requiring quick stringent measures (Martínez-Torrón 2021: 2). Both jurists and religious believers understood the exceptional circumstances they were in, considering that a lot still needed to be scientifically decided. In that regard the restrictions were necessary and not just convenient, especially in their attempts to "flatten the curve" in a period of great uncertainties (Dandara et al. 2021: 210).

Of particular importance for the 2020 Ramadan edition was the absence of the communal *iftar*, which terminated fasting in the evening, pulling together large groups to share meals together. This comradeship had been an indelible mark of Ramadan for centuries. Muslims generally increased mosque attendance during Ramadan to do marathon prayers known as *taraweeh* and *qiyam*. Such attendance increased in the last ten days as Muslims spent consecutive days and nights at mosques for the *i'tikaf* prayers (WHO 2020: 1). Muslims in Zimbabwe missed these acts of comradeship with the understanding that they were following divine law prohibiting deliberate facilitation of epidemic diseases. Being "particularly attuned to the exhortations by religious scholars" during Ramadan (Ndzovu 2020: 1), Zimbabwe Muslims found themselves in reception of numerous messages of caution. Homes were turned into temporary mosques, which the leadership of the Zimbabwe National Zakat Fund said had the enhanced function of developing family ties. The Supreme Council of Islamic Affairs worked closely with the Zimbabwe COVID-19 Muslim Taskforce, overseeing enforcement of council decisions on the closure of mosques and compliance with national statutes (Moyo 2020). The council noted that it was permissible under Islamic law to forgo certain obligatory rituals to serve lives. Muslims in Zimbabwe avoided both insistence on worshiping in groups despite the ban (Cilliers 2020: 1), and taking the legal route to challenge confinement as happened in neighbouring South Africa (South African High Court, April 30, 2020; Friedman 2020). That court upheld the ban stating that the pandemic threatened to collapse an already overwhelmed South African healthcare system (Ibid). Such "clear instructions" in favour of "national policies" were considered paramount (WHO 2020: 1).

The severity of the SARS-Vov-2 virus meant that mere analysis of the regulatory frameworks "without an appropriate consideration of their application" was inadequate (Guzzo 2020: 20). Admittedly, its world impact has been estimated at more than the dreaded Spanish Influenza of 1918 which resulted in the demise of nearly 50 million lives (Martínez-Torrón 2021: 1). It was equally in adequate to consider only secular application apart from religious law for which sheikhs and imams were invaluable.

Such acute cooperation was required where new fast spreading strains had developed (Consorti 2020a: 7), as one entering Zimbabwe from South Africa. That is particularly invaluable when divine law contains such a statute as: "If an epidemic may appear in a land, don't go there; and if you are in that land, don't escape from it." The religious leadership may securely use it to stay believers home in contentment, especially as the Muslim tradition adds that "one should keep away from a leper [one with a contagious disease] as one keeps away from a lion" (Consorti 2020a: 10). Sheikh Henry Balakaz, the secretary general of the Zimbabwe Muslim *Zakat* Fund, told Studio Seven that Muslims prayed at home in line with the lockdown rules, which gave them prime time with their families (Studio 7a). Such an interpretation of a crisis as an opportune time for enjoyment of family relations had the obvious tenacity of facilitating "adaptation to the disease or the restrictions resulting from it" (Kowalczyk et al. 2020: 2672). That was more important considering fear had gripped people of all ages and faith communities as the ultimate "hospitals for the soul" (Ibid). It was important that faith communities further regulate apart from the state (Sulkowski & Ignatowski 2020: 2).

Imam Isa explained to the same station that the idea of lockdowns was long prescribed by Al-Bukhari, as already highlighted above (Studio 7b). The idea was to show that history was already aware that in the past religious communities were able to adapt their religious practices to the demands of the epidemics in order to defeat them (Sulkowski & Ignatowski 2020: 2). Ibrahim told the same station that those who were sick could fast later, if only that was possible before the next Ramadan (Studio 7b). The Gutu and Chinhoyi congregations noted that they had no fear of contracting COVID-19 through consumption of public food, because they ate in their own homes at dawn and broke the fast back home at dusk. In Mashonaland East, Muslims gave out Ramadan groceries on 4 May 2020, at Chitekwe Primary School north of Mutoko growth point. The groceries comprised steri milk, cremora, cooking oil, instant porridge, matemba, sugar, rice, salt, spaghetti, maize meal, bars soap, soya chunks and a three-litre paraffin stove. Those acts of charity were done with full realization that acts of want  might put many people in danger of contracting COVID-19. It was similarly noted that minority faith communities in the United Kingdom "over-represented in areas of material deprivation" were "disproportionately affected by COVID-19" (Barmania & Reiss 2021: 16). Despite the ban on movement and gathering in Zimbabwe, the Muslim welfare groups did not forget the needy, and the government did not prohibit food assistance which was extremely necessary in that period of general cessation of work. As most of the professional work was brought into the obit of home, those managing that adaptation and creating more gave a hand to those whose means could not be thus adjusted. It was particularly difficult to bring to fruition those blue collar jobs that required one to get to the work place for inputs. It was generally observed, even then, that the restrictive regulations were in line with the Zimbabwe constitutional order with respect to health emergencies (Constitution 2013: Section 86 [2b]). By proscribing the normal flow of life, however, such laws always gave rise to certain painful limitations directly or indirectly (Androutsopoulos 2021: 1). The sanctity of the said regulations lay in the fact that they were short term, temporary and liable to revision from time to time.

## Muslims in Zimbabwe and the cancellation of *umrah* and *hajj*

Both Sunni and Shia Muslims in Zimbabwe accepted the cancellation of *umrah,* a minor pilgrimage to Mecca which normally runs throughout the year (Abdo & Jacobs 2020). The cancellation was not just in line with the theory of the spread of COVID-19 through human contact, "respiratory droplets and contact with contaminated surfaces" (WHO 2020: 1), but had a concrete foundation in the research works surrounding early pilgrims to Qom and Mashhad (Barmania & Reiss 2021: 16). The Shia shrines in Iran and Iraq, which ordinarily drew millions of pilgrims, were eventually closed due to such research works. The Shia kissed the walls of shrines where the religious figures were buried, which often bred diseases in ordinary times, raising fears that it would be worse with the more contagious COVID-19 (Abdo & Jacobs 2020).

Muslims initially hoped that the major *hajj* event, which takes place in Dhu al-Hijjah, might have a chance of surviving the pandemic (Chitwood 2020), but that did not happen. The traditions of kissing and sheer numbers running into millions made *hajj* authorities cancel it for the year 2020. During the *hajj* those closest to the Kaabah kissed the black meteorite during *hajj* circumambulations, which was risky with respect to COVID-19. Historical knowledge of previous cancellations and public health perceptions helped Muslims appreciate the multiple cancellations of pilgrimages to the holy shrines. In 1858, *hajj* was disrupted by cholera, while in 2012–2013 it was affected by outbreak of the Middle East Respiratory Syndrome (MERS) in Saudi Arabia (Chithood 2020). Such wisdom of 'staying away from the sick' also proved efficacious in the Bubonic Plague that broke out in Germany in 1527 (Consorti 2020: 9a). The main focus was the preservation of the sanctity of life as demanded by the Holy Scriptures and the sacred Muslim traditions. For the year 2020, however, a negligible number of Saudis was allowed into the Meccan shrine, observing the WHO benchmarks for the non-spread of COVID-19 (Barmania & Reiss 2021: 19). Cognizant of the safety traditions, however, Zimbabwean Muslims were content with their exclusion from the major Muslim shrines together with the rest of the world. So they were not only prevented by the statutory regulations, but were generally not prepared to take any risks as they were content that their stay was in line with the divine law of safety. Contrary to the positive stance taken by the Zimbabwe *ummah*, misguided believers in some places "may understand the physical health risks of meeting with others but still wish to attend communal worship on a regular basis" (Barmania & Reiss 2021: 20). Such blatant disregard for personal and collective safety with respect to Zimbabwean Muslims and Muslims domicile in Zimbabwe was partial noted with respect to funeral rites of one popular fitness trainer discussed below.

## Muslim funeral rites during COVID-19

As noted earlier, improperly handled funeral rites had led to the inadvertent spread of COVID-19 in South Africa and Indonesia among other nations (Barmania & Reiss 2021: 18). The faith communities felt obliged by context to follow certain procedures endorsed by the leadership, which even held the honour to recommend obliging funeral parlours to the faithful (Business Reporter 2015). Locally such an honour was reserved for the ambassador of Islam who vetted compliance with Muslim requirements. COVID-19 statutory instruments sought to control the volume of mourners to forestall the possibility of virus spread due to congestion. More so, all deaths were to be treated as suspected COVID-19 fatalities, and the accompanying rituals to be conducted with utmost restraint in the earliest time possible. But where there is religious competition and unverified suspicion fanned by the social media numbers are difficult to regulate (Karombo 2021). Reference is made here to a single funeral service which drew headlines at the end of November 2020. It was the funeral of Mitchell (Moana) Amuli, a socialite and fitness trainer of repute, with estranged parents – a Muslim father and a Christian mother. She died in a car-crash that killed three other passengers (Karombo 2021). Each parent claimed her body intending to bury it according to a specific tradition. When the High Court eventually decided in favour of the father, the case had already attracted sympathizers on either side (Kafe 2020; Karombo 2021). To try and narrow the gap the two families then agreed that the body would pass through the mother's Christian home enroute for burial.

Though the relevant law limited ritual to a hundred mourners with masks and maintaining social distancing, this particular funeral ceremony ran into quite a few hundreds (Mandivengerei 2020). Many mourners disregarded both masks and social distancing attracting this Facebook comment: "The picture here shows over 100 people not observing social distancing. What is really wrong with us? Where is the police?" (Kafe 2020). Although religious leaders had been at the forefront encouraging compliance with the rules, the faithful were not always meticulous in following the rules, courting the ire of the authorities. In some places people were actually dispersed with water cannons (Barmania and Reiss 2021: 17), while in others they were issued with "fixed penalty notices" (Hill 2020: 6). For Africans this might be a result of *unhu/ubuntu* requiring spontaneity in offering compassion in times of bereavement. Such a tradition makes it difficult to hold people back from expressing their heartfelt condolences in persons, even in the face of breaking a prohibition law as in the case of these mourners.

First mourners crowded the mother's residence in a high density Harare suburb known as Highfield, disregarding the mask notice the gate. The strategic placement of the plaque – 'NO MASK NO ENTRY' – served no purpose for the enthusiastic mourners (Mandivengerei 2020). Its regulatory authority as required by WHO standards was ineffectual in the absence of security authorities enforcing the said law. The police could have made the men manning the sanitizer stand more relevant in the midst of the COVID-19 storm, but in their absence the men were equally ignored to the point of giving up. A relevant component of the ritual (sanitizers) felt disempowered, further putting the mourners who literally jostled to get a clear view of the metal coffin on the hearse of a Muslim funeral parlour at risk. It was not immediately clear whether any risk assessment had been done for the smooth running of the rite of passage, and to enable contact-tracing if needed afterwards.

At the mosque *hijabs* were purposefully converted into masks for female Muslims, leaving a large section of male Muslims and non-Muslims to risk their lives without the protective masks. Then the mob moved on to Warren Hills Cemetery where they crowded the grave in a ritualistic manner with some holding the body and others shielding it with a green cloth as it was being lowered into the grave. The crowded scene has been frozen by *The Sunday Mail* photographer, Innocent Makawa, among others (Kafe 2020). The picture shows disregard for security despite a spike in the new cases with an average of 85 new infections a day, at the heels of 275 deaths (Mandivengerei 2020). Morality would dictate caution, but as Wildman et al. (2020:116) contend: "knowing that people are religious does not tell us as much as we might imagine about their ethical judgments." The obvious religious convictions of the mourners visible in pertinent regalia were insufficient to influence safety standards. Some had even invited non-Muslim observers, to dispel peddled myths about Muslims' burials (Mandivengerei 2020).

## Conclusion

Muslim perceptions on public health have been quite influential to Muslim reactions to statutory laws prohibiting gatherings for the purposes of worship during Ramadan as well as pilgrimages. Studies had confirmed the risky nature of undertaking pilgrimages that included the rituals of "touching and kissing," but without open support for the subsequent prohibitions by sacred traditions and divine laws, the outcome might be different. Funeral rituals, as elsewhere proved difficult to regulate despite supportive sacred scriptures. Secular law enforcement seemed best placed to assist in the implementation of statutory instruments in cooperation with religious leaders struggling to achieve the same from a religious perspective.

## Note

1 Schacht (1986: 34) defines *hadith* as "a formal tradition deriving from the Prophet." The capitalised word refers to a book containing several *hadiths* (traditions). Each tradition is called a *hadith*, and the book containing several *hadiths* is called *Hadith*.

## References

Abdalati, H., 1986, *Islam in Focus,* NOPP, Riyadh.

Abdo, G. & Jacobs, A. L., 2020, Are COVID 19 restrictions inflaming religious tensions? *Brookings*, April 13, Doha Center, viewed 20 June 2020, from https://www.brookings.edu/blog/order-from-chaos/2020/04/13/are-covid-19-restrictions-inflaming-religious-tensions/

Al-Bukhari, M., 1996, *Sahih,* Darussalam, Riyadh.

Al-Khayat, M. H., 2004, 'Health as a Human Right in Islam', *WHO Regional Office for the Eastern Mediterranean,* Harmony, Cairo.

Androutsopoulos, G., 2021, 'The Right of Religious Freedom in Light of the Coronavirus Pandemic: The Greek Case', *Laws* 10 (14), 1–9. https://doi.org/10.3390/laws10010014.

Ayatollahi, S. M. T., 1992, 'Nutrition from the point of view of Islam', *Medicine Journal of the Islamic Republic of Iran* 6 (2), 115–122.

Business Reporter, 'Doves launches Muslim funeral package', *Newsday* 22 May 2015.

Chitwood, K., 2020, '*Hajj* cancellation wouldn't be the first- plague, war, and politics disrupted pilgrimages long before coronavirus', *The Conversation,* viewed 21 July 2020, from www.theconversation.com

Cilliers, C., 2020, 'Malema defends cops asking Muslims defying lockdown in South Africa: "Muhammad is bigger than the president?"', viewed 28 July 2020, from https://citizen.co.za/news.

Consorti, P., 2020a, 'Introduction', in P. Consorti (ed.), *Law, Religion and Covid-19 Emergency*, pp. 7–11, DiReSom, Pisa.

Consorti, P., 2020b, 'Religions and Virus', in P. Consorti (ed.), *Law, religion and covid-19 emergency,* pp. 15–18, DiReSom, Pisa.

Dandara, C., Dzobo, K. & Chirikure, S., 2021, 'COVID-19 Pandemic and Africa: From the Situation in Zimbabwe to a Case for Precision Herbal Medicine', *OMICS, A Journal of Integrative Biology* 25(4), 209–212. https://www.liebertpub.com/doi/10.1089/omi.2020.0099.

Friedman, H., 2020. 'South African court upholds COVID-19 ban over objections of mosque and imams', *Religion Clause.* May 5.

Guzzo, L. M., 2020, 'Law and Religion During (and after) Covid-19 Emergency: The Law is Made for Man Not Man for Law', in P. Consorti (ed.), *Law, Religion and Covid-19 Emergency*, pp. 19–27, DiReSom, Pisa.

Hill, Q. C. M., 2020, 'Coronavirus and the curtailment of religious liberty', *Laws* 9(27), 1–19.

Kafe, E., 2020, 'Moana finally rests', *The Sunday Mail* 29 November 2020.

Karombo, T. A., 2021, 'Social media star died, then a battle over her burial rites reached Imbabwe's high', *Religion Unplugged.* 4 February 2021.

Kowalczyk, C. O., Roszkowski, K., Montane, X., Pawliszak, W., Tylkowski, B. & Bajek, A., 2020, 'Religion and faith perception in a pandemic of COVID-19', *Journal of Religion and Health* 59, 2671–2677. https://doi.org/10.1007/s10943-020-01088-3.

Mandivenga, E. C., 1983, *Islam in Zimbabwe,* Mambo Press, Gweru.

Mantineo, A., 2020, 'I have a dream: Restarting, but going where?' in P. Consorti (ed.), *Law, Religion and Covid-19 Emergency*, pp. 29–34, DiReSom, Pisa.

Martínez-Torrón, J., 2021, 'COVID-19 and religious freedom: Some comparative perspectives', *Laws* 10 (39), 1–16. https://doi.org/10.3390/laws10020039.

Mandivengerei, P., 2020, 'Zimbabwe: Mourners defy covid-19 regulations to bury Moana', *AllAfrica* 29 November 2020, viewed 31 May 2021, from https://allafrica.com/stories/202011300356.html.

Moyo, J., 2020, 'Zimbabwe: Villagers cancel ritual of meeting dead spirits', *AA World-Africa* 21 April 2020, viewed 31 May 2021, from https://www.aa.com.tr/en/africa/zimbabwe-villagers-cancel-ritual-of-meeting-dead-spirits-/1812480

Muslim, I. N., 2010, *Sahih,* Pustaka Azzam, Jakarta.

Ndzovu, H. J., 2020. 'Women's stories of breaking the mould as Muslim preachers in Kenya', *The Conversation,* 23 April 2020.

Picciaredda, S., 2020, 'Religions, Africa and COVID-19', in P. Consorti (ed.), *Law, Religion and Covid-19 Emergency,* pp. 109–118, DiReSom, Pisa.

Rahman, A. A. & Mahmud, A., 2014, 'A review of the Islamic approach in public health practices', *International Journal of Public Health and Clinical Sciences* 1(2), 1–13.

Rivers, J., 2006, 'Proportionality and variable intensity of review', *The Cambridge Law Journal* 65, 174–207.

Schacht, J., 1986, *An Introduction to the Islamic Law,* Clarendon Press, Oxford.

Shaban, A. R. A., 2020, 'Ramadan 2020: Muslims Straiten rows for the locked down fasting', *Africa News,* 21 March 2020, viewed 10 July 2020 from http://www.africanews.

Studio 7, *Voice of America.* 2020. 1900 Bulletin [a 26/04/2020], [b 21/05/2020] [c 24/05/20], Viewed from www.voashona.com.

Sulkowski, L. & Ignatowski, G., 2020, 'Impact of COVID-19 pandemic on organization of religious behaviour in different Christian denominations in Poland', *Religions* 11(254), 1–15. https://doi.org/10.3390/rel11050254.

Wildman, W., Bulbulia, J., Sosis, R. & Schjoedt, U., 2020, Religion and the COVID-19 pandemic. *Religion, Brain and Behavior* 10, 115–117. https://doi.org/10.1080/2153599X.2020.1749339.

Winiger, F., 2020, '"More than an intensive care phenomenon": Religious communities and the WHO guidelines for Ebola and Covid-19', *Spiritual Care* 9(3), 245–255. https://doi.org/10.1515/spircare-2020-0066.

World Health Organisation, 2020, 'Safe Ramadan practices in the context of COVID-19', viewed 22 May 2021, from https://www.who.int/emergencies/diseases/novel-coronavirus-2019/technical-guidance/points-of-entry-and-mass-gatherings

# 15 Repositioning the agency of Rastafari in the context of COVID-19 crisis in Zimbabwe and Malawi

*Fortune Sibanda*

## Introduction

Globally, the raging coronavirus (COVID-19) pandemic caused by the SARS-CoV2 virus has created an unprecedented health crisis affecting over 80 million people and claiming over 1,750,000 lives (Kovalchuk, Wang, Li, Rodriguez-Juarez, Ilnytskyy, Kovalchuk, & Kovalchuk 2021). First detected in Wuhan in China, the World Health Organisation (WHO) declared it a public health emergency on 30 January 2020 (Nhamo, Dube & Chikodzi 2020:4; WHO 2020). The SARS-CoV2 mainly spreads through human-to-human transmission particularly via airborne and contact routes. Research has shown that "COVID-19 has a rather broad spectrum of clinical manifestations, ranging from asymptomatic, to mild flu-like disease, to pneumonia, that in some cases can further progress to acute respiratory distress syndrome (ARDS), major organ failure and death" (Kovalchuk et al. 2021:1571). In addition, Kovalchuk et al. (2021) observed that approximately 20% of COVID-19 cases are serious or severe, and death rate is currently estimated to be around 10%. In all this, whilst the elderly and individuals with pre-existing conditions are among the most affected, it has recently become thread-bare that no one is completely safe from the ferocity of the disease across the class, gender, age, race and national divides. This makes COVID-19 pandemic a serious health crisis that requires urgent action by individuals, private and public institutions as well as religious players.

This chapter examines the Nyabinghi Rastafari communities' responses to COVID-19 crisis in Zimbabwe and Malawi. The chapter argues that Rastafari, an often stigmatised, misunderstood, demonised and criminalised minority religious movement located on the margins (Afari 2007; Sibanda 2017a), has navigated around hegemonic attitudes, *politricks* and conspiracy theories of 'Babylon' system in order to reposition its agency in the context of COVID-19 crisis in both Zimbabwe and Malawi. Rastas consider 'Babylon' to be Western hegemony in general terms, but the term also refers to any system of oppression, both by whites or blacks who are never trusted because they are full of tricks – *'politricks'* (Edmonds 2003). In other words, 'Babylon' is life-denying and de-humanising, which has resulted in

DOI: 10.4324/9781003241096-15

Rastafarians protesting against the endemic Western epistemological hegemonic tendencies detrimental to human flourishing. The Rastafari Afrocentric counter-cultural perspective echoes what the Nigerian literary artist, Chimamanda Ngozi Adichie, described as "the danger of a single story" (Adichie 2009). Therein, it has to be asked: To what extent can Rastafari agency provide an alternative narrative in the context of COVID-19 crisis in Zimbabwe and Malawi? Before delving into the nuts and bolts of these issues, focus is first placed on the theoretical framework and research methodology that informed the study.

## Theoretical framework and research methodology

The chapter was informed by the Afrocentric theoretical framework and a qualitative research methodology. Also known as Afrocentricity, the Afrocentric theory is the study and examination of phenomena from the standpoint of Africans as subjects rather than objects calling for "collective consciousness" among African people (Asante 1998, 2007; Johnson 2001:408). Popularised by Molefi Kete Asante and a group of other Temple University scholars, Afrocentricity regards history, culture and philosophy of African people as critical in determining one's approach to reality and the understanding of the world. Put differently, Afrocentricity implies that there is a distinct African worldview anchored on three basic tenets, namely, (a) harmony with nature, which emphasises the uniqueness and right-to-be of every group and species; (b) survival of the tribe, which suggests a reciprocal relationship between the individual and the community; (c) and foremost, spiritual conscientiousness, which reveals that the spirit is invested in everything (Johnson 2001:409; Setiloane 1986:4). These tenets are said to be expressed in the thoughts and behaviours of most African people and could therefore inform their responses to emergency disaster situations such as COVID-19. The broader intellectual aim of Afrocentricity is to challenge and to deconstruct Western denial and misrepresentation of African history, knowledge systems and culture (Asante 1998; Sibanda 2017b:191), which could foreground the agency of Rastafari.

With Rastafari being an Afrocentric movement in its orientation, the Afrocentric theory is helpful in exploring Rastafari responses to COVID-19 pandemic in Zimbabwe and Malawi. The Afrocentric theory is beneficial because it can stand as "both a corrective and a critique" (Asante 2007:27) to the attitudes and actions of current and future generations pertaining to the coronavirus disease. The corrective features of the Afrocentric theory targets the stigmatised, exploited, underutilised, underdeveloped, misused and abused Rastafari lifestyle, philosophy and spirituality that could be harnessed to combat COVID-19 crisis in Zimbabwe and Malawi. As a critique, the Afrocentric theory could challenge Africans to express their agency seeking home-grown solutions tailored to the public health needs and predicaments of Zimbabwe, Malawi and the African continent at large.

Afrocentricity challenges the white "racial superiority" that places Western culture at the centre, whilst African heritages are marginalised. This explains why Asante and other scholars developed Afrocentricity in order to "obliterate the mental, physical, cultural and economic dislocation of African people by thrusting African people as centred, healthy human beings in the context of African thought" (Asante 2007:120). Therefore, the Afrocentric theory is relevant to this study as it challenges the *politricks* of Western epistemology and racism by placing the agency and action of African people at the centre in the fight against COVID-19 pandemic in Zimbabwe and Malawi.

The chapter utilised a qualitative phenomenological research design that provided a description of the experiences of participants from an insider perspective. The study corroborated insights from the phenomenological and historical approaches to describe and analyse data. The historical method involves a hermeneutics and is important in tracing the origins, development and impact of the COVID-19 pandemic and to bring out how Rastafari communities perceived the disease in Zimbabwe and Malawi. The research used the phenomenological principles such as *epoche* (bracketing out), descriptive accuracy, *eidetic* intuition (establishing the meaning) and comparison (Cox 1996; Sibanda 2017b:192). The two approaches were used in a complimentary way. In order to collect data, the study conducted unstructured in-depth telephonic interviews with 14 purposively sampled information-rich Nyahbinghi Rastafari elders in Zimbabwe and Malawi. Of the 14 interviewees, nine of them were based in Zimbabwe whilst the remaining five were based in Malawi. In Zimbabwe, of the nine study participants, two were women Rastas and seven were male whereas in Malawi one participant was female out of the five participants. In addition, besides the telephonic method, the in-depth interviews were enhanced through social media conversations, especially WhatsApp. Along the same lines, the study used Documentary Analysis of the print and electronic media of newspapers, Rastafari music, archival documents and social media text messages. Essentially, social media analytics was used for studying texts and songs, which were gateways to understanding Rastafari responses to COVID-19 pandemic in Zimbabwe and Malawi. On ethical matters, the study uses "fire names" of some of the informants with the consent of such participants and remained anonymous where it was suitable.

## The hegemonic rivalries surrounding COVID-19 crisis

The devastating effect of COVID-19 pandemic is wreaking havoc and humbling every country, economy, society, and social class such that many governments were caught unprepared or underprepared by coronavirus (Zeleza 2020). It is notable that initially China covered up on the COVID-19 outbreak and only notified WHO after hundreds had been infected. This created an environment of fear, class struggles and anxiety, which propelled racism and xenophobia (Nhamo et al. 2020:12). In addition, COVID-19 pandemic exposed social and political fault lines in the community with those marginalised on the receiving end. Put differently, the pervasive structural and social inscriptions of differentiation still cast their formidable and discriminatory capacities for prevention and survival including disparities on health care access. This is comparable to Sen's (1981) observation about poverty and famines where "it was not lack of food per se but the inability to access it that lay at the root of many famines". The availability of COVID-19 vaccines also had similar trends of inequitable distribution, with Africa being the most affected. This further confirms a warning against the hypocrisy of dominant powers attributed to the former Libyan leader, Muammar Gaddafi, when he stated, thus: "They will create the viruses themselves and sell you the antidotes. Thereafter, they will pretend to take time to find the solution when they already have it". This makes COVID-19 to be regarded by some Afrocentrists (Rastas included) as a planned genocide and a scandal of great magnitude.

In fact, the coronavirus was regarded as a foreign pathogen, a 'Chinese virus' in the eyes of the former American President, Donald Trump and his Republican followers (Zeleza 2020). Indeed, at the beginning of the coronavirus outbreak, China bore the brunt of both victims and victimization. The entire world feared the contagion spreading from China and other Asian countries such as South Korea, Taiwan, Singapore, and Iran where the disease quickly diffused. This triggered anti-Chinese and anti-Asian racist bashing in Europe, North America, and even Africa. Pertaining to Africa, Zeleza (2020, n.p.) notes that

> For many Africans it was a source perverse relief that the coronavirus had not originated on the continent. Many wondered how Africa and Africans would have been portrayed and treated given the long history in the western and global imaginaries of pathologizing African cultures, societies, and bodies as diseased embodiments of sub-humanity.

This shows the Western hegemonic tendencies that created an imbalance in society from time immemorial.

There is a long and shameful history of unethical drug testing on communities of colour across the globe (Pailey 2020). For instance, the white "racial superiority" reared its ugly head in early 2020 when two French doctors proclaimed on their national television that Africa would be the most appropriate location for a coronavirus vaccine trial. The paradox at that time was that Africa had the lowest recorded number of cases globally (Pailey 2020). This shows that black bodies could be used or abused for the convenience of some hegemonic forces that evoked their Conradian and Hegelian racist approaches to black bodies.

The hegemonic rivalries were further noted when Tanzania and Madagascar were caught up in the COVID-19 controversies. The then Tanzanian

President, John Magufuli, requested the military to test the genuineness of the donated COVID-19 test kits which he suspected were faulty. Furthermore, Magufuli ordered that Madagascar COVID Organics treatment be brought and used in Tanzania (Nhamo et al. 2020:13). The COVID Organics was a herbal remedy made out of Artemisia plant prepared by the Malagasy Institute of Applied Research. What is critical to note is that WHO initially dismissed the COVID Organics saying that it was not a cure for COVID-19 but later changed its position indicating the possible benefits of alternative medicines to treat the disease (Nhamo et al. 2020:13). This resonates with Nhemachena (2021:1) who observed that Africa as a region "has ever since not been allowed to reclaim anything original". Essentially, it echoes the idea that Africa and other regions of the Global South have demonstrated that they are not passive centres for medical experimentation but are sites of home-grown solutions which should be transmitted globally (Pailey 2015, 2020). Therefore, there is a lot of politics surrounding the origins, development and possible solutions to COVID-19 pandemic, which has triggered conspiracy theories, even among Rastafarians in Zimbabwe and Malawi.

## History of Rastafari in Zimbabwe and Malawi

Historically, the emergence of Rastafari is traced to Jamaica among the ex-black slaves partly due to the influence of Garveyism, Ethiopianism and Pan-Africanism. Marcus Garvey was an early 20th-century Jamaican black nationalist and evangelical preacher who popularised the 'Back to Africa' movement stressing black pride. As "successors of Garvey" (Tafari 1980:1), Rastafarians were told to look to Africa for the crowning of a black King who would be their Redeemer. Therefore, the coronation of Emperor Haile Selassie I on 2 November 1930 as Negus of Ethiopia was important in the history of Rastafari as it was perceived by Rastas as a fulfilment of Garvey's prophecy (Afolabi 2004; Sibanda 2012). The crowning of Selassie was a foundation to both Ethiopianism and Pan-Africanism as Rastafarians regard Ethiopia as their 'Zion' and source of inspiration.

Partly through roots reggae music popularised by Bob Marley, Rastafari spread from Jamaica to the rest of the world, including Southern African countries such as Zimbabwe and Malawi. The revolutionary element of Rastafari was anchored on black people's experiences of social, political and economic marginalisation due to colonialism. The Rastafari communities in Zimbabwe and Malawi shared a common colonial history under the British-instituted Federation of Rhodesia and Nyasaland. Under the federation, Zimbabwe was Southern Rhodesia, Zambia was Northern Rhodesia whilst Malawi was Nyasaland. Therefore, the emergence of Nyahbinghi Rastafari communities in Malawi and Zimbabwe occurred within the context of the revolutionary struggles against oppressive "Babylon" systems and the euphoria of independence (Sibanda 2019:371).

Malawi got its independence from the British rule in 1964 under the leadership of Hastings Kamuzu Banda. The following year, His Imperial Majesty Emperor Haile Selassie I, had a three-day visit to Malawi at a time when there were ethnic wars for leadership amongst the Ngoni, Yao and Tonga (Sibanda 2019). During that visit, Haile Selassie went to Zomba, Blantyre, Chiradzulu and Cholo districts, which stimulated the growth of Rastafari movement in Malawi. It is not surprising that today, Malawi is home to thousands of Rastas of the Nyahbinghi tradition religiously following a natural *livity* encompassing *Ital* vegetarian dietary practices (Sibanda 2019:371). The legacy of Selassie's visit is notable in 'Zomba Emperor's View', a piece of land on the Zomba plateau in the Southern region of the country. The Nyahbinghi Rastafari experience in Malawi is comparable to that of Nyahbinghi Rastafari in Zimbabwe.

The emergence of Rastafari in Zimbabwe is also anchored in the revolutionary and ideological roots associated with Pan-Africanism and Ethiopianism that preceded the independence of the country in 1980 (Sibanda 2019). During the colonial period, Rastas operated as a subculture in Zimbabwe but were invigorated by the songs of freedom from roots reggae music. The euphoria of freedom from colonial rule stimulated by the historic Bob Marley show and his message at independence eve, on 17 April 1980, promoted a fresh perspective among the black populace, which further prompted the emergence of Rastafari as a significant movement in Zimbabwe. Today, Zimbabwe is home to several Nyahbinghi Rastafari houses mainly located in the urban areas (Sibanda 2019). Nyahbinghi Rastas follow an organic and vegetarian dietary pattern encompassing a wholistic natural herbalism and environmentalism as enunciated in the next section.

## Rastafari beliefs and practices in Malawi and Zimbabwe

In light of the foregoing historical milestones of the development of Rastafari in Malawi and Zimbabwe, I will now provide an overview of Rastafari beliefs and practices. The Nyahbinghi Orders in Malawi and Zimbabwe recognise the divinity of Emperor Haile Selassie I, whom they regard as the head creator, black messiah, Christ in his kingly character – Jah Rastafari (Sibanda 2015a, 2017a). Rastas also believe in the Bible as a holy book from which they draw their dietary patterns, make use of *ganja/marijuana* as a herb, and observe the cultivation of dreadlocks, among other teachings and practices. Indeed, Rastas believe that *ganja* is a natural sacred herb with multiple roles identified by Afari (2007:89) as "medicinal, nutritional, pharmaceutical, industrial, biological, cosmetological, cosmological, spiritual, intellectual and therapeutic properties for the benefit of all humanity". This shows that in light of the COVID-19 crisis, the Rastafarians do not shy away from advocating the invaluable properties of this natural sacred herb.

Rastafarians in both Malawi and Zimbabwe regard dreadlocks, a natural hairstyle, as a distinctive marker of their identity and pride in response to the colonial legacy that inferiorised black people. This is borne out of a Nazarene tradition and vow anchored in the Bible (cf. Lev.21:5; Num. 6.5), emulating the lion's mane (Chitando and Chitando 2004:1; Sibanda 2017a:414). In addition, Rastas follow a strict vegetarian diet that avoids ingestion of meat guided by Leviticus 11:41–42. This special diet is known as *Ital* (vital) food and is relevant to the Rastafari interventions in COVID-19 contexts in Malawi and Zimbabwe. Rasta music, also known as "Jah Music" encompasses roots reggae music and Nyhabinghi music vital in cascading Rastafari messages and advocacy for love, peace, justice, tolerance and harmony (Sibanda 2017a). "Jah music" is handy in propagating public health messages in the context of COVID-19 pandemic.

In line with the above, Rastas respect the symbolic colours of red, gold and green as important to their lifestyle. The colours are inspired by the Ethiopian flag, given that Ethiopia escaped colonial rule and therefore stands as an emblem of African freedom and independence. For Rastas, Ethiopia is their 'promised land' or 'Zion' and a basis for Afrocentricity. The green colour is very significant in Rastafari cosmology as it mirrors Rastafari green philosophy, vegetarian diet, growth and life (Sibanda 2015b, 2017a). These ideals are relevant to the COVID-19 crisis in Zimbabwe and Malawi, where health and being in harmony with nature are perceived through the prism of natural *livity* (lifestyle). The Rastafarians in Malawi and Zimbabwe make use of "dread-talk" that bastardises conventional English language, which thrives on "word, sound and power" (Afari 2007; Dolin 2001). Using dread-talk, Rastas have stood their ground in defying the "Babylon" system and to express their agency in the face of COVID-19 crisis.

## Grappling with COVID-19: Rastafari perspectives and experiences

This section explores the Rastafari perspectives, experiences and strategies they developed in response to COVID-19 crisis in Zimbabwe and Malawi. The data on the first aspect pertaining to Rastafari perspectives on the causes and interventions by the state and the international community to prevent and manage the spread of COVID-19 were gathered through in-depth interviews and documentary analysis. Next, the section focuses on Rastafari experiences and strategies for responding to the COVID-19 crisis in Zimbabwe and Malawi.

## Rastafari perspectives on the causes of COVID-19

The Rastafari participants in both Malawi and Zimbabwe had similar views on the causes of COVID-19 pandemic. The participants emphasised that Rastafari in general is a very diverse movement with free thinkers on the many aspects of life including the issue COVID-19 pandemic. However, the most dominant position of Rastafari communities in Malawi and Zimbabwe pertaining to the causes of COVID-19 pandemic is epitomised by one Rastafari Elder of Zimbabwe who was interviewed at the onset of the disease in early 2020 stating, thus:

> It is not clear enough what the causes of the disease are. We are still looking for answers for its cause. However, as Rastas we are convinced that it is a man-made virus not only designed to kill but to instil prolonged fear, increasing anxiety and chaos forcing social instability, economic reconstruction resulting over a period of time. A cashless society with the majority of the world population living on credit and vouchers would emerge because without jobs and businesses people would be totally dependent on state handouts. In the new world order, the virus is used as a weapon. This is an Armageddon germ or biological warfare.

The above perspective is also shared by some Rastafarians in Malawi as testified by one of the Rastafari Elders, Ras Sakara, who belongs to the Kambalowa Binghi, Chikwawa in Southern part of Malawi. In a comparable position to that of Rastas in Zimbabwe, this Malawian Rastafari Elder upheld the view that the disease is man-made. In his words, the Elder stated, thus:

> We are very worried about the fruits of Evils some minds of people produce toward other people's lives. COVID-19 pandemic and any disease that causes pain and misery in life … anything that pains our bodies is from Evil. We regard them as Evil and Evil comes from bad minds. So COVID-19 pandemic is from evil minds and a fruit of Evil minds, but pain is not our wish.

In a follow-up interview, Ras Sakara asserted that the source of Evil was 'Babylon'. From these excerpts, it can be deduced that the Rastafari communities in Zimbabwe and Malawi regard COVID-19 pandemic as a ploy to eliminate some sections of humanity through a biological warfare. From a telephone interview with a Zimbabwean participant, Man Soul JAH, reference was made to the biblical causes of pestilence and disease after humanity errs in one way or another. For instance, Man Soul JAH said that the unbridled abuse of nature, experimentation and scientific view of the world have resulted in humanity crossing its boundary to infringe the animal kingdom, which is possibly the source of the virus. He added that although the Coronavirus disease could be natural in its cause, but it is compounded by humanity's mischievous experimentation and chicanery. Therefore, there is *politricks* in the entire subject on this pandemic.

In Rastafari worldview and ideology, the selfish actions of humanity can result in Armageddon, which is the earth's final battle between good and evil. Rastas believe that good will triumph in the end. Rastafarians in both Zimbabwe and Malawi asserted that JAH Rastafari never created them in order to destroy them. He will defend, protect and nourish them in time of sickness. Along the same lines, JAH Rastafari and Ancient elders have warned of Armageddon. History tells of past experiences from slavery and colonisation. Therefore, for Rastas, the COVID-19 pandemic is a man-made disease.

## Rastafari and the COVID-19 intervention strategies

A number of precautionary and intervention strategies were implemented in response to the COVID-19 pandemic in both Zimbabwe and Malawi as will be explored below:

### Self quarantine and hand hygiene

Rastafarians took measures that promoted public health guidelines. The Rastafari lifestyle was reinforced as a response to some state interventions such as lockdown rules and the guidelines for hygiene in both Zimbabwe and Malawi. Basing on a biblical text from the book of Isaiah 26:20, which says: "Come, my people, enter your inner chambers, and shut your doors behind you; hide yourselves for a while until the wrath is past" (RSV), Rastafarians reasoned that self quarantine was a divine advice. Rastas also said they practiced social distancing when in public as well as washing up to maintain hand hygiene. The participants said the issue of hygiene was part of Rastafari teaching, which stressed that cleanliness was next to Godliness. One Rasta Elder in Zimbabwe pointed that well before COVID-19, the standard Rasta greeting was a 'lion paw greeting', where clenched fists, as opposed to an open handshake, were used in a gesture that implied 'touch my blood'. This was claimed to have had an advantage of reducing the spread of communicable diseases such as typhoid and now, COVID-19 pandemic, particularly where some are transforming to an 'elbow greeting' style. These hygiene standards show that Rastas have been pacesetters despite the fact that most people in society never noticed it. Such public health practices could reposition the agency of Rastas from the margins to the centre.

In addition to the above observations, Rastas are also acting to promote public health protocols through social distancing and avoiding large gatherings to prevent the spread of the disease. Rastas in both Malawi and Zimbabwe affirmed that since COVID-19 pandemic is a contagious disease, physical (social) distancing must be practiced so as to avoid the spread of the virus. They asserted that it is better to practice the COVID-19 regulations than to die or to cause more spread of the disease. However, for Rastas, the physical (social) distancing strategy also produced its own challenges from an Afrocentric perspective. For instance, one Key Informant from Zimbabwe presented a communal position of the Nyahbinghi Rastafarians stating that

> the impact of social distancing (among Rastas), first as Afrikan people, becomes disrespectful in various ways and forms. We are a very much

hands-on and embracing people, living, eating and sleeping, just as a family. We are very communal in the way we do our daily runnings. So, the call to implement social distancing will create stress in various ways and forms.

It other words, this practice is contrary to the standard African norms and values of *Ubuntu* (humanness). This Rastafari Elder of Zimbabwe further noted:

> The lockdown will seriously impact on the enterprising ventures of most Rastafarians because they are self-employed and the majority of them are in the informal sector. Rastas in the 21st century argue that they are still very much discriminated against and marginalised by the state/government. On this basis, most Rastas will not register for state handouts as they perceive it to be an entrapment for manipulation by egocentric politicians.

The above views show that Rastas have not remained unscathed by the effects of the lockdown, which forced them to discontinue "Jah works" to earn a living. The statement also reveals Rastafari scepticism about state handouts, which they perceive within the framework of *politricks*, despite the misery associated with COVID-19 pandemic on their *livity*.

### Rastafari Ital foodways

The study established that in both Zimbabwe and Malawi, Rastafari sought to promote health and human flouring through Ital foodways. The Ital foodways consisted of the use of natural foods and medicines in their natural diet including fresh vegetables and fruits. Authentic Rastafarians follow a strict vegetarian diet that avoids junk food and meat products. As Sibanda (2019:374) notes, Rastafarian lifestyles are confirmed by statements which say: "You are what you eat" and "Let your food be your medicine and your medicine be your food". Through right *livity* anchored on Ital food, Rastas could prevent and manage the impact of COVID-19 pandemic in both Malawi and Zimbabwe. As stated by Elder Ras Jahbulani Trevor Hall of Zimbabwe, "the true pure *livity* of the Ras Tafari is maintaining a wholistic natural herbalism, which is vegetarian and a spiritual and physically balanced life." Rastas maintain a strong nutrition and live as natural as possible through an Afrocentric culinary heritage relevant to public health interventions in COVID-19 pandemic contexts.

In addition, Ancient Abuna Bondomali and the Royal Nazarene family of Zimbabwe also echoed the importance of *Ital* foodways and diet in COVID-19 contexts. The Royal Nazarene family said they follow a totally vegan diet because the body should be nourished through herbs and organic diet. In fact, from narratives of Rastas in both Malawi and Zimbabwe, the Rastafari food consisted of vegetarian diet and alkaline food such as moringa tea, zumbani tea, artmizia tea, marijuana tea, tansy tea, neem tea, pawpaw leaf tea, ginger tea and garlic tea. All these are herbal teas that reflect food-medicines. In the face of COVID-19 pandemic, the herbal teas were much in use among Rasta families and non-Rastas alike. The researcher established through interviews and also observed that in most retail shops, the shelves sold these processed herbal teas (except for marijuana tea).

Rastafari communities in Zimbabwe and Malawi were convinced that Jah Rastafari, His Imperial Majesty, was in control as He taught them to live healthy living and follow healthy eating habits, which consist of an alkaline state of living. Given that human nutrition is put into the relationship between acids and alkalis, there is need to maintain them in proper balance of 80% alkaline and 20% acid, thereby avoiding acid ash. As Afrika (1998:89) notes, "The normal ratio for acid-alkaline varies with the type of diet. The junk food, animal flesh eater's diet is the highest acid diet. It is the most destructive and numerous dis-eases." An alkaline state of living consists of a high content of magnesium, sodium, calcium and potassium. This is consistent with the views of Rastas in both countries whose lifestyles promote a largely vegetarian diet that would most likely keep the coronavirus at bay. Essentially, Rastas reasoned that acidic foods are a catalyst for the virus. Therefore, for Rastas, a good immune system means good health. Rastafari dietary consciousness shunned Genetically Modified Foods, which were foods artificially preserved and "polluted" by modern technologies and Western consumerism (Sibanda 2019). Elder Ras Sakara of Malawi's conclusion aptly captures this Rastafari perspective, thus:

> As a remedy for COVID-19, eat natural foods. Natural foods are alkaline. They make our cells to have a conducive environment. Unnatural foods give our bodies frequencies, which denature our cells. This causes pain and early deaths than planned by the Most High, the Mighty of mighties. Remember, the Bible wrongly said that people acquired death by eating a prohibited fruit. No! But [through] eating unnatural foods, which give the bodies frequencies that do not tally with the body's nature. The nature of a thing is and must be our baseline. In everything we do, we must refer to the nature base.... In conclusion, stay natural, eat natural, drink more water – it's an alkaline.

From a list of these mitigation measures, one cannot miss the positive proactive agency of Rastafari communities in both Malawi and Zimbabwe, through Ital foodways under the shadow of COVID-19 pandemic.

### Rastafari herbal remedies

In both Zimbabwe and Malawi, Rastafarians stressed the importance of indigenous natural herbs as a strong measure to promote human flourishing.

The vitality of herbal healing in the context of the COVID-19 pandemic was strongly affirmed by one Rastafari Elder who stated: "Life is in herbs because herbs give strength and natural healing." Top on the list of herbs used by Rastas is marijuana/ganja/cannabis, which is a miracle plant to enhance health and well-being. This resonates with the Rastafari belief in the supremacy of life, partly reflected in the life-affirming values of marijuana. Informed by the Bible, Rastas in both Malawi and Zimbabwe have the conviction that marijuana is the tree of life for the healing of the nations (Revelation 22:2). This resonates with Hewitt's (2018) observation that among Rastafarians this 'holy herb' (marijuana), is a free gift from God ushered through God's creation. Therefore, the Rastafari use of indigenous herbs (including marijuana) is critical, against the backdrop of challenges facing bio-medicine in the context of COVID-19 pandemic in Malawi and Zimbabwe.

Basing on my previous studies on Rastafari communities in the pre-COVID-19 era, the use of marijuana/ganja/cannabis for therapeutic effects are extant, where members of this movement called for its legalisation (Sibanda 2014). In the current study the Key Informants in Zimbabwe and Malawi further confirmed the medicinal and herbal therapeutic effects of cannabis in the context of COVID-19. The informants were unanimous at claiming that Cannabis Sativa has compounds like THC and CBD, which can be used to treat various symptoms, including those associated with the coronavirus. Apparently, this claim has a contemporary scientific basis as research into 'medicinal marijuana' are becoming prevalent and popular because of their health benefits, encompassing pain relief, improved anxiety, and reduced inflammation (Simpson 2021). In other words, cannabis products have extensive therapeutic benefits, which may offer help in the fight against COVID-19, a disease associated with severe acute respiratory distress and lung fibrosis. This shows that Rastafari is a positive force in the quest for health and healing in response to COVID-19 pandemic, though this sometimes goes unnoticed by the larger populace.

The study also established that Rastas in Malawi and Zimbabwe upheld the need to steam and bath with various indigenous herbs such as zumbani and marijuana as a precautionary measure or for managing the dis-eased, on a regular basis. The herbs clear the bronchitis and breathing system. Therefore, for Rastafarians, steaming and bathing could keep the coronavirus at bay because of the high temperatures and the herbal therapy. On the use of marijuana, the mainstream view is that the consumption of cannabis is most commonly done by inhaling the smoke of cannabis flower (Simpson 2021). However, this is not the only way cannabis's therapeutic compounds can be utilised. For instance, alongside using it in bathing and steaming, cannabis oil extracts, like CBD oil, also come to the fore, among other uses. As Simpson (2021:n.p.) notes, "Cannabis oil can be consumed through ingestion, vaping, nasal sprays, or topical application. Many delivery mechanisms don't involve the lungs and leave out potentially harmful substances that come with smoke inhalation." This observation shows that there is a lot of potential in the use of cannabis in the fight against COVID-19 pandemic, among Rastafarians.

### Chi Gong: the call for regular physical exercise

Besides surviving on a healthy lifestyle characterised by Ital food and diet, Rastas in Malawi and Zimbabwe expressed the need to do physical exercises regularly. This is a promotion of human flourishing through art therapy comprising "meditation, physical work (Jah works) and exercise" (Sibanda 2019:378). These exercises are based on the 'Chi Gong' bodily movement, which is a physiotherapy and yoga philosophy traceable to Kermetic knowledge. Literally, "Chi" is control of breath, whilst "Gong" means "master" (Sibanda 2019). For Rastafarians, 'Chi Gong' is meant to cleanse, heal and energise the body. The ability to control ones breath through 'Chi Gong' physiotherapy is relevant in addressing COVID-19 pandemic, an acute respiratory distress syndrome. Building up on this, Elder Ras Sakara of Malawi, who has mastered the art of 'Chi Gong', stated:

> Apart from eating natural food-medicines [as remedy for COVID-19], we must do physical exercises. These exercises open the 12 gates in our body to be filled up with enough Ang Els (airs) like oxygen, hydrogen, among others, which sustain our life....Have rest and relax. Walk on earth barefoot in the sunlight to receive and be charged with their frequencies. Our melanin convert those frequencies into into energy, which fight body disorders.

The skills and philosophy of 'Chi Gong' show that Rastafarians are Afrocentric. They are prepared to heal themselves through this art of physiotherapy that thrives on the individual's effort. This confirms the Rastafari view that health is not injected but earned. For Rastas, 'Chi Gong' is helpful for the health and well-being of people under COVID-19 crisis in both Malawi and Zimbabwe.

### Rastafari environmentalism and COVID-19

Rastafari communities are super environmentalists informed by an I-consciousness and Rastafari 'green philosophy' that is in harmony with nature (Sibanda 2015, 2019). In this way, the Rastas in Malawi and Zimbabwe are convinced that the global trend of lockdown and quarantine have made the global environment to reset and improve its health. In the words of one Key Informant: "The rivers, oceans, lakes are getting strength from no pollution of pollutants due to the fact that industries are on lockdown. Even the air is getting more fresh because aeroplanes are not flying. The climate is on reset!" There is a critical need for a balance of things in the created order. One Key Informant from Malawi stated:

> Because of the climate change crisis, viruses that were dormant erupted and proliferated. Mother Earth is saying I have had enough pollution of carbon emissions that is depleting the Ozone layer and the world came to a stand still through lockdown. For two months Mother Earth had a well deserved sigh under the new normal. COVID-19 is a new strain that could be linked to environmental changes.

Thus, an environmental stewardship is called for to abate the current trends of the Anthropocene whose causes are linked to anthropogenic factors of the most industrialised nations. A Zimbabwean Elder echoed these sentiments saying:

> All what is going on is interrelated, the Coronavirus is said to thrive during cold climate. And now wreaking havoc in all nations. The virus is climate related. Humanity is shooting itself in the foot. The erratic change we have in our climactic cycle isn't normal and in many instances looking as if it's being controlled by man (the order) for their own benefits, but with detrimental effects to the environment.

This reminds us that in the face of COVID-19 pandemic, Rastafarians remained conscious to live a purposeful life where the environment/Mother Earth are protected. A Zimbabwean Rastafari Elder, Ras Jahbulani, added his voice by stating, thus:

> It is important to strike a balance between humanity and nature. [As human beings] no other strategy is needed than to maintain a unified thinking embracing our diversity and practice of One Love, One People, One human race. Jah Ras Tafari!

With Just One Earth, collective consciousness is required to attack the 'elephant in the room' – COVID-19 pandemic. From the Malawian perspective, Elder Ras Sakara said: "Plant more trees and herbs, which purify air that make our environment more habitable." This echoes the advice from His Imperial Majesty that Rastas must plant a million trees every year (Sibanda 2012, 2015), the planting of which is crucial to provide food-medicines and fresh air for promoting human flourishing.

### Coping with COVID-19 crisis through reggae music

The study established that in both Zimbabwe and Malawi Rastafari communities utilise 'Jah music', that is, roots reggae music and Nyahbinghi music in two main ways: (a) to promote public health messages in response to the COVID-19 pandemic (b) as a tool to warn people about 'conspirational thinking' and bio-medical warfare manifesting in the form of COVID-19 pandemic. The messages that come through music make Rastafari a significant social force in society.

## Promotion of public health messages

In the two countries under focus, COVID-19 awareness campaigns through music were done. For instance, on the first point, I refer to one of the songs on COVID-19 by a group of Zimbabwean Rastafari artistes: Toggyman, Mama Ithiopia and Ancient Abuna Bondomali who collaborated on an awareness campaign song. In the collaboration, Toggyman was on the lead vocals whilst Mama Ithiopia featured on the backing vocals and Ancient Abuna Bondomali did the poetry. The message was that COVID-19 was a very dangerous disease. Music becomes a handy tool, thriving as 'word, sound, power'. It shows the power of oral art where the musicians sing about, *inter alia*, "misery in people and people in misery" (Muwati 2018:xiv). In the context of COVID-19, 'Jah music', particularly reggae music, provided "a mode of reasoning that offers an alternative to the established way of doing and looking at things" (Karenga 1993:7). Therefore, playing and listening to reggae music is a coping strategy that Rastas use in their interventions. Reggae music has the potential to endear Rastafarians to people of all walks of life since its popularisation by Jamaican Rastafari reggae icons such as Bob Marley and the Wailers. In the context of COVID-19, Rastafarians could easily occupy the centre from their usual social location at the margins in both Zimbabwe and Malawi thereby confirming Lucky Dube's observation that "Nobody can stop reggae 'cause reggae is strong" (1989). Reggae music enhances Rastafari resilience as a minority and marginalised religion in the face of global challenges like COVID-19 pandemic.

## 'Conspirational thinking', bio-medical warfare & vaccination apathy

On this second point, we find the ambivalence of Rastafari contribution to issues of public health and development in the context of COVID-19 crisis. The Rastafarian communities in both Zimbabwe and Malawi expressed their open reservations about the safety of vaccines to prevent the spread of COVID-19 pandemic. In fact, Rastas have no trust in the whole inoculation exercise. For Rastas, the inoculation programme is a Western ploy to wipe out the Black race. Therefore, resistance to vaccination efforts by Rastas is due to the fact that historically, previous epidemics saw black people being used as guinea pigs both on the African continent and in the West. From existing literature, some French doctors suggested that COVID-19 vaccines needed to be tested on the African continent (Pailey 2020). The Social Media was also awash with stories that claimed that the mortality rate of the vaccinated people out-weighed the non-vaccinated (Wolfe & Nierenberg 2021). This has created a 'vaccination hesitancy' and conspiration theories globally, thereby entrenching Rastafari scepticism in both Zimbabwe and Malawi.

In line with the above, Elder Ras Jahbulani Trevor Hall used music to warn fellow Rastas about the sinister plans of 'Babylon' pertaining to biological warfare. He produced two songs related to these issues, namely, 'Third world war inna Afrika' and 'It's a Conspiracy'. In his words, Elder Ras Jahbulani stated: "My 2 songs I had written and recorded a couple of years ago warning people of the conspiracy and the third world war, are being confirmed since we're in the midst of that right now." Commenting on the relevance of the message in his songs, Elder Ras Jahbulani Trevor Hall added that:

> Most Ras Tafari sons and dawtas I know see the COVID-19 pandemic as part of the planned genocide by the new world order to eliminate a large portion of the world population during this 4th Industrial Revolution (the Armageddon), which has been part of their long term plan as seen in the way they had constructed the collection of books to create their bibliography scriptures called the King James Version of the Holy Bible. This started their spiritual subduance of mostly our Black Afrikan people and people of colour.

In this way, it is this type of ideological struggles that keep people immobilised in the context of vaccination programme in COVID-19 pandemic times. To further hammer this Rastafarian view on vaccination, Elder Ras Jahbulani added:

> It's not just the Ras Tafari community asking these questions about COVID-19. The conspiracy is now a harsher reality. How and why in your right mind would you be willing to take vaccination if your *livity* is pure and there's no proof it's preventative or a cure to the disease?

This is a similar position held by Rastas in Malawi as confirmed by an Empress from that country who expressed it through a Reggae song chanting down the 'Bumbo Klaat' in COVID-19 contexts. This Rastafari stance may be mistaken by mainstream society not only to be anti-society and counter-cultural, but also extreme, unreasonable and counter productive. The Rastafarians in Zimbabwe and Malawi risk being regarded as a movement minimising the threat of COVID-19 pandemic.

## Conclusion

At the beginning of this chapter, I made reference to Adichie's concern over the dangers of a single story. The common single narrative is to regard the dominant and more established religions such as Islam and Christianity as the only key development agents that most African governments could work with in the fight against COVID-19 pandemic. In this way, minority religions such as Rastafari are excluded at the discussion platforms for policy formulation on, *inter alia,* health and other development initiatives. As the chapter has demonstrated, the Rastafari communities in Zimbabwe and Malawi are a force to reckon with in the quest for health and well-being in response to COVID-19 and the development agenda through their cultural identities. Indeed, Rastafari cultural identities such as music, Ital foodways, holistic natural herbalism and environmentalism as well as spiritual and physically balanced lives engender creative and unique parameters that promote public health and human flourishing in both Zimbabwe and Malawi. Through a labour of love and resistance not to die in the face of COVID-19 (Calvo 2020), Rastafarians are defying the western approaches to health and healing enmeshed in hypocrisy and *politricks.*

The chapter further demonstrates the "danger of a single threat" (Redfield 2020) where COVID-19 pandemic eclipses all other threats, in both Zimbabwe and Malawi. Through 'conspirational thinking', Rastafarians defy Western epistemological hegemonic tendencies and biomedical warfare approaches thereby concentrating the cause of their misery around a singular threat – the *politricks* of Babylon system. In this way, despite being a significant social force, the Rastafarian total resistance to Western biomedical technology (including COVID-19 vaccines), influenced by an Afro-epistemological standpoint, is tantamount to counter-productivity, once "stupid deaths" (Paul Farmer's phrase cited in Redfield 2020) begin to be recorded among their rank and file. Yet, against the backdrop of a lingering medical imperialism, Rastafarians need to reposition their agency by exercising a judicious integration of Afrocentric knowledge systems and strategies with any progressive Western-engineered biotechnology. This is especially critical given that Rastafari foregrounds the embracement of human diversity and the practice of One love, One aim, One people and One human race in order to drive positive complementary actions in the face of pandemics in Malawi and Zimbabwe.

## References

Adichie, C.N. (2009) "The Danger of a Single Story", TED Global, Retrieved from https://www.ted.com/talks/chimamanda_ngozi_adichie_the_danger_of_a_single_story?language=en, Accessed: 20 July 2020.

Afari, Y. (2007) *Overstanding Rastafari: Jamaica's Gift to the World*, Jamaica: Senya Cum.

Afolabi, J.A. (2004) "By the Rivers of Babylon: The Bondage Motif in the Performing Arts, Life and Aesthetics of Rastafarians" *Tinabantu: Journal of African National Affairs*, 2(1): 37–49.

Afrika, L.O. (1998) *Afrikan Holistic Health: Your Guide to Health and Well-Being*, Brooklyn, NY: A&B Publishers Group.

Asante, M.K. (1998) *The Afrocentric Idea*, Philadelphia, PA: Temple University Press.

Asante, M.K. (2007) *An Afrocentric Manifesto: Toward an African Renaissance*, Malden: Polity.

Calvo, D. (2020) "'They Agreed To Kill Us, We Agreed Not To Die': Acts of Love and Resistance to Confront Covid-19 by Members of Afro-Brazilian Religions" https://anthrocovid.com/2020/06/05/they-agreed-to-kill-us-we-agreed-not-to--die-acts-of-love-and-resistance-to-confront-covid-19-by-members-of-afro-brazilian-religions/, Accessed: 20 July 2020.

Chitando, E. and Chitando, A. (2004) "Black Female Identities in Harare: The Case of Young Women with Dreadlocks" *Zambezia*, 31 (1&2): 1–21.

Cox, J.L. (1996) *Expressing the Sacred: An Introduction to the Phenomenology of Religion*, Harare: University of Zimbabwe Press.

Dolin, K.Q. (2001) "Words, Sounds and Power in Jamaican Rastafari" MACLAS Latin American Essays, Retrieved from https://www.questia.com/library, Accessed: 28 May 2020.

Dube, L. (1989) "Reggae Strong" from Album Prisoner, Produced by Shanachie Label, https://www.dancehallreggaeworld.com/lucky-dube.html

Edmonds, E.B. (2003) *Rastafari: From Outcasts to Culture Bearers*, Oxford: Oxford University Press.

Hewitt, R.R. (2018) "For the Healing of the Nations: Rastafari Dialogical Narrative Discourse on the Decriminalization of Marijuana/Ganja" in Okyere-Manu, B. and Moyo, H. (Eds). *Intersecting African Indigenous Knowledge Systems and Western Knowledge Systems: Moral Convergence and Divergence*, Pietermaritzburg: Cluster Publications, 116–134.

Johnson, V.D. (2001) "The Nguzo Saba as Foundation for African American College Student Development Theory" *Journal of Black Studies*, 31(4): 406–422.

Karenga, M. (1993) *Introduction to Black Studies*, Los Angeles: University of Sankore Press.

Kovalchuk, A., Wang, B., Li, D., Rodriguez-Juarez, R., Ilnytskyy, S., Kovalchuk, I., & Kovalchuk, O. (2021) "Fighting the Storm: Could Novel Anti-TNFα and anti-IL-6 C. sativa cultivars tame cytokine storm in COVID-19?" *Aging*, 13(2):1571–1590.doi:10.18632/aging.202500.

Muwati, I. (2018) "Introduction: Singing Nation: Music and Politics in the Decade of Crisis" in I. Muwati, T. Charamba and C. Tembo (Eds). *Singing Nation and Politics: Music and the 'Decade of Crisis' in Zimbabwe 2000–2010*, Gweru: Midlands State University Press.

Nhamo, G., Dube, K., & Chikodzi, D. (2020) *Counting the Cost of COVID-19 on the Global Tourism Industry*, Cham, Switzerland: Springer Nature Switzerland AG.

Pailey, R.N. (2020) "Africa does not need saving during this pandemic", Al Jazeera, 13 April 2020, Retrieved from https://www.aljazeera.com/indepth/opinion/africa-saving-pandemic-200408180254152.html, Accessed 5 June 2021.

Pailey, R.N. (2015) "Treating Africans with an Untested Ebola Drug" Retrieved from https://www.alijazeera.com/indepth/opinion/2014/12/treating-africans-with-an-unte-2014123195838317148.html, Accessed: 20 August 2020.

Redfield, P. (2020) "COVID-19: The Danger of a Single Threat" Retrieved from- https://culanth.org/fieldsights/the-danger-of-a-single-threat, Accessed: 20 July 2020.

Sen, A. (1981) *Poverty and Famines: An Essay on Entitlement and Deprivation*, Oxford: Clarendon Press.

Sibanda, F. (2019) "Promoting Human Flourishing through Rastafari Ital Foodways in Africa" in M.C. Green (Ed). *Law, Religion and Human Flourishing in Africa*, Stellenbosch: AFRICA SUN MeDIA, 363–381.

Sibanda, F. (2017a) "Praying for Rain?: A Rastafari Perspective from Zimbabwe" *The Ecumenical Review*, 69(3): 411–424.

Sibanda (2017b) "Rastafari Perspectives on Land Use and Management in Postcolonial Zimbabwe" in M.C. Green, R.I.J. Hackett, L. Hansen and F. Venter (Eds). *Religious Pluralism, Heritage and Social development in Africa*, Stellenbosch: SUN MeDIA Stellenbosch, 189–203.

Sibanda, F. (2015a) "'Legalize it!': Re-thinking Rastafari-State Relations in Postcolonial Zimbabwe", in Pieter Coertzen, M.C. Green & L. Hansen (Eds). *Law and Religion in Africa: The Quest for the Common Good in Pluralistic Societies*, Stellenbosch: SUN MeDIA Stellenbosch, 185–204.

Sibanda, F. (2015b) "Rastafari Green Philosophy for Sustainable Development in Postcolonial Zimbabwe: Harnessing Eco-theology and Eco-justice" in F.H. Chimhanda, V.M.S. Molobi & I.D. Mothoagae (Eds). *African Theological Reflections: Critical Voices on Liberation, Leadership, Gender and Eco-justice*, UNISA: Research Institute for Theology and Religion, 187–206.

Sibanda, F. (2014) "Quest for Identity: Rastafari Cultural Identities as Expression of Liberation in Postcolonial Zimbabwe" Unpublished Doctor of Philosophy Thesis submitted to the Department of Religious Studies, Classics and Philosophy, Harare: University of Zimbabwe.

Sibanda, F. (2012) "The Impact of Rastafari Ecological Ethic in Zimbabwe: A Contemporary Discourse" *The Journal of Pan African Studies*, 5(3): 59–76.

Simpson, K.W. (2021) "Cannabis as a treatment for COVID-19" Retrieved from https://www.openaccessgovernment.org/cannabis-as-a-treatment-for-covid-19/106833/, Accessed: 7 July 2021.

Tafari, I.J. (1980) "The Rastafari – Successors of Marcus Garvey" *Caribbean Quarterly*, 26 (4): 1–12.

WHO. (2020) Coronavirus disease 2019 (COVID-19) Situation Report – 51. Retrieved from https://www.who.int/docs/default-source/coronavirus/situation-reports/20200225-sitrep-36-covid-19.pdf?sfvrsn=2791b4e0_2. Accessed 20 August 2020.

Wolfe, J. & Nierenberg, A. (2021) "The Delta Misinformation Loop", *The New York Times*, August 10.

Zeleza, P.T. (2020) "The Coronavirus: The Political Economy of a Pathogen" Retrieved from https://www.linkedin.com/pulse/coronavirus-political-economy-pathogen-paul-tiyambe-zeleza/?trackingId=fr9iQ29QSr2Ui9M57n7VWA%3D%3D, Accessed: 25 March 2020.

# 16 'When a pandemic wears the face of a woman'

## Intersections of religion and gender during the COVID-19 pandemic in Zimbabwe

*Molly Manyonganise*

### Introduction

The novel COVID-19 pandemic has created exceptional circumstances that have altered nearly all facets of society (Kofman & Garfin, 2020:S198). Within scholarship focusing on the effects of the pandemic, there has emerged a wealth of commentary on the gendered implications of COVID-19. This chapter is premised on the view that as with any global crisis, women have been hardest hit by COVID-19 within the Zimbabwean context. The question that may arise from this assertion is how has that happened? It is understood that the pandemic came unannounced to the extent that people did not have time to really prepare for its coming. It, therefore, becomes imperative for academic scholars to pay attention to how the response in particular to the pandemic has had a lot of effects on women throughout the world in general but for purposes of this chapter, on Zimbabwe in particular. As a pre-emptive measure, I should hasten to declare that this analysis is by no means exhaustive because the study is being carried out when the pandemic is still on-going. Secondly, I may not have witnessed all that women have/ are experiencing in the period of this pandemic. What the chapter intends to do is to start conversations around the impact of COVID-19 especially on women. This is because historic crises have always had dire effects on women and girls and the level of gender equality in general and the spread of the new coronavirus disease [is] not different unless immediate action is taken by integrating a gender-sensitive lens to all COVID-19 response (UNHR, 2020). This is not to say men have not been affected by the pandemic but as a gender academic who is very much interested in the intersections of religion and gender, I am almost always forced to disaggregate the impact of any crisis in order to see how it affects men and women differently. The focus of the chapter is on how COVID-19 has/is affected/affecting women though being cognizant of the fact that there are other ways that men have also been impacted upon by the pandemic. This chapter is going to focus on the various areas that women have found themselves to have been affected by the pandemic. It analyses the social, economic, religious, governance as well

DOI: 10.4324/9781003241096-16

as how women have been impacted upon in the area of health. The aim is to find out the various ways in which the pandemic has influenced religious attitudes towards gender as well as the pandemic's impact on patriarchy. This should assist in establishing the intersection of religion and gender in the context of the COVID-19 pandemic.

## Mapping the COVID-19 pandemic context

The corona virus was first discovered in China, Wuhan Province in December 2019 and after affecting countries beyond China's borders, the World Health Organization (WHO) declared it a pandemic on March 11 2020 (Murphy, 2020:495). It was not long before the virus hit the African borders despite the false myths that had done the rounds on social media presenting the virus as a disease that could not affect black people. Zimbabwe registered its first case and fatality in March 2020. While there had been uncertainty and disorganisation coupled with lack of political will effecting a national response to the pandemic, the death of Zororo Makamba and the accusations levelled by the family against the government as well as public outcry jostled the government to eventually declare a lockdown which started on 30 March 2020 while schools and institutions of higher learning had been closed on 24 March 2020. Both air and ground travel was banned. Professionals in various sectors that were defined as essential needed clearance or exemption letters to be allowed to move around during the lockdown. A dusk to dawn curfew was put in place. The purpose of the lockdown was to ensure that people stayed at home and were to come out only for essential services such as getting health care, food or attending funerals in cases where this could not be avoided. People were encouraged to always sanitise and wash their hands regularly as well as masking up when going out. While the lockdown was gradually eased after 90 days, due to the spike in those infected by the virus caused the government to call for another hard lockdown on 2 January 2021. The home was and continues to be viewed as providing safety from the pandemic but later became a source of other challenges that were not foreseen. These and others are going to be discussed below. It is important to note that the paper will focus mainly on the challenges faced due to the initial lockdown in the 2020 year.

## Women in the midst of COVID-19: a religion and gender analysis

An analysis done by Archambeault (2020:2) shows that COVID-19 is exposing and exacerbating the existing inequalities that put among other groups girls and women at increased risk of Gender- Based Violence (GBV). The international and local media ran many stories exposing how the pandemic has created an enabling environment for (GBV) Archambeault (2020:2) further notes that COVID-19 pandemic is projected to drive 31 million new cases of GBV by the end of 2020 and cause a one-third reduction in progress towards ending GBV by 2030. Early evidence and expert projections show that COVID-19 is already and will continue to drive incidences of GBV across the globe (Archambeault, 2020:2). In South Africa, in the first week of March when the first lockdown was effected, the police recorded 2,300 complaints of GBV (Crux, 2020). This resonates with the Zimbabwean context. Within the Zimbabwean context, women have been/are experiencing all forms of violence be it physical, emotional, psychological, and verbal during the lockdown period. Men and women have been used to live separately especially the stay-at-home women/mothers, and men have been going out to try and eke out a living. However, because of the lockdown, they have been forced to be staying for long periods of time together. As a result, in those homes where women have been exposed to domestic violence, this has escalated. Within a week of the lockdown, Musasa Project reported receiving 592 calls from women and girls who were experiencing GBV compared to 500 calls they used to receive prior the lockdown period (UNCT, Zimbabwe, 2020). When GBV data was collated in July 2020, it indicated that between March and June 2020, 2,768 cases related to violence against women and girls were reported across the country which was a 70% increase (WILDAF, 2020). It was further noted that of these cases, 94% were women who were being exploited sexually, economically and physically. Intimate Partner Violence (IPV) accounted for 90% in these cases (WILDAF, 2020). The lockdown closed alternatives of escaping violence such as seeking shelter with relatives or seeking recourse through the traditional-set structures. While the lockdown was meant to make people safe from infection, the prevalence of GBV showed that "not everyone is safe at home" (Sarson & MacDonald, 2020). For Sarson and MacDonald (2020), women are being caught in these dual pandemics of COVID-19 and GBV.

The other type of violence that women are experiencing during this lockdown is Sexual Gender-Based Violence (SGBV). For vulnerable households, there have been reports of women encountering demands for sexual favours in return for food especially in those areas where food relief is being distributed. It is a pity that for those vulnerable households, women are being asked to engage in sexual intercourse by the men distributing this food. In this case, food is being used as a tool to abuse women. Also of concern is how women were being forced into sexual encounters at times by their own husbands. Sexual encounters during lockdown may have increased to the extent that women became concerned. Buttel and Ferreira (2020:S197) argue that important public health imperatives like lockdowns, stay-at-home orders, social isolation and social distancing have had a profound impact on families experiencing intimate partner violence." Kofman and Garfin (2020:S199) observe that in pursuit of large-scale mitigation efforts to protect public health, the vulnerabilities of some-at-risk populations have been magnified. I have had discussions with women who complained that they were failing to put their uteruses on lockdown during the lockdown period.

The issue of forced sexual encounters among married couples is an area that has not received much attention in religious circles in Zimbabwe. When it then happens in lockdown contexts, it puts women at risk of sexual violence from their husbands or intimate partners. This obviously is an area that faith communities and the church in Zimbabwe in particular need to start conversations on, in the post-COVID-19 lockdown era. Religious leaders need to rethink their construction of sexual intercourse as an activity that women should always be ready to take part in even when the odds are against them.

Still on SGBV, in mid-June, three MDC Alliance young women were abducted, tortured and sexually abused, probably by their political opponents when the lockdown was in force. The reason that was given was that they did not observe the lockdown rules by participating in an 'illegal' demonstration. However, when one looks at the picture showing the composition of the demonstrators, one notices that it was not an all-women demonstration. Men were also present. One then wonders why only women were targeted for abduction, torture and sexual abuse. Such occurrences allow us to nuance how "gender dynamics interact with traditionally patriarchal political processes and institutions" (Oxford Research Encyclopedia, n.d) being so explicitly interwoven in the COVID-19 context as a way of silencing female political voices.

It has also been noted with concern how the girl child has been put at risk by the closure of schools. The fact that everyone was at home made the girl child become vulnerable to child predators and they were being sexually abused. A month and a half into the lockdown, there was a story that circulated on social media of a mother lamenting how during the lockdown, two of her daughters were impregnated by their blood brother. Maybe this brother used to engage in sexual activities with other women before the lockdown, but due to the fact that our society constructs men as sexual animals, this brother may have felt that he could not abstain during this lockdown and he ended up engaging in sexual activities consensually with his sisters and they got pregnant. While there is need to collate exact figures on child pregnancies, unofficial reports from schools in Zimbabwe indicate that quite a huge number of girls fell pregnant during the pandemic-induced lockdown. Some of the girls are as young as Grade fours (taking into cognisance that some girls are starting to menstruate at the age of nine). Burzynska and Contreras (2020:1968) note that "with schools closing throughout the developing world where stigma around teenage pregnancies prevails, we will probably see an increase in drop-out rates as teenage girls become pregnant or married." Thus, the coronavirus is intensifying the many gender inequalities as existing discriminatory and harmful norms continue or worsen (Align, 2020).

Furthermore, the girl child is at risk of being forced into early marriage. When schools around the world began closing their doors in March, child protection experts predicted that large numbers of children in the poorest parts of the world might never return to the classroom (Grant, 2020). From

UNESCO's estimation, 89% of students enrolled in education globally including nearly 743 million girls were out of school because of COVID-19 closures (Grant, 2020). It is generally agreed that schools provide 'safe' spaces for girls by shielding them from being married off as children (Norgah, 2020). In the COVID-19 induced lockdown, they could have provided safety nets for girls who are likely to be married off especially as a way to circumvent the corona-induced poverty. A good case is what happened in Mhondoro Ngezi, a rural area in Zimbabwe's Mashonaland West province. A 14-year girl was married off to a 65-year old businessman by her parents (the businessmen and the parents are members of the Johane Marange apostolic sect) who claimed that their livelihoods had been frozen by the coronavirus induced lockdown (Chiduku, 2020). Hence, they had to sacrifice their daughter so that they could survive. In this case, marrying off young girls is seen as a survival mechanism during the COVID-19 pandemic lockdown. However, Nenge (2013) has provided a hermeneutical analysis of child marriages within the Johane Marange church and argues that this challenge needs to be understood as stemming from their erroneous interpretation of the biblical text as well as the traditional religio-cultural attitudes towards women as inferior beings. We, therefore, need to see the pandemic as an enforcer of already existing religious attitudes towards women.

Women have also been affected economically by the pandemic. It was noticeable that due to the lockdown, a lot of women lost their livelihoods that has resulted in the economic disempowerment of women because of the closure of the informal sector where women are the majority. Women have also failed to adequately feed their families during the lockdown. Complains are coming through of how hunger has become more dangerous than the virus itself in the absence of safety nets from both religious institutions and government. When the lockdown started, human transporters were also stopped from operating. Hence, it was reported in the media how women from Epworth (a high density suburb in Harare) were walking to and from Mbare (a high density suburb in Harare where the vegetable market is located) carrying loads of vegetables for resale. This shows how fending for one's family had become a burden for women in Zimbabwe during the lockdown. In addition, women who depended on their children or husbands in the diaspora faced a number of challenges in trying to access remittances sent to them. Companies dealing in this business were closed at the onset of the lockdown. Even when they were opened, women could not get the money because they did not have exemption letters which would enable the security sector to allow them to get into towns. As such women failed to feed their families due to this restriction. It was noted that the high prevalence of GBV was directly linked to the economic difficulties that were induced by the lockdown. As stated by UNCT Zimbabwe (2020), the COVID-19 pandemic had a tremendous effect on GBV due to the resultant socio-economic stresses. In addition, Archambeault (2020:8) notes that apart from GBV, the socio-economic impacts the COVID-19 mitigation measures will exacerbate

other risks such as economic insecurity as well as food and water shortages. Therefore, when analysing socio-economic impacts as causal factors
of GBV, one needs to factor in the way the pandemic has challenged African masculinities. It is unfortunate that most of the non-governmental organisations that are dealing with GBV cases and its causal factors in the
COVID-19 context seem to be turning a blind eye on the religio-cultural
factors; yet these could be central and could be useful in guiding responses.
Within the realm of African hegemonic masculinity, men are constructed as
sole providers of their families. The lockdown challenged this construction
as most men found themselves failing to provide for their families. In some
instances, the use of violence needs to be understood as a way of hiding
away from this vulnerability of failing to fulfil a socially constructed role.
Kabeer (2007) cited in Pasura and Christou (2018:532) argues that men respond to the loss of their hegemonic status in different ways, with some
studies showing that some men resort to domestic violence among other
viles. It becomes imperative, therefore, to understand this violence as being
informed in part by historically and culturally specific social constructions
of masculinity (Shefer et al., 2010). In addition, women who are working
from home are burdened by performing double roles of being professionals
and homemakers at the same time

Despite these negatives, we also need to examine how the pandemic-
induced lockdown may have influenced a reconfiguration of African masculinities. Reports on social media have shown how men during the lockdown
have been negotiating their way into those spaces that are traditionally designated as feminine, for example, the kitchen. Mwiine (2020) has termed
these 'lockdown masculinities' and argues that self-isolation and the general
stay-at-home campaign challenged most of the everyday ways of being men
and meant that men and some women have had to 'learn' new ways of being
and doing gender. Many a time, men found themselves helping out in the
kitchen because of the long periods they were 'stuck' at home. In this case,
both men and women were able to resist the cultural restrictions placed
upon them. From Mwiine's analysis, it is through such kinds of resistances,
negotiations animated by COVID-19 stay-at-home campaigns that there is
the potential to disrupt gendered norms which provides new ways of forging
new forms of masculinities and femininities as well as enacting them within
the domestic sphere (2020).

Women's Sexual Reproductive Health (SRH) was also affected by the
lockdown. For example, women failed/are failing to access contraceptives
due to the lockdown. It was anticipated that the COVID-19 lockdowns
which went on for about six months would have reduced access to contraceptives for approximately 47 million women in 114 low and middle-income
countries, contributing to an additional 7 million unintended pregnancies
(Eghtessadi et al., 2020:287). A study in Ethiopia showed that the pandemic
was having adverse effects on the supply chain for contraceptive commodities by disrupting the supply chain and by delaying the transportation of

contraceptive commodities (Feyissa et al., 2020:24). In Zimbabwe, the lock-down restricted women from accessing contraception. For example, if one wanted to get into the city centre, they needed clearance letters from the employer stating why it was necessary for them to be granted permission to travel. Alternatively, for those seeking to buy medication, they needed to show their prescriptions to the police manning roadblocks. Yet women do not get clearance letters or prescriptions for contraceptives. As a result, they were denied access to the much needed contraceptives. Simply because the police wanted to see a letter of clearance exposed the women to unwanted pregnancies. Those women who depend on injections for contraception were in danger of getting pregnant if the injection expired during the lock down. A lot of women were joking on social media saying by December 2020, they would give birth to 'Covid children'. On the other hand, men who used to condomise had their access to condoms restricted, hence, exposing women to unwanted pregnancies as well as STIs if the men were engaging in extra-marital relationships before the lockdown. The interconnectedness of SRH, gender and governance was clearly put to the test during the first lockdown, when a woman in labour had her husband made to pay a bribe for her to be allowed to pass through a police roadblock in Harare on her way to a Maternity hospital (Ncube, 2020). The policemen who were male would not empathise with the woman in pain not only for a few pieces of sil-ver but because they were men and she was a woman. This lays bare the fact that corruption is not neutral but gendered. Hence, women and girls under stringent lockdown rules have limited access to social protection threaten-ing their SRH rights (Eghtessadi et al., 2020:287).

Furthermore, the religio-social construction of women as carers puts women at greater risk of contracting the virus. For women, especially in Africa, social distancing becomes a luxury. How do they social distance from those that are close to them? Even those who may be infected by the virus? It was saddening to hear the story of a Zimbabwean woman in the United Kingdom, who when her daughter was dying due to the virus admin-istered CPR having the full knowledge that she was infected which even led to her own infection. So how do we tell women who traditionally have been constructed as carers and nurturers of households to social distance? How practical is it in the African context? In fact, a lot of women are getting in-fected because they are trying to fulfil that role of themselves as carers of the infected. This is embedded in African religio-social construction of women as carers and as nurturers of societies and even households. Such a con-struction has exacerbated the pain that women go through during this time of COVID-19 because the pandemic has altered the way women mourn their dead. The demand for social distancing and wearing of masks meant that the funeral night vigils were no longer possible. At the peak of the virus, the dead were taken from the mortuary straight to the graveyard. Yet, cultur-ally, bodies would lie in-state at home allowing relatives particularly women to perform the necessary funeral rites. The perceived contagiousness of the dead body of a person who succumbed to the virus prohibited women from bathing the body or viewing it which traditionally allows them to bid proper farewell to the departed. Limits to the number of those who could attend funerals also brought heartache to a lot of women who could not bid farewell to their close relatives. A lot of these women together with the rest of the people continue to suffer from this pain of altered funeral procedures as they continue to seek for closure.

The other way that women have been affected by the virus is in the area of their spirituality. The closure of religious buildings has had an effect on religious women. Women are the majority within faith communities. In this case, the physical church has a special place in the hearts of the majority of women. How then can these women be told that they can no longer visit that physical structure? A place where they feel they can offload their burdens. How do they survive without hearing the sermons of their spiritual leaders, messages from those they believe provide a link between themselves and the supernatural? I have read quite a number of messages from pastors on WhatsApp platforms telling their congregants that the place they were used to go to is not the church, but that the congregants are the church. That may not have been the right time to be telling congregants because they were never prepared for it. Such a message is only relevant if all members are coming from believing homes. However, there is need to understand that at times, women in particular, are coming from homes where the husband is a non-believer, and they may not have the permission to be the church at home. Some religious leaders have resorted to the virtual church. This has been very innovative and creative. However, to the majority of women, the virtual church is not helping much especially considering that the majority of the women do not have the gadgets that would enable them to connect to the virtual church. They do not have smart phones or laptops. Those that have may find the cost of internet data inhibitive.

### Looking the beast in the eye: equipping faith communities to confront gender inequality in the COVID-19 context

What then is the role of faith communities in dealing with the above-mentioned challenges? For a long time, faith communities have been described as gender-insensitive as well as gender incompetent. It is encouraging though that we have begun to see them grappling with the destructive legacy of patriarchal styles of authority and subordination of women. They have begun to feel uncomfortable with among others, 'All-men's gatherings'. However, it is also because of the calls that gender activists and academics have been making demanding that there should not be anything for women without them. From a gender perspective faith communities need to do the following if they want to be effective in any pandemic situation (this is not presented in any order of importance): First faith communities need to interrogate and challenge their underpinning theologies which tend to leave out or to trivialize women's experiences and concerns. This would create space for more conversations on the role of women both in these communities and society at large. Women in faith communities are the ones experiencing all the gender vices of the pandemic; thus, there is need to provide spaces where they tell their stories of hurt and resistance. Nadar (2012:274) notes that while telling their stories places women in a position of vulnerability, the stories also become authoritative dialogical texts. That is the reason why establishing gender desks within religious organisations is of paramount importance. Such desks should be able to deal with women's issues in times such as the one we find ourselves in due to COVID-19.

Second, faith communities are called upon to condemn the underlying culture of violence against women since GBV and abuse are realities for members within these communities. This condemnation should be a lived reality within faith communities and not just a confessed one. Such condemnation calls upon leaders of faith communities not to be violent against women themselves so that they lead by example. Faith communities in Zimbabwe can take a leaf from what the Catholic Church in South Africa on 28 August 2020 did. It held a national day of prayer over women's plight in the COVID-19 era. The theme of the prayer was 'I Can't Breathe' which was reminiscent of George Floyd's murder by police in the United States of America. The prayer was meant to reflect on the hardships that were being faced by women in South Africa and across the world which for the church had been worsened by months of COVID-19 lockdowns. Sister Hermenegild Makoro aptly explained the experiences of women during COVID-19 lockdown when she said at this prayer meeting,

> The effects of COVID-19 during the lockdown period made us all feel like walking zombies, the 'dry bones' of whom the Prophet Ezekiel spoke...The pandemic has made women feel they were captured in a concentration camp. For some, it might have felt like they were in 'gas chambers'...
>
> (Crux Staff, 2020)

A recognition of the negative experiences of women needs to be accompanied by a clear condemnation of GBV. While organisations like the World Council of Churches as well as the Zimbabwe Ecumenical bodies have been visible in speaking out against GBV, there is need to encourage local churches within communities to do the same. There is need for more voices from faith communities to converge in speaking out against the scourge.

A rereading of the sacred text in ways that are life-giving to women is another significant way in which faith communities can deal with gender inequality. Oduyoye (1997:494) writing from an African Christian theological perspective argues that women in Africa view God as the source of their oppression since he has been presented to them as a male God. From her

analysis, "the androcentric Bible and Church have not been able to warp women's direct experience of God as a living liberator" (1997:494). For Oduyoye (1997:495), rereading scripture and especially the stories of women in the Bible helps to bring God closer and enhance his presence around women. Hence, a rereading of scripture in life affirming ways makes it easy to uphold the humanity of each gender during a crisis such as COVID-19 pandemic if faith communities continually teach positively about both genders. For this to be successful, there is need to rethink the way boys and girls are socialised within faith communities. How sustainable is the way faith communities and societies have been socializing our boys and girls? Can we continue to promote dangerous masculinities and femininities? Or it is time to find other ways of socialization; ways that will ensure that our boys and girls value the humanity of the other so that during a crisis such as COVID-19, they are not thinking of abusing each other but they look out for each other.

## Conclusion

The intention of this chapter was to show the gendered effects of the COVID-19 pandemic. The paper has highlighted the various ways in which women have been affected by the pandemic. The paper has shown that religions are also institutions and systems of power interacting with others in the gender order of society (The Church of Scotland, n.d). It has been shown how religion can challenge and contribute to change rather than reinforce traditional dynamics of gendered power. As such, the chapter has provoked faith communities to start serious conversations around the effects of pandemics such as COVID-19 on women. Unless myths around certain topics which affect women but which faith communities feel they are not comfortable to talk about are dealt with, the abuse and marginalisation of women will continue. It is important to note that the men who perpetrate violence against women are members within faith communities and they remain comfortable for as long as we do not talk about it. Women who are the majority of the victims are also members in our Faith communities. What this means is that the membership of faith communities has both perpetrators of violence and victims. This, therefore, justifies the need to start these conversations so that gender-sensitivity starts in the house of faith.

## References

Align, 2020. Gender norms and the coronavirus. At https://www.alignplatform.org/ [Accessed on 06 January 2021].

Archambeault, L. 2020. *Beyond the Shadow Pandemic: Protecting a Generation of Girls from Gender-Based Violence through COVID to Recovery*. Georgetown: Save the Children.

Burzynska, K. & Contreras, G. 2020. Gendered Effects of School Closures during the COVID-19 Pandemic. *Lancet.* At https://doi.org/10.1016/s0140.6736(20)31412.14. [Accessed on 06 January 2021].

Buttel, F. & Ferreira, R.J. 2020. The Hidden Disaster of COVID-19: Intimate Partner Violence. *Psychological Trauma: Theory, Research, Practice and Policy,* 12(S1): S197–S198.

Chiduku, C. 2020. 'COVID-19 lockdown spawns child marriages'. *Newsday.* At https://www.newsday.co.zw/ [Accessed on 06 January 2021].

Crux Staff. 2020. *South Africa Catholics Stage Day of Prayer over Women's Plight in COVID Era.* At https://cruxnow.com/church/ [Accessed on 28 August 2020].

Eghtessadi, R., Mukandavire, Z., Mutenherwa, F., Cuadros, D. & Musuka, G. 2020. Safeguarding gains in the Sexual and Reproductive Health and AIDS Response amidst COVID-19: The Role of Civil Society. *International Journal of Civil Society,* 100: 286–291.

Feyissa, G.T., Tolu, L.B. & Ezeh, A. 2020. Impact of COVID-19 Pandemic on Sexual and Reproductive and Mitigation Measures: The Case of Ethiopia. *African Journal of Reproductive Health* (Special Edition on COVID-19), 24(2): 24–26.

Grant, H. 2020. *Why COVID School Closures Are Making Girls Marry Early.* At https://www.theguardian.com/ [Accessed on 06 January 2021].

Kabeer, N. 2007. Marriage, Motherhood and Masculinity in the Global Economy: Reconfigurations of Personal and Economic Life. IDS Working Papers, 290, Institute of Development Studies, Brighton, United Kingdom.

Kofman, Y.B. & Garfin, D.R. 2020. Home is Not Always a Haven: The Domestic Violence Crisis Amid the COVID_19 Pandemic. *Psychological Trauma: Theory, Practice and Policy,* 12(S1): S199–S201.

Murphy, M.P.A. 2020. COVID-19 and Emergency eLearning Consequences of the Securitisation of Higher Education for Post-Pandemic Pedagogy. *Contemporary Security Policy,* 41(3): 492–505.

Mwiine, A.A. 2020. *Men in the Kitchen and the (Re)configurations of Masculinity in Domestic Space during COVID-19 Lockdown in Uganda.* At https://www.genderandcovid-19.org/ [Accessed on 06 January 2021].

Nadar, S. 2012. 'Feminist Theologies in Africa'. In Bongmba, E.K. (ed.) *Wiley-Blackwell Companion to African Religions,* 269–278. New Jersey: Wiley-Blackwell.

Ncube, A.L. 2020. *Shocker as Police Force Expecting Mom to Pay Bribe for Safe Passage to Labour Clinic.* At https://www.iharare.com/ [Accessed on 06 January 2021].

Nenge, R.T. 2013. 'A Hermeneutical Challenge in the Fight Against HIV and AIDS in the Johanne Marange Apostolic Church'. *Exchange,* 42(3): 252–266.

Norgah, S. 2020. *Shattered Dreams: From the Impact of COVID-19 on Girls' Education.* At https://www.globalpartnership.org. [Accessed on 06 January 2021].

Oduyoye, M.A. 1997. 'The African Experience of God through the Eyes of an Akan Woman'. *Crosscurrents,* 47(4): 493–504.

Oxford Research Encyclopedia. n.d. Violence, Politics and Gender. At https://www.ifes.org/sites/ [Accessed on 04 January 2021].

Pasura, D. & Christou, A. 2018. Theorising Black (African) Transnational Masculinities. *Men and Masculinities,* 21(4): 521–546.

Sarson, J. & MacDonald, L. 2020. *Pandemics: Misogynistic Violence against Women and Girls and COVID-19.* At https://nsadvocate.org/2020/ [Accessed on 15 August 2020].

Shefer, T., Stevens, G. & Clowes, L. 2010. Men in Africa: Masculinities, Materiality and Meaning. *Journal of Psychology in Africa*, 20(4): 511–518.

The Church of Scotland, n.d. Living a Theology that Counters Against Women. At www.sidebysidegender.org [Accessed on 07 January 2021].

United Nations Country Team. 2020. *Providing Services to Survivors of gender-based Violence during COVID-19*. At https://reliefweb.int/ [Accessed on 29 December 2020].

United Nation Human Rights Report. 2020. *Confronting COVID-19 from the Prism of Faith, Gender and Human Rights. United Nations.*

Women in Law and Development in Africa. 2020. *Zimbabwe: COVID-19 Lockdown – Gender-Based Violence Cases up by 70 Percent.* At https://www.wildaf-ao.org/ [Accessed on 29 December 2020].

# 17 Religion and COVID-19 in Southern Africa

## Implications for the discourse on religion and development

*Ezra Chitando*

### Introduction

The interface between religion and COVID-19 in Southern Africa (as indeed in other parts of the world), provides a valuable opportunity for gleaning insights for the discourse on religion and development. This is because the different religions' responses to COVID-19 are a useful pointer to how they respond to other development initiatives. Methodologically, the chapter is informed by the important role of Sustainable Development Goal (SDG) 3, namely, "Ensure healthy lives and promote well-being for all at all ages." Thus, sound health (such as responding effectively to COVID-19) provides the platform for achieving all the other SDGs. Further, the COVID-19 pandemic has had a major impact on the quest to achieve the SDGs in Africa (Ekwebelem et al. 2021), hence the need to examine how chapters on religion and COVID-19 can be interpreted in the context of the SDGs.

Chapters in this volume contribute towards reflections on religion and development, as they confirm how faith communities have been responding to COVID-19. They show how religion responds to a pressing health emergency, thereby providing useful indications on how religion interacts with development, more broadly defined. This will contribute towards clarifying the critical relationship between religion and development. It is my conviction that the lessons learnt from religion's engagement with COVID-19 in Africa will be deployed more strategically to prepare for future emergencies and to strengthen other development initiatives on the continent.

The relationship between religion and development is attracting the attention of scholars in diverse disciplines, globally. This includes scholars in anthropology, religious studies, gender, security, economics, and others. Further, where development practitioners previously did not think that religion was a major factor in development, they have begun to pay more attention to the interface between religion and development. Thus, Katherine Marshall (2001), in an article, "Development and Religion: A Different Lens on Development Debates," writes as follows:

> The world of religion has been an unacknowledged and often unseen force for many development practitioners in the past. Many reasons,

DOI: 10.4324/9781003241096-17

good and bad, explain this divorce; long traditions of separation of state and religion are deeply engrained and deliberately place a remove between development and faith issues. Institutions like the multilateral development banks which interact with governments as a matter of basic institutional structure may find limited vehicles to interact with a broad range of civil society institutions, religious institutions among them. The vocabulary and approach of spirituality seemed, often though not always, inimical to the technical, hard-nosed approach of development practice.

(Marshall 2001: 243)

If Marshall could refer to a "divorce," between religion and development, it is now possible to refer to a "re-marriage" and, as the chapters in this volume confirm, a dynamic one at that! Indeed, there is a sense in which religion and development have gone from a rocky divorce into a blissful honeymoon period. Whereas only about a decade ago there were limited publications within the sub-field, the recent overviews by Ignatius Swart and Elsabé Nell (2016), Emma Tomalin (2018, 2021), Barbara Bompani (2019), and Chitando et al. (2020) have shown that there is growing interest in religion and development. This has effectively made it an expanding sub-field within the academic study of religion more broadly defined. What the interaction between religion and COVID-19 does is to avail an opportunity to review the religion and development discourse more closely, utilising a specific case study. However, before engaging in such an undertaking, it is helpful to provide an overview of how the religion and development "re-marriage" has come about. This will assist in placing the review of the chapters on religion and COVID-19 in parts of Africa into their proper historical and theoretical context.

## Religion and development: summarising key issues in the "re-marriage"

The responses to COVID-19 by different religious actors confirm the complex role of religion in the face of different social challenges. Ascertaining how religion interfaces with these multiple social challenges constitutes the major focus of research within the sub-field of religion and development. One would be keen to ask the following question: "why is the interest in religion and development increasing?" A longer study is required to do justice to this theme, but I will draw attention to what I see as some of the major issues.

First, the limitations of the secularisation thesis have become apparent. The assumption that as modernity advanced, the status of religion would diminish, has been shown to be severely limited (see for example, Stark 1999; Clark 2012; Müller 2020). Writing from an African perspective, Mustafa H. Kurfi (2013) strenuously maintains that religion remains a major factor of life and needs to be factored in development discourses in Africa. Religion has stubbornly persisted and remains vibrant across diverse contexts, including the so-called 'developed' countries where it was expected to become less influential. In particular, the COVID-19 pandemic precipitated an increase in some religious activities, such as prayers (see for example, Boguszewski et al. 2020). This resilience of religion has generated or deepened scholarly interest in establishing whether and how it has a bearing on development.

Second, the increased visibility of religion in global affairs has led to growing interest in exploring its interface with development. Some scholars have highlighted how religion remains a significant force in international relations (see for example, Fox 2001; Haynes 2021). This role of religion in international relations remained clear during the COVID-19, with some faith-based organisations such as the World Council of Churches (WCC) calling upon particularly governments in the global North to share vaccines with the Global South. Interest in the theme of religion in international relations has precipitated the focus on religion and development, including paying attention to how this would influence relations between Europe and Africa, for example (Ellis and Ter Haar 2006).

Third, the global religion and human security nexus, particularly the rise of militant versions of religion and their implications for development, has increased interest in the field of religion and development. It has become clear that religion is available for mobilisation and deployment by various political actors. This has led to studies on religion and violence (see for example, Munson 2005). However, to balance the scales, there have been publications on religion and peace building and development (Flanigan 2013). This close relationship between religion and security also features in reflections on radicalisation within religions and COVID-19 (Avis 2020).

Fourth, the contributions of faith-based organisations to community transformation, particularly as complementing the efforts of the state in the Global South, have attracted the attention of some scholars. Thus, for example, the prominent role of faith-based organisations in development efforts have justified the interest in religion and development (Cooper 2019). Further, global development efforts through the United Nations Millennium Development Goals (2000–2015) and the Sustainable Development Goals (2015–2030) have reinvigorated interest in the interface between religion and development (see for example, Tomalin et al. 2019).

Fifth, there is an effort by scholars of religion to shake off the critique that their discipline lacks practical relevance and only concentrates on abstract or theoretical issues. Focusing on religion and development offers them an opportunity to claim that they are engaged in a critical undertaking. There is justification in this claim, however. As chapters in this volume confirm, scholars of religion were needed to analyse the role of religion in the COVID-19 pandemic. There is an emerging appreciation that scholars in the scientific study of religion can assist with clarifying how religion either promotes or impedes health (and other development) initiatives (Wildman et al. 2020).

These developments have given the sub-field of religion and development a new lease of life, with a number of scholars, particularly in Europe, providing valuable insights. On the other hand, scholarship on religion and development in Africa remains less studied, especially outside South Africa. Chitando et al. (2020) provide a detailed review of the growth of the sub-field in Africa. Chapters in this volume are making a valuable addition to this discussion in Africa by analysing how religion has responded to the COVID-19 pandemic in parts of Southern (and East) Africa.

## The central argument of this chapter

Having outlined the context in which research and publication on religion and development is being undertaken, in this section I outline the central argument of this chapter. This chapter contends that reviewing how religions have responded to COVID-19 in parts of Africa has definite implications to the discourse on religion and development, both in Africa and globally. Its central argument is that there is no single and simplistic interpretation of the role of religion in responding to COVID-19 (and, by extension, to development). The responses are dynamic and complex and may not be exhausted by using descriptive words such as "positive" or "negative." As I argue below, scholars will probably need to coin potentially confusing labels such as, "positive-while-negative" when describing religion's interface with COVID-19 (and development).

Whereas commentators on religion and development often proffer sharply divided perspectives, the chapters in this volume confirm the need to revise this trend. Often, the dominant argument is over whether religion facilitates or frustrates/threatens development. Thus, the suggestion is that religion does one thing or the other, but not both. This can be seen from the titles of some previous/earlier publications. For example, the volume co-edited by Gerrie ter Haar and James J. Bussutil (2005) has the title, *"Bridge or Barrier?"* The subtitle of Jeffrey Hayne's (2007) book on religion and development is, *"Conflict or Cooperation?"* The volume edited by Kenneth Mtata is entitled, *Religion: Help or Hindrance to Development?* (2013). All these titles suggest that religion can only be either positive or negative, but not both.

My central argument is that the responses by religions to COVID-19, as expressed by chapters in this volume, confirm that this "either or" approach to the interface between religion and development might not be the most effective or productive one. I am arguing that a "both and" perspective will give us a more rounded picture about the relationship between religion and development. I will argue that this position, which maintains that religion is both a positive and negative force in the quest for health (for example, in responding to COVID-19) and development, is more sustainable.

## Positive responses by religion to COVID-19 in Southern Africa

The chapters in this volume provide clear evidence of the critical role of religion in responding to COVID-19 and promoting development in Southern Africa. In this section, I shall highlight some of the key themes that have emerged from the chapters. I must hasten to add that the analysis in this section is more indicative than exhaustive, due to space and thematic considerations.

### *The contribution of indigenous knowledge systems and African traditional religions to the COVID-19 response*

One of the major challenges characterising the global discourse on religion and development is the marginalisation of indigenous knowledge systems (IKS) (see for example, Noyoo 2007). Chapters in the first part of this volume highlight the extent to which individuals and communities utilised indigenous knowledge systems in their responses to COVID-19. Chapter 2 on Ubuntu (a widespread concept in diverse African contexts) by Beatrice Okyere-Manu and Stephen N. Morgan shows the potential of concepts from the long past to remain relevant in responding to contemporary challenges such as COVID-19. Similarly, Chapter 3 by Tenson Muyambo on indigenous systems relating to social distancing, and Macloud Sipeyiye on resources from Ndau traditional religion, confirms the value of broadening coverage when debating religion and health (COVID-19), and development. Bernard P. Humbe's call for a more inclusive approach to the debate between science and religion (Chapter 5) can also be located in this scheme where African indigenous knowledge systems and religions are taken into account because they provide the spectacles that the majority of citizens use to frame their understanding of disasters or development initiatives.

### *Resilience by minority or marginalised religions*

Linked to the marginalisation of indigenous knowledge systems and religions is the exclusion of minority religions such as Rastafari. Most scholarly publications on religion and development tend to focus on established missionary religions such as Christianity and Islam. These religions have had a longer presence on the continent and have become more established, thereby enabling them to own schools and health centres. However, younger religions such as Rastafari must be included in discourses on religion and development. Chapter 15 by Fortune Sibanda shows how Rastafari cultural identities such as music, Ital foodways, holistic natural herbalism and environmentalism as well as spiritual and physically balanced lives engender creative and unique parameters that promote public health and human flourishing.

This brings a radical dimension to the discourse on religion and COVID-19 (and development). Development should not only be approached from the perspective of initiating practical projects aimed at improving the welfare of people, or alleviating suffering. A broader perspective is required to appreciate that development is also related to deepening consciousness and expanding individual and communal sense of identity. Thus, the chapter by Sibanda on Rastafari and COVID-19 challenges us to look beyond the "usual suspects" (read Christianity and Islam) when reflecting on the impact of religion in Africa. More work is required to interrogate the contribution of new religious movements to identity and social cohesion in Africa.

### *Effective collaboration with public health and political authorities*

Many of the chapters in this volume demonstrate the remarkable flexibility of the religions and their willingness to collaborate with public health and political authorities in response to COVID-19 in the region. Against the stereotype that religions are rigid systems that are characterised by a fundamentalist slant, many chapters confirm how religious leaders were quick to embrace and popularise public health messages. Thus, Chapter 8 by Paskas Wagana highlights the positive role of the churches in Tanzania, a country that had a difficult response to the pandemic due to the stance of its late former President, John Magufuli. Chapter 10 by Sonene Nyawo describes the positive role of the churches in responding to COVID-19 in Eswatini, while Nelly Mwale and Joseph Chita (Chapter 11) draw attention to the collaboration to respond to the pandemic by the main church umbrella bodies in Zambia. Tshenolo Madigele and James Amanze describe some of the positive responses by the churches in Botswana in Chapter 12, while Edmore Dube demonstrates the flexibility shown by Muslims in Zimbabwe in the face of the pandemic in Chapter 14. This dimension is important, as the Islamophobia propagated by some sections of the media (particularly in relation to the theme of religion and violence that I alluded to earlier) creates the impression that Islam is a rigid religion.

The dominant trend that emerges from the descriptions provided in the chapters referred to in the foregoing paragraph is that of religion acting to promote public health messages such as observing social distancing, sanitising and avoiding large gatherings. This was also the experience of religion in other parts of the world, albeit with some challenges (see, for example, Tan et al. 2021 in relation to Malaysia; and Osei-Tutu et al. 2021 in the context of Ghana). To a large extent, many religious leaders sought to echo the messages disseminated by public health officials and politicians to prevent the spread of COVID-19 and to mitigate its impact. Although most of the chapters in this volume cover the period before the full-scale drive towards promoting COVID-19 vaccination, one could add that many religious leaders were also supportive of the move and some were keen to lead by example by being publicly vaccinated, while putting on their religious regalia.

### *Religions and COVID-19: flexibility, adaptability and rationality*

Aligned to the foregoing descriptions of religion working systematically with public health officials and politicians, chapters in this volume also underscore the flexibility, adaptability and rationality of religion in the face of COVID-19. Chapter 7 by Lucia Ponde-Mutsvedu and Sophia Chirongoma confirms the shift from physical meetings to online services by different religious bodies. Although this shift has been uneven, with mostly Pentecostal churches that were already utilising online platforms enjoying an upper hand, it is fair to say that many religions were quick to adjust. Once again, this runs contrary to conventional wisdom that casts religions as intrinsically conservative systems that are unable to move quickly or adjust to changing realities.

Many chapters in this volume illustrate the flexibility, adaptability and rationality of religious actors in the face of COVID-19. Although there was what one might call, perhaps uncharitably, the extremist fringe (whose dimensions I discuss below), the majority of religious actors were willing to be guided by the health experts. They operated with an open theological or religious system that did not pit faith and science as being locked in mortal combat. Instead, they contended that all the knowledge that those working in the health sector had was from the same source that inspired religion. This confirms the position reached earlier by Stark et al. (1996) that the idea that religion is non-rational stems from bias against the phenomenon and is not borne by evidence. Thus, some religious people might take up fundamentalist and unreasonable positions. However, this does not imply that religion is non-rational, as the responses to COVID-19 in different contexts in Southern Africa confirm.

## Negative responses by religion to COVID-19 in Southern Africa

Whereas there were many positive responses to COVID-19 by religions, as outlined above, it is also important to acknowledge that there were a number of negative responses. Once again, space considerations mean that I can only summarise these negative responses in this section. These related mostly to theological interpretations that either minimised the pandemic or deepened fear, resistance to public health messages and the marginalisation of specific groups such as people with disability and failure to act decisively to respond to increased violence against women.

### *Immobilising theological positions in relation to COVID-19*

Some theological positions had the effect of immobilising individuals and communities in the face of COVID-19. In Chapter 9, Julius Gathogo reviews the challenges emerging from some 'prophecies' in Kenya in the face of the pandemic. In Chapter 6, Helena Van Coller and Idowu A. Akinloye adopt a legal perspective and show how the state's lockdown measures could be justified in the face of some religious leaders who were absolutizing freedom of movement and worship (see also Tengatenga et al. 2021 with reference to Malawi). These examples highlight the capacity of religious actors to sometimes adopt positions that can present religion as unreasonable and extreme, particularly in the face of a major threat such as COVID-19.

Ponde-Mutsvedu and Chirongoma (Chapter 7) and Nyawo (Chapter 10) also bring out some problematic aspects of religion. Ponde-Mutsvedu and Chirongoma draw attention to the cyber bulling that characterised the lockdowns in Zimbabwe, while Nyawo highlights the problematic character of some interpretations of COVID-19 that characterised it as God's punishment for sin. Similarly, some indigenous knowledge systems that readily identified COVID-19 with earlier sicknesses ran (and still run) the risk of minimising its threat to health and well-being. It is this dimension of promoting a fatalistic worldview that has led some critics to challenge the positive rating of religion in discourses on development.

### *Cultural conservatism, resistance to science and COVID-19 prevention strategies*

Across most chapters, the notion of religion struggling with the full implementation of COVID-19 prevention strategies runs through. While highlighting the flexibility of the Muslim approach to the pandemic, in Chapter 14 Dube shows how observing funeral rites was a challenge for many Zimbabwean Muslims. This aspect was also noted by Muyambo in Chapter 3 in the context of indigenous burial practices. This strategic rite of passage emerged as a contentious issue in the wake of COVID-19. Thus, it appeared the established mourning and burial patterns largely struggled to conform to the guidelines handed down by the health authorities. Perhaps this has to do with the finality associated with death and the need to avoid the consequences associated with angering the dead. Thus, while I noted the flexibility that religions demonstrated in responding to COVID-19, it is important to admit that there were limits to such flexibility.

Chapter 5 by Humbe shows how some religious positions seek to challenge science. Indeed, there are some fundamentalists in the different religions who seem determined to counter science and whose highest selling point is resistance to science. Such religious actors emerged as stumbling blocks in efforts to mobilise religious communities to counter COVID-19 and its negative effects. Other religious actors in different countries sought to project themselves as martyrs by refusing to accept the public health messages. They positioned themselves as more faithful than those who cooperated with the public health authorities. This position became more entrenched when some led resistance to the vaccination efforts, particularly in 2021 when vaccines became more widely available. Ideas relating to Africans being used as guinea pigs (see for example, Samarasekera 2021) and theological ideas linking vaccination with having the mark of the beast (Letšosa 2021) promoted vaccine hesitancy and slowed down the vaccination drive by governments in the region (as it did in other parts of the world). The interface between religion and conspiracy theory (Dyrendal et al. 2019) emerged as a major negative force in efforts to respond effectively to COVID-19 in Africa, as in other parts of the world.

### *Struggling to address increased violence against women and girls during the pandemic*

Religions, having patriarchal foundations, have generally struggled to address violence against women. These patriarchal foundations inform religion's tacit (and active) support for men's violence against women (see for example, Johnson 2015) and to promote the general silence in the face of violence against women (Chitando and Chirongoma 2013). The COVID-19 induced lockdowns in the region resulted in increasing cases of violence against women and girls. In Chapter 16, Molly Manyonganise highlights religion's struggle to address the increase in violence against women in the wake of COVID-19. She draws attention to how religion needs to be more alert in responding to violence against women, including during emergencies.

In discourses on religion and development, religion's role in holding back women features prominently. Manyonganise's chapter is a reminder that religion needs to be more purposeful in addressing gender inequality, holding men to account and to promote justice. COVID-19 has exposed the high levels of sexual and gender-based violence that women experience, globally. Her chapter also underscores the fact that pandemics are gendered (Marindo 2017). Thus, religion needs to be more proactive in addressing violence against women if it is to become a valuable resource for social transformation.

### *Overlooking persons with disability*

Religions have struggled to address the rights of persons with disability (see for example, Schumm and Stoltzfus 2011). In Chapter 13, Makomborero A. Bowa discusses the marginalisation of persons with disability by faith communities during COVID-19 in Southern Africa. Bowa contends that churches have struggled to read the Bible positively in relation to the rights of persons with disability. This has resulted in the systematic exclusion of persons with disability in churches and society. His chapter serves to draw attention to the interaction between religion and persons with disability in the face of pandemics.

### Religion and COVID-19 in Southern Africa in the context of religion and development

The foregoing sections have drawn attention to the achievements and struggles of faith communities in parts of Africa in the context of COVID-19. In this section, I seek to summarise some insights for the discourse on religion and development.

First, the analysis above shows that no single story is possible in relation to religion and COVID-19 in Southern Africa. The chapters confirm that the pattern is complex, with religion being a positive factor in some instances, and a challenge in others. For example, while it possible to regard religious leaders' acceptance of the lockdowns as positive, their failure to respond to violence against women is negative. Another example would be the religious leaders' flexibility in moving to online platforms being a positive development. However, some of the messages being proclaimed on the online platforms were negative. This generates the idea of being "positive-while-negative" that I referred to above.

Second, it is helpful to invest in researching into factors that shape a religion to be a positive, negative or "positive-and-negative" factor in responding to a pandemic or contributing to development in a specific context. Thus, contextual sensitivity must be prioritised in research works into religion and COVID-19 or development. Chapters in this volume have sought to uphold this dimension by emphasising the specific local, denominational, national or regional contexts in which religion sought to respond to COVID-19. This implies the need to privilege lived religion ahead of theoretical constructs of what a specific religion ought to be (see, for example, Knibbe and Kupari 2020).

Third, from the onset of COVID-19, religion has been visible on the frontlines in different African countries. Religious leaders have largely been encouraging their followers and the larger society to observe public health protocols, adjust rituals and observances and prevent the spread of COVID-19. This has exploded the myth that religions are intrinsically conservative and not flexible. African Traditional Religions and Rastafari, for example, promoted indigenous herbs in the face of the challenges facing biomedicine during COVID-19. Although debate will continue to rage over the efficacy of these herbs, what remains clear is that religion remains a highly significant social force in Africa (and elsewhere). Serious development practitioners must, therefore, be serious about religion!

Fourth, it is very strategic for research works into religion and development to include focusing on specific themes in order to generate more sustainable conclusions. Chapters in this volume have concentrated on religion's response to COVID-19 in Southern (and parts of East) Africa. Other studies could focus on key thematic areas such as religion and: gender equality, climate change, education, peace building, food security, sustainable consumption and other development goals, with special reference to Africa.

## Conclusion

The COVID-19 pandemic caught the world unawares. It instigated panic and affected lives in very profound ways. In the middle of this uncertainty, religion stepped up to respond. As chapters in this volume demonstrate, some of these interventions were quite progressive and contributed towards mitigating the impact of the pandemic. However, the chapters also show that some of the interventions were counterproductive. Approaching the theme from the perspective of the discourse on religion and development, this chapter has sought to summarise the trends that are discernible in this volume. The chapter has illustrated how the interface between religion and COVID-19 in Southern Africa enriches the debate on religion and development in very clear ways. In conclusion, it is anticipated that when future generations will reflect on the COVID-19 pandemic (particularly in Africa), they will do well to integrate the story of religion's response in order for their narratives to be more comprehensive.

## References

Avis, William. 2020. The COVID-19 pandemic and response on violent extremist recruitment and radicalisation. Helpdesk Report, K4D. Available at: https://reliefweb.int/sites/reliefweb.int/files/resources/808_COVID19%20_and_Violent_Extremism.pdf, accessed 5 August 2021.

Boguszewski, Rafal et al. 2020. "The COVID-19 Pandemic's Impact on Religiosity in Poland," *Religions* 11(12), 646. https://doi.org/10.3390/rel11120646.

Bompani, Barbara. 2019. "Religion and Development: Tracing the Trajectories of an Evolving Sub-Discipline," *Progress in Development Studies* 9(3), 171–185.

Chitando, Ezra and Sophia Chirongoma. Eds. 2013. *Justice Not Silence: Churches Facing Sexual and Gender-based Violence*. Cape Town: Sun Media.

Chitando, Ezra, Masiiwa R. Gunda and Lovemore Togarasei. 2020. "Introduction: Religion and Development in Africa," in Ezra Chitando, Masiiwa R. Gunda and Lovemore Togarasei, eds., *Religion and Development in Africa*. Bamberg: University of Bamberg Press, 13–35.

Clark, J. C. D. 2012. "Secularization and Modernization: The Failure of a "Grand Narrative," *The Historical Journal* 55(1), 161–194.

Cooper, Rachel. 2019. Faith-based organisations and current development debates. Helpdesk Report, 4KD. Available at: https://opendocs.ids.ac.uk/opendocs/bitstream/handle/20.500.12413/15397/624_Faith_Based%20Organisations_Synthesis.pdf, accessed 5 August 2021.

Dyrendal, Asbjørn, David G. Robertson and Egil Asprem. Eds. 2019. *Handbook of Conspiracy Theory and Contemporary Religion*. Leiden: Brill.

Ekwebelem, Osmond C. et al. 2021. "Threats of COVID-19 to Achieving United Nations Sustainable Development Goals in Africa," *American Journal of Tropical Medicine and Hygiene* 104(2), 457–460.

Ellis, Steve and Gerrie Ter Haar. 2006. "The Role of Religion in Development: Towards a New Relationship between the European Union and Africa," *The European Journal of Development Research* 18(3), 351–367.

Flanigan, Shawn T. 2013. "Religion, Conflict and Peacebuilding in Development," in Matthew Clarke, ed., *Handbook of Research on Development and Religion*. Cheltenham, UK: Edward Elgar, 252–267.

Fox, Jonathan. 2001. Religion as an Overlooked Element of International Relations. *International Studies Review* 3(3), 53–73.

Haynes, Jeffrey. 2007. *Religion and Development: Conflict or Cooperation?* Basingstoke: Palgrave Macmillan.

Haynes, Jeffrey. 2021. Religion and International Relations: What Do We Know and How Do We Know It? *Religions* 12: 328. https://doi.org/10.3390/rel12050328

Johnson, Andy J. Ed. 2015. *Religion and Men's Violence against Women.* New York: Springer.

Knibbe, Kim and Helena Kupari. 2020. "Theorizing Lived Religion: Introduction," *Journal of Contemporary Religion* 35(2), 157–176. https://doi.org/10.1080/13537903.2020.1759897

Kurfi, Mustapha H. 2013. "Secularization and Development in Africa: A Terrific Façade," *Global Journal of Human Social Science, Sociology and Culture* 13(6), 15–19.

Letšosa, Rantao. 2021. "What Has the Beast's Mark to do with the COVID-19 Vaccination, and What is the Role of the Church and Answering to the Christians?" *HTS Teologiese Studies/Theological Studies* 77(4), a6480. https://doi. org/10.4102/hts.v77i4.6480

Marindo, Ravayi. 2017. "Gendered Epidemics and Systems of Power in Africa: A Feminist Perspective on Public Health Governance," *Africa Development* 42(1), 199–219.

Marshall, Katherine. 2001. "Development and Religion: A Different Lens on Development Debates," *Peabody Journal of Education* 76(3/4), 339–375.

Mtata, Kenneth. Ed. 2013. *Religion: Help or Hindrance to Development?* Leipzig: Evangelische Verlagsanstalt.

Müller, Tobias. 2020. "Secularisation Theory and Its Discontents: Recapturing Decolonial and Gendered Narratives: Debating Jörg Stolz's Article on *Secularization Theories in the 21st Century: Ideas, Evidence, and Problems,*" *Social Campus* 67(2), 315–322.

Munson, Henry 2005. "Religion and Violence," *Religion* 35(4), 223–246.

Noyoo, Ndangwa. 2007. "Indigenous Knowledge Systems and Their Relevance for Sustainable Development: A Case of Southern Africa." In Emmanuel K. Boon and Luc Hens, eds., *Indigenous Knowledge Systems and Sustainable Development: Relevance for Africa.* Delhi: Kamla-Raj, 167–172.

Osei-Tutu, Annabella et al. 2021. "The Impact of COVID19 and Religious Restrictions on the WellBeing of Ghanaian Christians: The Perspectives of Religious Leaders," *Journal of Religion and Health* 60: 2232–2249.

Samarasekera, Udani. 2021. "Feelings towards COVID-19 Vaccinations in Africa," *The Lancet* 21 (March), 324.

Schumm, Darla and Michael Stoltzfus. Eds. 2011. *Disability and Religious Diversity: Cross- Cultural and Interreligious Perspectives.* New York: Palgrave Macmillan.

Stark, Rodney. 1999. "Secularization, R. I. P," *Sociology of Religion* 60(3), 249–273.

Stark, Rodney, Laurence Iannaccone and Roger Finke. 1996. "Religion, Science, and Rationality," *American Economic Review* 86(2), 433–437.

Swart, Ignatius and Elsabė Nell. 2016. "Religion and Development: The Rise of a Bibliography," *HHTS Teologiese Studies/Theological Studies* 72(4), a3862. http://doi.org/10.4102/hts. v72i4. 3862.

Tan, Min M., Ahmad F. Musa and Tin T. Su. 2021. "The Role of Religion in Mitigating the COVID-19 Pandemic: The Malaysian Multi-Faith Perspectives," *Health Promotion International.* doi:10.1093/heapro/daab041

Tengatenga, James, Susan M. T. Duley and Cecil J. Tengatenga. 2021. *"Zimitsani Moto*: Understanding the Malawi COVID-19 Response," *Laws* 10(2), 20. https://doi.org/10.3390/laws10020020

Ter Haar, Gerrie and James J. Busuttil. Eds. 2005. *Bridge or Barrier: Religion, Violence and Visions for Peace*. Leiden: Brill.

Tomalin, Emma. 2018. "Religions, Poverty Reduction and Global Development Institutions," *Palgrave Communications* 4, 132. DOI: 10.1057/s41599-018-0167-8.

Tomalin, Emma. 2021. "Religions and Development: A Paradigm Shift or Business as Usual?," *Religion* 51(1), 105–124. DOI:10.1080/0048721X.2020.1792055

Tomalin, Emma, Jörg Haustein and Shabaana Kidy. 2019. "Religion and the Sustainable Development Goals," *The Review of Faith & International Affairs* 17(2), 102–118. DOI:10.1080/15570274.2019.1608664

Wildman, Wesley J. et al. 2020. "Religion and the COVID-19 Pandemic," *Religion, Brain & Behavior* 10(2), 115–117. DOI:10.1080/2153599X.2020.1749339

# Index

abuse 174, 178, 183
advocacy 164, 179, 182, 183
African culture 27, 28, 34
African ethics 27, 28, 33, 34, 104; *see also* Ubuntu
African traditional religion 73
African value(s) 25, 27, 32, 34
Afrocentric theory (Afrocentricity) 214, 215

*Biripiri* (measles) 42, 43
Botswana Network of Christian Communities 172, 175–177
Bronfenbrenner's ecological model 104–105, 110, 111, 113

*Chi Gong* 225; *see also* Rastafari
*chigubhu-giya* 67–68
Christian healing 77
Church (Christian), the 120, 175–177, 180–183
Church mother bodies (Zambia) 155, 156, 161, 163, 165–166
Church umbrella bodies (Zambia) 155, 156, 158, 159–170
community, communitarian 27, 29–33, 104, 111
coronavirus (COVID-19): as bio-medical warfare 227, 228; causes/origins of 213, 219–220, 233; containment measures 126–130; definition of 54, 55; and diaconia 180; dying, death and burial of victims 82; epidemiological paradigm of 74; as fulfillment of end time prophecies 145–146, 151; as God's punishment for sin 143–144, 149–150; impact of 131, 132; modes of transmission 55; pandemic 25,

26, 28, 32, 33, 155–162, 164–169, 186–188, 193–196, 198–199, 232–241; and prophecies 134–138; as a spiritual warfare 144–145, 150; symptoms of 52–55, 61, 67
culture 29–31
cyberbullying 108, 109

death 89, 90, 92
diaconia 180
disability(ies): interpretation of biblical texts on 187–189, 190–193, 196–199; persons with 186–199; positive perspectives on 187, 189, 196–199; and social exclusion 192, 193; and social ideology of inclusion 193, 196, 198; social model of 187–188, 198
Disaster Management Act 92

ecumenical bodies 142, 143
elderly people 172–174; respect to 32, 33
end time prophecies 145, 149, 151
environmentalism 225
Eswatini 141
ethics of *Ubuntu* 28, 33, 34; *see also* humanness; *Ubuntu/Unhu*

family 25, 27, 28, 30–33
family power 83
fasting 112, 143, 150
femininity 237, 241
food: insecurity 66–67; *ital* foodways 222–223
freedom: of association 89, 95; institutional right to 91; of movement 89, 95; of religion 89, 90–92, 95, 98
funeral rites 92, 94–95, 97, 202, 209–210, 121, 122

gender (inequality) 232, 233, 239
gender-based violence 173, 178, 182, 233, 234–240
governmentality, theory of 116, 117
grief 110, 111, 121
grieving 179

*Hadith* 19, 204–205
*hajj* 205, 208
health: multi-sectoral approach to 66; public 4, 7, 155, 159
humanness 27–34; *see also* Ubuntu
hut on fire, theory of 5

Indian variant (Delta) 126
indigenous communities: challenges of 59–62; promises of 63–68
influenza pandemic of 1918 127, 128; *see also* Spanish Flu
Information and Communication Technology 103, 105, 108, 113
injustices 181
interconnectedness 28, 104, 110, 113

kingdoms, two 144, 145, 149, 150
Kenya 126
*kutanda botso* 47

leaders: African Pentecostal 11, 12, 136; traditional 67, 68; *see also* religious leaders
leprosy (*Maperembudzi*) 41, 42
lockdown 172–175, 203, 205, 207, 233, 234, 235, 236, 237, 238
lockdown regulations 89, 90–98, 147, 148

Malawi 213, 214, 218, 220
masculinity (men) 232, 234, 235, 237, 238, 241
media (social) 107, 108, 155, 160
Medicine Control Authority of Zimbabwe 79
Ministry of Health and Child Care (MoHCC) 77
Mosque 92, 95, 112
Mother Earth 226

Nairobi Metropolitan Area 130
National Hygiene Programme 130
National prayer 143, 150
Ndau indigenous religio-cultural resources 63–68
Ndau social history 56–59

negative and discriminatory perspectives on disability 186–187, 189, 191, 193, 196, 199
new normal 104, 109

online religion 103

pandemic (s) 27–34, 75, 155–169, 186–188, 193–196, 198–199, 203, 205, 232–233, 236–237, 240–241
pastoral care 120, 165, 166
person 26, 28–30
phenomenology of religion 54, 215
politics: of biblical interpretation 3, 4; as exercise of power /hegemonic rivalries 3, 4, 215–217; of gender 9, 10; of (public) health 4, 6, 9, 10; and religion 5
poverty 186–188, 192, 193–199
prayer(s) 7, 13, 92, 94–95, 112, 120, 122, 178
preventive and containment measures 53, 66
public health 4, 5, 7, 9, 10; Muslim perceptions on 203–205; *see also* health
public health education 164–165
public worship 160, 163, 166
punishment for sin 143, 149

quarantine 33, 61, 66, 107

Ramadan 205–208, 210
Rastafari: beliefs and practices 218–219; causes of COVID-19 (perspectives on) 219–220; environmentalism 225–226; herbal remedies 224–225; history of 217–218; intervention strategies 221–228
rationality 96–97
reggae music 226–228; *see also* Rastafari
regulations and restrictions 146
religion(s): in combating COVID-19 119–122; as a coping mechanism/ resource 121, 142, 143, 152, 159; definition of 2, 3; and development 4, 245, 246, 253; interface with public health and politics 4, 7, 9, 249, 155, 159; as a meaning-making framework 12, 13, 121; minority 248; overlooking persons with disability 252; and (resistance to) science 72, 251; role in society 4, 75

religious: fraternity 175; gatherings (and ban on) 89, 90–98, 90, 92, 94–95; leaders (and politicians) 7, 8, 9, 119–123; organizations 120, 121; pilgrimages 122; resource(s) 159, 163–168; responses 155–160, 164, 167–169, 221–228; services 121; symbols/objects 122; *see also* religion(s)
remedies: (traditional) herbal 81, 224–225; traditional home 81
rights: human 90–91, 98; limitation of 90–91, 95, 98

Sankofa, perspective (theory of) 38, 39
second coming of Jesus 145, 147
self-isolating (isolation) 32–33, 61, 65, 66, 107, 118, 120, 121, 221, 222; *see also* self-quarantine
self-quarantine 33, 104, 105, 221, 222
Shia 19, 202, 208
social distancing 39, 40, 45, 61, 111, 234, 238
social power 118
solidarity 29, 30, 34, 160–162
South Africa 89, 90–93, 98; Constitution of 91
Southern Africa: church in 186–187, 189, 191, 193, 196–199; context 188–189, 191, 194, 197, 244; delimitations of 5
Spanish Flu 128
spiritual capital theory 53, 63, 66
spirituality 239
spiritual warfare 143, 144, 147, 148, 151
State of Public Emergency 172
stewardship of creation 133

stigmatization and marginalisation 187, 189–190, 192, 196, 198
*Sunnah* 19, 203
Sustainable Development Goals 245

Tanzania 116–124
tele-evangelism 10, 103, 105, 108, 113; *see also* online religion
tele-health 10, 103, 105, 107

Ubuntu 25–34, 104, 105, 109, 110; concept of 27, 28–34; ethical principles of 28–33
*Ubuntu/Unhu* 45, 48, 104, 105, 109, 110, 113
*ummah* 208
*umrah* 208
unconstitutional 93, 95–97
unreasonable 93–95

vaccine(s): conspirational thinking on 227–228; resistance to 8; skepticism/hesitancy 8, 12, 77, 227, 228
violence against women and girls 252; *see also* gender-based violence

women 232–241
World Health Organization 72
worldview (analysis) 2, 3, 148, 149, 150, 151, 152
worship places 92, 94
Wuhan (China) 1, 127, 155, 233

Zambia 155, 156, 158, 160–162, 164, 166, 169
Zimbabwe 37, 73, 103, 202, 210, 213, 214, 218, 232

For Product Safety Concerns and Information please contact our EU
representative GPSR@taylorandfrancis.com
Taylor & Francis Verlag GmbH, Kaufingerstraße 24, 80331 München, Germany